ACCLAIM FOR

THE CALORIES IN, CALORIES OUT COOKBOOK

"I like *The Calories In, Calories Out Cookbook* because it's not a fad diet book and no food groups are eliminated. It encourages us to really look at what we're eating—and in so doing to take the first step to making healthy lifestyle changes."
—GEORGE L. BLACKBURN, MD, PHD, S. Daniel Abraham Professor of Nutrition,
Harvard Medical School/Beth Israel Deaconess Medical Center

"*The Calories In, Calories Out Cookbook* provides a unique, innovative way to a healthier lifestyle. It helps people understand what calories are all about, how to determine daily calorie needs, and how to balance caloric intake with calorie expenditure through exercise. And it provides terrific recipes to satisfy even the heartiest appetite. All told, a first-rate guide!"
—MALCOLM K. ROBINSON, MD, Metabolic Support Service,
Brigham and Women's Hospital, Division of Nutrition, Harvard Medical School

"A real winner! *The Calories In, Calories Out Cookbook* is an excellent way to eat wonderful, real food and manage your weight. It does not contain long lists of 'do's' and 'don'ts'; instead, it helps guide you in making smart decisions to optimize your health. Its clear user-friendly guidelines and tips will help anyone interested in adopting a healthier lifestyle."
—KATHY MCMANUS, MS, RD, LD/N, Director of the Department of Nutrition,
Brigham and Women's Hospital, Boston, Massachusetts

"Losing weight is all about calories and *The Calories In, Calories Out Cookbook* gives you all the information you need to keep it off FOREVER. Don't miss this one!"
—CAROLINE APOVIAN, MD, author of *The Overnight Diet*,
Director of the Center for Nutrition and Weight Management at Boston Medical Center,
and Professor of Medicine at Boston University School of Medicine

"Do you want to understand what calories are, where they are found, how to burn them, and how to prepare delicious healthy recipes that will help you stay within your calorie needs? Then USE and ENJOY *The Calories In, Calories Out Cookbook*. This is a must-have in every household and for all adults and children seeking to live healthier lives!"
—RAFAEL PEREZ-ESCAMILLA, PHD, Professor, Yale School of Public Health

"Finally, an up-to-date and scientifically rigorous approach to sustainable weight management coupled with exceptional recipes! Forget the fads and instead enjoy a diverse and healthy diet while feeling more vibrant and reducing your risk of many chronic diseases impacting our population."
—STEVEN K. CLINTON, MD, PHD,
Professor, College of Medicine, The Ohio State University

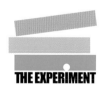

THE EXPERIMENT

BECAUSE EVERY BOOK IS A TEST OF NEW IDEAS

"For anyone who is trying to balance energy intake and output, *The Calories In, Calories Out Cookbook* really fills a gap. In addition to providing calculations of calories and nutrients per serving, it also gives readers a count of how much physical activity it will take to balance what's taken in. It offers tasty pairings to make delicious meals plus lots of helpful cooking tips, and an appendix filled with useful nutritional facts and figures. All in all, this is an outstanding book—one that many of us who are dietitians and nutritionists can recommend to our patients and clients without reservation."

—JOHANNA DWYER, DSC., RD, Professor of Medicine,
Tufts Medical School, and Director of Frances Stern Nutritional Center at New England Medical Center

"*The Calories In, Calories Out Cookbook* is my new go-to guide for clients, colleagues, and friends. Long overdue, it embraces what dietitians and researchers have been touting for decades: for optimal health, eat smarter and move further. This wonderful resource has it all—solid evidence, healthy tips, caloric and physical activity recommendations, shopping lists, and of course, fabulous recipes. Readers are sure to enjoy, eat well, and prosper!"

—COLLEEN SPEES, PhD, MEd, RD, LD, Assistant Professor,
The Ohio State University Medical Center

"*The Calories In, Calories Out Cookbook* is *the* go-to book for healthy living. Catherine Jones and Elaine Trujillo not only deliver tasty and easy recipes but also provide readers with expert knowledge and guidance on what calories are and how the body uses them. They weave a delicate balance of calories in and calories out without depending on dieting. I can't wait to share this book with my friends, colleagues, and clients."

—JULIE SCHWARTZ, MS, RDN, CSSD, LD, Certified Wellness Coach,
Chair of the Weight Management Dietetic Practice Group, Academy of Nutrition and Dietetics

"This book presents an incredibly practical tool that will help everyone understand what really matters when it comes to attaining and maintaining a healthy body weight. Thinking in calories can be a challenge, but everyone can understand what 30 minutes of jogging entails!"

—SUZANNE DIXON, MPH, MS, RD, Health & Nutrition Consultant,
The Health Geek, LLC, www.NoNutritionFear.com

"This intelligent book explains the elusive calorie—both friend and foe of women around the globe. It teaches us how to keep our bodies energized with healthy—and not empty—calories. The recipes are delicious crowd-pleasers, and the many tips peppered throughout are a boon for busy moms. Finally, an intelligent and indispensable guide for healthy living and not fad dieting."

—CAROLINA BUIA,
coauthor of *Latin Chic*, and mother of two sets of twins

THE CALORIES IN, CALORIES OUT
COOKBOOK

THE CALORIES IN

CALORIES OUT

COOKBOOK

200 Everyday Recipes That Take the Guesswork Out of Counting Calories—Plus, the Exercise It Takes to Burn Them Off

CATHERINE JONES and
ELAINE TRUJILLO, MS, RDN

Introduction by **Malden Nesheim, PhD**

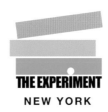

THE EXPERIMENT

NEW YORK

THE CALORIES IN, CALORIES OUT COOKBOOK: *200 Everyday Recipes That Take the Guesswork Out of Counting Calories—Plus, the Exercise It Takes to Burn Them Off*
Copyright © Catherine C. G. Jones, 2014
All photographs except those on pages 65, 67, 79, 123, 129, 210, 215, 219, 237, 263, 266, and 330, or otherwise noted copyright © Law Soo Phye, 2014
Photographs of Catherine Jones on pages xiv and 409 and of Elaine Trujillo on page 409 copyright © Andrew Markowitz Photography

The Experiment, LLC
220 East 23rd Street, Suite 301
New York, NY 10010–4674
www.theexperimentpublishing.com

This book contains the opinions and ideas of its authors; it is not intended to take the place of medical or dietary advice. Please consult with a physician, dietitian, or other health care professional before beginning any diet, exercise, or health program. The authors and publisher expressly disclaim responsibility for any liability, loss, or risk—personal or otherwise—which is incurred as a consequence, directly or indirectly, of the use and application of any of the contents of this book.

The views of this book do not necessarily represent the views of NIH and/or DHHS, or the Federal Government.

The Experiment's books are available at special discounts when purchased in bulk for premiums and sales promotions as well as for fundraising or educational use. For details, contact us at info@theexperimentpublishing.com.

Many of the designations used by manufacturers and sellers to distinguish their products are claimed as trademarks. Where those designations appear in this book and The Experiment was aware of a trademark claim, the designations have been capitalized.

Library of Congress Cataloging-in-Publication Data

Jones, Catherine Cheremeteff.
 The calories in, calories out cookbook : 200 everyday recipes that take the guesswork out of counting calories : plus, the exercise it takes to burn them off / Catherine Jones and Elaine Trujillo, MS, RDN ; introduction by Malden Nesheim, PhD.
  pages cm
 Includes bibliographical references and index.
 ISBN 978-1-61519-104-8 (pbk. : alk. paper) -- ISBN 978-1-61519-105-5 (ebook : alk. paper)
1. Reducing diets--Recipes. 2. Low-calorie diet--Recipes. 3. Food--Caloric content. I. Trujillo, Elaine B. II. Title.
 RM222.2.J6166 2014
 641.5'63--dc23
    2013050755

ISBN 978-1-61519-104-8
Ebook ISBN 978-1-61519-105-5

Cover design by Susi Oberhelman
Front cover photographs: EVERYONE'S FAVORITE VEGGIE BURGER (recipe appears on page 212): Matthew Greenland; WOMAN: rubberball/Getty Images; MAN Maartje van Caspel/Getty Images
Text design by Pauline Neuwirth, Neuwirth & Associates, Inc.

Manufactured in the United States of America
Distributed by Workman Publishing Company, Inc.
Distributed simultaneously in Canada by Thomas Allen and Son Ltd.

First printing May 2014
10 9 8 7 6 5 4 3 2 1

*For Mark, who inspired this book,
and the rest of my family, with
love and gratitude.*
CJ

*To those who inspire me in their
quest for better health,
and to my family, for their love
and encouragement.*
ET

*Texts on Ayurveda and on Yoga
give us this advice. That half
the stomach should be full of
food. Space should be left in one
quarter of the stomach for water,
and one quarter should be left for
breath.*

—Swami Veda Bharati,
Five Pillars of Sadhana

CONTENTS

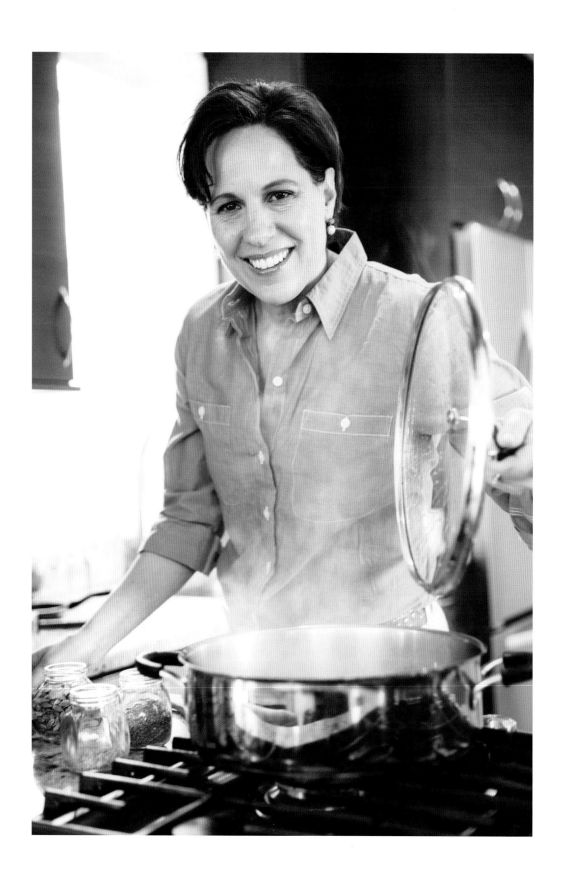

A COOKBOOK FOR EVERYONE

By Catherine Jones

ONE NIGHT WHILE I was visiting my younger brother, Mark, in Los Angeles, we were discussing what to make for dinner. He looked me straight in the eyes, and in a slightly exasperated voice said, "All I want is a cookbook with really good recipes that won't make me fat. And, I want to know how many calories I'm eating, so I can burn them off in the gym. Do you think you can do that?"

This calorie-and-exercise-focused cookbook is my gift to Mark, my family, you and your family, and anyone else you happen to be cooking for. My unique approach is designed to be sustainable and practical, with enough options to feed families whose members have a range of different calorie and nutritional needs.

While I was developing and testing the recipes, compiling nutritional breakdowns, and calculating exercise values with my coauthor, Elaine Trujillo, MS, RDN, I became slimmer. A lot slimmer. In fact, I had people asking me what I was doing to lose so much weight. I told them that I was keeping track of how many calories I consumed daily and how many I burned off.

Doing this caused me to eat less—about 10 percent less—and to exercise more. I was not dieting: I was eating smarter and healthier, and the results were amazing.

This is not a fad diet book, one that occupies the hot seat for a year and then fades away when the next trendy diet comes along. It's a supremely practical health-based cookbook for everyone, singles and families, looking to improve on what they eat, how much they eat, and how many calories they burn off. My plan is not low-carb—it's smart carb. It's not low-fat—it uses healthy fats in moderation. And it's not high-protein—it advocates for lean proteins in appropriate amounts, with lots of vegetable protein sources. No food groups were eliminated.

You will also see that there are no strict menus or diet plans that need to be adhered to. The goal is for you to create your own menus to suit your and your family's individual calorie needs and eating habits. I've read my share of diet books, followed the prescribed diets for two to three weeks (usually while cooking separate meals for my family), and then shelved the books, leaving them to collect dust. Yes, I lost a bit of weight each time, but as most folks have experienced, after stopping the diet, a few weeks later the weight came right back on. This cookbook offers a lifestyle plan, one that will empower you to make the smartest choices possible every time a food decision needs to be made.

My main goal with *The Calories In, Calories Out Cookbook* is to change the way you cook, eat, drink, and exercise. Admittedly, it takes some time to produce a homemade meal, to pack lunch for work or school, and to go to the gym, jog, walk, or practice yoga or Pilates. But your efforts will pay off. I guarantee they will. Every positive lifestyle change you make is an investment in your health and overall well-being.

WHO AM I FEEDING?

When it comes to food, I divide the world into two general camps: those who feed themselves and those who get fed. Julia Child summed it up beautifully with these words: "I was thirty-two when I started cooking; up until then, I just ate."

If you do not or cannot cook, for whatever reason, but you are extremely lucky (extremely lucky!), you get fed healthy, delicious home-cooked meals every day by someone who loves you. My family is an example of this extremely lucky group. They are thankful, which I appreciate. If, on the other hand, you eat out for most of your meals, you fall into the second camp, and you run a much higher risk of losing control of your calorie intake and general health. All this said, most people fall somewhere between the two camps. My goal is to get you to move more toward the first camp of cooking most of your meals and, once you are there, to keep you there.

So, who am I feeding every day?

Let's start with myself. I am fifty, slim, and generally fit and flexible. I practice yoga almost daily and exercise at least three times a week. Because I am a food writer, cookbook author, cofounder of the nonprofit Share Your Calories, and an ambassador's spouse with myriad social obligations, my life orbits around food. I spend many hours in the kitchen, cooking for my family, recipe developing and testing, and, when I am living overseas, organizing and attending official functions.

At my desk, I write about food, often salivating as I retaste dishes in my mind. I love healthy, fresh, simple food bursting with flavor. The more flavorful the meal is, the less I tend to eat, and the more satisfied I feel. I follow a mostly vegetarian diet. I eat seafood and some white meat, but almost zero red meat. I will have a bite of steak or lamb just to try it. And, yes, I do splurge every once in a while. Homemade cupcakes, cookies, and ice cream are my sweet-tooth downfalls.

My husband, Paul, follows a very healthy diet. While he has mastered the art of diplomacy, his kitchen skills are remedial at best. He eats his big meal at lunch and dines on toast and a wedge of cheese or pasta, accompanied by a glass of wine, for dinner. A few years ago, he switched to a midday main meal, which he claims has resulted in his feeling more energized throughout the day and sleeping better at night. He exercises at least one hour every day, almost without fail. Weight has never been an issue for Paul. He eats mostly fish and chicken, though on a rare occasion, he likes a good grilled steak or lamb chop.

Feeding my daughter, Allie, is where things begin to get a little tricky, but it's a challenge I've wholeheartedly embraced. She's seventeen and a tennis player, and since the age of thirteen, she has been a pescetarian—a vegetarian who eats seafood. Because she wants to stay in shape, my biggest challenge is making sure that every calorie she eats is nutrient dense. She has embraced good health and shows amazing discipline for a teenager. She does some form of exercise every day, either tennis, running, or yoga. Simply put, she inspires me, and her friends, too. They used to playfully tease her about her salads, veggie burgers, sprouts, and whole-grain lunches; now they ask her to share.

My teenage son, Hale, is active in sports and loves fried foods, but with a bit of grumbling, he's learned to forgo the greasy stuff and instead to eat baked or grilled chicken, sautéed shrimp, grilled salmon, and other healthy dishes the rest of us enjoy. Occasionally, greasy foods come into play. I included a crispy fish stick recipe just for him (and possibly for your finicky fish eaters, too). I want Hale to eat fish, and this is his preferred way of eating it for now. He also likes the Crab Cakes with Super-Easy Tartar Sauce (page 119). Because he's growing rapidly, he can afford the highest calorie intake in the family, so he's the only one who eats dessert daily. He claims that he has a special compartment in his stomach for dessert that never gets full.

As I've shown here, feeding a family can be a complicated and frustrating business, even for a professional cook. Children's calorie requirements continually change as they grow, and their tastes change, too. Parents have their own calorie needs, trending downward as the years go by. So, with all of those age groups in mind, I have come up with a collection of 200 appealing recipes that will satisfy a broad range of tastes and calorie needs. I hope you, your family, and everyone else around your table enjoys them.

WHY CALORIES COUNT

One day, long before I mentioned this cookbook idea to anyone in the publishing business, I got an e-mail from my publisher-friend Matthew Lore. He suggested I get my hands on a copy of *Why Calories Count: From Food to Politics* by Marion Nestle and Malden Nesheim. I did, and that book changed my life. It gave me permission to finally (yes, finally!) stop dieting forever. Instead, my focus turned to counting my daily calories and burning them off. I eat less but better, and I exercise more. I don't make a big deal about it. I just do it.

I am thrilled that Malden Nesheim, PhD, professor emeritus of nutrition at Cornell University, agreed to write an introduction to calories for this book, called Understanding the World of Calories (page 1). He's a calorie expert, and his introduction will teach you how food provides energy, what calories are, how they are measured, and how our bodies use them. His words will help clarify this complicated subject, and motivate you to pay closer attention to your diet and overall health. You may need to read this section twice to absorb all of the information—it took me a while to fully grasp it. Donny Bliss, a talented medical illustrator, contributed some creative images that will help you better understand the concepts.

In the section Determining Your Calorie and Exercise Needs (page 11), my coauthor, Elaine, helps you do just that. Using a simple four-step formula and the Harris-Benedict equation, she guides you to the magic number of calories your body needs daily. Once you know your Total Daily Calorie Needs, you can better stay within your limits by tracking how many calories you consume and burn off.

Elaine, Malden, and I would love to see the United States become a nation of predominantly healthy and fit people again. I say "again," because in the past, Americans were healthier. Statistics prove it. In fact, the whole world was healthier. Heart disease, diabetes, cancer, autoimmune and inflammatory diseases, and obesity were nowhere near the steadily climbing rates that we see today, especially among the young. There was a time when people used to walk, bike, and simply move around more. Kids played outside without being told to. We weren't all glued to our multiple screens for endless hours. It was the era before fast food, junk food, and supersized everything. We ate less and exercised more.

The bottom line is that you can't ignore bad health. It eats at your wallet, your time, your work, and your energy. It lessens your ability to do the fun things in life. Parents have an additional obligation to keep their children healthy. Setting a good example and offering healthy options at the earliest possible age will prepare children for the future, when they will have to make their own decisions. It is one of the most worthwhile investments you can make.

COOKING AT HOME

The fact remains, we require food to fuel our bodies. Choices have to be made at least three times a day, if not more. Nothing beats homemade meals, especially nourishing ones. That said, with my unique approach in *The Calories In, Calories Out Cookbook,* I've tried to make your life in the kitchen as painless—and productive—as possible.

At the front of the book, in a section called About the Recipes, Plus Shopping and Cooking Tips (page 21), I share my kitchen philosophy and give you guidance on shopping and cooking. I list the How-to Tips scattered throughout the text (page 28). These are tricks of the trade I've gleaned over many decades of cooking, both professionally and at home, as well as from my extensive travels around the globe. The Essential Pantry (page 29) is a record of every ingredient used in this book. I made sure that each ingredient appears multiple times in the recipes, so you don't buy a funky spice that you only use once a year. Essential Equipment (page 34) is a peek inside my kitchen. I share my equipment lineup and how I use my gizmos and gadgets. At the back of the book, Ingredient Notes and Recommended Brands (page 339) describes some of the less familiar items in the Essential Pantry. Frequently Asked Questions (page 350) addresses common issues, and in an awesome Appendix, compiled by Elaine, you'll find Calorie Values for nearly 1,000 common foods.

Every recipe comes with at least two important bits of information, Calories In and Calories Out, and most also include the added features of Calorie Combos and Calorie Cuts. Calories In offers a complete breakdown of the recipe's nutritional values; Calories Out tells you how much walking or jogging is needed to burn off the calories in that dish. Calorie Combos list serving suggestions and their caloric values. And Calorie Cuts tell you how to cut calories from the recipe if you want or need to. (Elaine and I go into more detail on each of these sections in Determining Your Daily Calorie and Exercise Needs, below).

I wrote this book with my brother Mark in mind, and you, too. My guiding principle while developing the recipes was to focus on taste first and foremost, and then to reduce calories and fat as much as possible. The calorie and exercise values accompanying each recipe, and the Calorie Values in the Appendix, are not intended to make you feel guilty, not at all. Please don't regard them with a sense of dread. They are there to empower you, to increase your calorie awareness so you can better meet your optimal calorie intake.

I would love to hear your stories about your positive lifestyle changes, improved eating habits, portion control tricks, motivation secrets, exercise tips, and anything else. It would give me tremendous pleasure and satisfaction to know that you are cooking and enjoying my recipes. Please drop me a note at www.caloriesinandcaloriesout.com.

Working together, we can all inspire each other for a healthier tomorrow. As the ancient Chinese philosopher Lao-tzu wrote, "A journey of a thousand miles begins with a single step." It's never too late to change. You can do it. You must do it. For yourself. For your children and grandchildren. And, for the health of future generations.

FIVE SIMPLE STEPS TO A HEALTHIER YOU

1. As much as possible, eat whole unprocessed foods.
2. Cook and eat at home as often as possible.
3. Keep track of your calorie intake and calorie output.
4. Walk, jog, or engage in some form of movement every day.
5. Close your eyes, lower your shoulders, and take a couple of deep, stress-relieving breaths through your nose. Relax and let go.

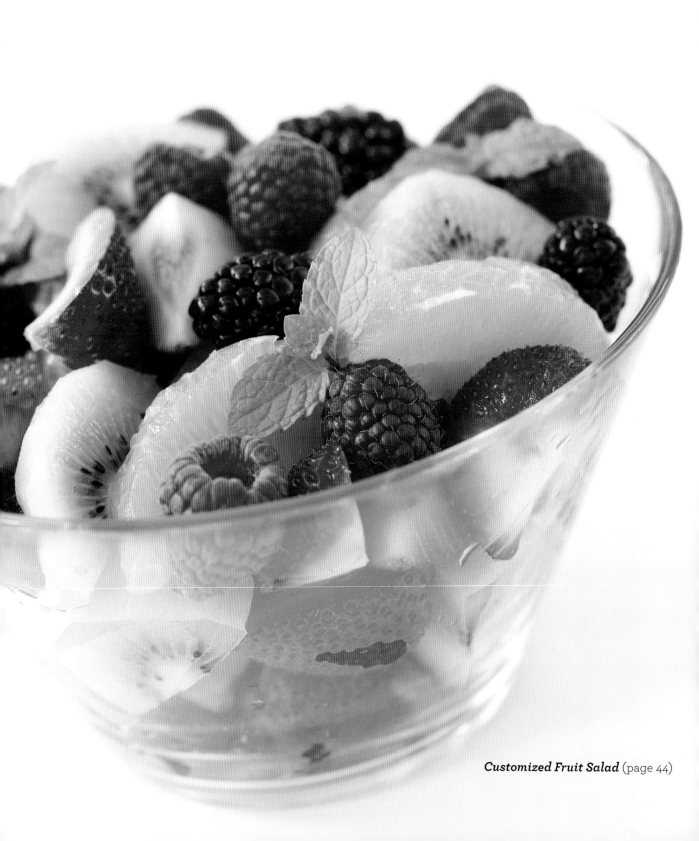

Customized Fruit Salad (page 44)

UNDERSTANDING THE WORLD OF CALORIES

By Malden Nesheim, PhD

WHEN CATHERINE SENT me the outline for this book, I was intrigued by her idea of writing a book that provided not only ways to prepare delicious food, but also a way to help connect what we eat and what we do for healthy weight management. Marion Nestle, professor of nutrition, food studies, and public health at New York University, and I had just published the book *Why Calories Count: From Science to Politics*. In it we discuss why we think the consumption of too few or too many calories is perhaps the most important cause of public health nutrition problems in the world today. Consuming too few calories can lead to malnutrition and susceptibility to infectious disease, while consuming too many can lead to overweight, obesity, and related health problems.

In the United States, about two-thirds of adults are overweight or obese, which we believe is related to the ways in which our food system encourages the consumption of too many calories, while our lifestyles cause us to expend too few. *The Calories In, Calories Out Cookbook* provides a tool to help you cope with this environment.

In this introduction, I explain what calories are, how we measure them, and how our bodies use them. I have spent my life studying, teaching, and carrying out research on aspects of human and animal nutrition. I grew up on an Illinois farm, studied agriculture at the University of Illinois, and obtained a PhD in nutrition and biochemistry from Cornell University, where I have spent my entire academic career. Early in my education, I had the opportunity to study with H. H. Mitchell at the University of Illinois, Champaign-Urbana. He introduced me to the principles of energy metabolism that are a foundation of the science of nutrition. Here I provide some of that background to help readers understand calories and to see how useful an understanding of energy concepts can be in planning our daily lives.

HOW FOODS PROVIDE ENERGY

Energy metabolism, the series of reactions that our bodies carry out to gain energy from our food, has been called the "fire of life." There are striking similarities between fire and energy metabolism. (This is where it gets a little scientific, so bear with me, please.) We obtain energy from food by a process of oxidation. Through metabolic reactions in our bodies, the oxygen in the air we breathe combines with the carbon and hydrogen atoms in the organic components of our food to form carbon dioxide and water. Energy is released in the process. If we burn food in a flame, the same process occurs. Oxygen is combined with the carbon and hydrogen atoms, and energy is released in the form of heat. That means we can estimate how much energy we can obtain from food by burning it in a flame and measuring the heat that is produced in units called *calories*.

In the 1800s, scientists developed devices called *calorimeters* to measure the calories

How a Calorimeter Measures a Food's Calories

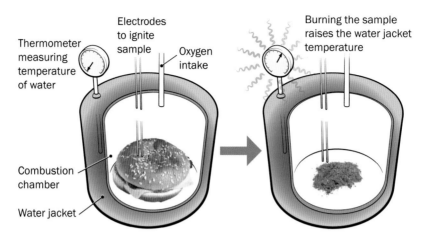

FIGURE 1. To determine a food's calories, food is placed in a calorimeter's combustion chamber. The test food gives off heat energy, and as it is completely burned that heat energy raises the temperature of the water in the water jacket surrounding the combustion chamber. The test food's calorie value is calculated from this rise in temperature of the water.

released when a food was burned, also called the *gross energy of the food*. A calorimeter can determine the calories provided by a food by burning it completely and, in the process, converting the food's calories to carbon dioxide and water in the presence of oxygen (see Figure 1, above). Living systems conform to the laws of physics, notably the first law of thermodynamics, which states that energy can neither be created nor destroyed, but can only change form. This precept explains how metabolism can convert energy from food into: 1) heat, 2) energy to build body tissue, 3) electrical energy for nerve transmission, and 4) the work of muscles. Energy not used for immediate purposes can be stored by the body, primarily as fat (see Figure 2, opposite).

What Is a Calorie and How Are Calories Measured?

If you search the Internet, you may find calories defined as those pesky, tiny creatures that live in your closet and sew your clothes a bit

tighter every night! Science, however, demands something more precise. The official definition of a calorie used by chemists is:

> One calorie is the amount of heat energy needed to raise the temperature of one gram of water by one degree Centigrade, from 14.5 to 15.5 degrees, at one unit of atmospheric pressure.

One gram is a very small unit, so nutritionists measure food calories in units 1,000 times greater, called *kilocalories*, which refer to raising the temperature of a kilogram of water one degree centigrade under the same conditions. This means that 100 kilocalories can raise the temperature of a liter of water (1.06 quarts) from 0 degrees Centigrade to the boiling point, 100 degrees Centigrade. This seems like a lot of heat, especially when a single cheeseburger can have 600 kilocalories. Our blood doesn't boil after eating a cheeseburger, because our metabolism doesn't release the heat all at once. We use that heat in small increments of energy to help us

How We Use Energy from Food

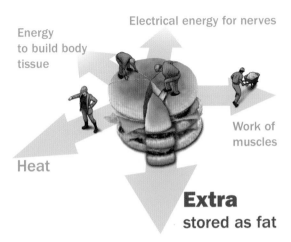

Energy to build body tissue

Electrical energy for nerves

Heat

Work of muscles

Extra stored as fat

FIGURE 2. Our metabolism converts the energy supplied by the food we eat in four ways (clockwise from lower left): Into (a) heat; (b) energy to build body tissue; (c) electrical energy for nerve transmission; and (d) the work of muscles. Extra energy is stored by the body, primarily as fat.

maintain body temperature, power the digestion of our food, make our brains function, build body tissue, and/or move our muscles. Any energy not used immediately is stored mainly as fat, which can be used later, when we are not eating.

To add to the confusion of the definition, the use of the term *calorie* is often inconsistent. The small-c calorie, sometimes called the gram calorie, is used mostly by chemists to describe chemical reactions, whereas the kilocalorie is the unit used to describe energy in foods. Often a kilocalorie is designated simply as a Calorie, with a capital C. However, in most uses with food, the term *calorie* is used to mean kilocalorie or Calorie. In this book, when we use the term *calorie*, we are referring to kilocalories—the ones you see on food labels.

In Europe and other parts of the world where the metric system is used, you may see the energy value of food described in terms of *joules*, the energy unit of the International System of Units based on the metric system. In this system, the terms kilojoules (1000 joules, kj) and megajoules (1000 kilojoules, Mj) are used to quantify food energy. A calorie is equivalent to 4.2 joules.

How Food Becomes Energy

Foods are made up of a large number of chemical components that to a large extent can be broadly classified as fats, carbohydrates, and proteins. These are known as *macronutrients*, and they are metabolized to provide the body with energy. The fats are the familiar vegetable oils or animal fats, such as lard or beef fat, that we consume when we eat animal products. Carbohydrates consist of sugars and starches and other plant components, such as fiber, while proteins consist of amino acids that the body can use for tissue synthesis. Other food components such as vitamins or mineral elements (known as *micronutrients*) do not provide energy in any significant amounts. Alcohol, though not a nutritional component of foods, can also be a source of calories.

But before food components can be used for energy, they must be absorbed into the body. The ingested food must be digested, a process whereby food is broken down into small molecules that can be absorbed from the intestinal tract and taken into the body.

Digestive enzymes found in the mouth, stomach, and small intestine carry out this process efficiently. Undigested food passes to the large intestine, where bacteria are able to further break down these food molecules into components that can be absorbed. Any food residue remaining after bacterial digestion, as well as sloughed-off intestinal cells and countless bacteria, are eliminated from the body as feces. Very small amounts of absorbed food components are excreted in urine and so are not available for body processes. The gross energy of the food must be corrected for these losses to determine just how

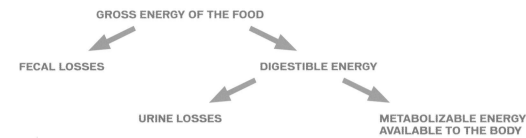

METABOLIZABLE ENERGY OF FOOD

GROSS ENERGY OF THE FOOD

FECAL LOSSES   DIGESTIBLE ENERGY

URINE LOSSES   METABOLIZABLE ENERGY
                      AVAILABLE TO THE BODY

much is available for our body to use. The process is summarized in the diagram above. The calories shown on food labels are estimates of the *metabolizable energy content* of the serving size listed. They are calculated from the amount of fat, carbohydrate, and protein in the food.

One way to determine the metabolizable energy content of a food relies on work done in the late 1900s by Wilbur Atwater, a professor of chemistry at Wesleyan University in Connecticut, who is considered the father of nutritional science in the United States. Atwater carried out large numbers of digestion experiments with human subjects, carefully measuring food intake and urine and fecal losses of energy with a wide variety of foods commonly used in diets of Americans at that time. He also summarized data from similar experiments published by laboratories throughout the world. He found that the metabolizable energy value of carbohydrates and proteins from typical diets of that time was about 4 calories per gram, while for fats, the value was about 9 calories per gram. He also determined that alcohol had an energy value of 7 calories per gram. The calorie values for carbohydrates (4), proteins (4), and fats (9) have come to be known as *Atwater values: 4,4,9*.

By knowing the carbohydrate, protein, and fat content of the foods in your diet, you can estimate the amount of usable energy by applying the Atwater values. Later, Atwater

and other investigators found that losses in digestion for some foods, especially those higher in fiber, were greater than for others, so the Atwater values were adjusted to account for the lower digestibility of specific foods. Using these principles, the United States Department of Agriculture has formulated food composition tables that provide estimates of the calories and other nutrients in more than 7,500 different foods. These tables, along with other nutrition databases, were used to calculate the calorie and nutrient content of the recipes in this book.

How Do We Use Calories?

When sugars (from carbohydrates), fatty acids (from fats), and amino acids (from proteins) enter the body, they can be completely oxidized to carbon dioxide and water, assembled into new body molecules, or stored, principally by converting them to fat. Scientists have generally divided calorie usage into three distinct categories: 1) calories used to power basal metabolism, 2) calories used to metabolize food, and 3) calories used for work or physical activity. These three uses can be readily measured, and their sum makes up the energy we must obtain from our diet to support life. Children who are growing, as well as pregnant or nursing women, have additional requirements to support the growth of body tissue, the fetus, or milk production.

THE BASAL METABOLISM

In the nineteenth century, physiologists devised instruments that could accurately measure the heat produced by a person who was resting or who was engaged in various activities. These researchers were struck by the predictability of the heat production of individuals when they were resting. This led to the concept of the *basal metabolic rate*, which has been considered the minimum energy expenditure compatible with life. The basal metabolic rate (BMR) is typically measured after an overnight fast when a healthy person is at rest, is in a comfortable environmental temperature, and is mentally tranquil.

The BMR is low in infants, rises quickly in the first year of life, and then declines through childhood and adolescence. From about ages 20 to 50, the BMR is fairly constant, but it declines by about 1 to 3 percent per decade after that. Women have a BMR that is about 6 percent lower than men throughout all life stages, probably because they have higher body fat levels. Fatty tissue is less metabolically active than lean tissue.

Your BMR can be estimated quite accurately by *prediction equations* developed by J. A. Harris and F. G. Benedict many years ago (see box below). You only need to input your height, weight, and age to get an estimate of your BMR. Most individuals' actual BMR will fall within a range of about 10 percent of the predicted value.

Using such equations, a 30-year-old woman who is 5 feet, 6 inches (168 cm) tall and 130 pounds (59 kg) is estimated to have a BMR of 1,390 calories per 24 hours, while a 60-year-old woman of the same height and weight will have a BMR of 1,250 calories. A 30-year-old man who is 5 feet, 10 inches (178 cm) tall and 170 pounds (77 kg) is estimated to have a BMR of 1,810 calories per 24 hours, while a 60-year-old man of the same height and weight will have a BMR of 1,610 calories. This decline in BMR with age is one of the reasons we can't eat as much as we get older if we want to maintain our body weight. Except for the most active people, the calorie cost of the BMR is the largest component of the energy requirement, and it is one that we can do little to change. In the section called Determining Your Daily Calorie and Exercise Needs (page 11), Elaine takes you through the steps of using the Harris-Benedict equation and your activity level to determine your daily calorie needs.

The Energy Cost of Metabolizing Food

The BMR is measured after an overnight fast because, as I've already noted, eating raises the heat production of a resting individual. The amount of heat produced depends on the amount and the type of food consumed, and it takes several

---

BASAL METABOLIC RATE BY HARRIS-BENEDICT EQUATIONS

WOMEN
BMR = 655 + (4.35 x weight in pounds) + (4.7 x height in inches) - (4.7 x age in years)

MEN
BMR = 66 + (6.23 x weight in pounds) + (12.7 x height in inches) - (6.8 x age in years)

hours for heat production to return to basal levels after a meal. This phenomenon is termed the *thermic effect of food* and represents heat produced due to the act of digesting and metabolizing a meal. We are experiencing food's thermic effect when we feel warm after ingesting a big meal.

The thermic effect of consuming a meal consisting of carbohydrates or fats is usually about 5 to 10 percent of the calories consumed. For proteins, on the other hand, the thermic effect may be as much as 20 to 30 percent of the calories consumed, due to the complexities of the metabolism of protein's amino acids after they are absorbed. Although the heat produced after eating is considered a loss of energy, some of the heat can be used to maintain body temperature.

The Use of Daily Calories Ingested by a Moderately Active Person

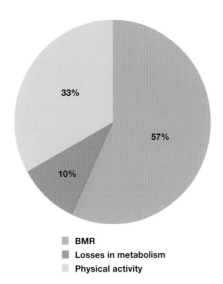

- ■ BMR
- ■ Losses in metabolism
- ■ Physical activity

The Energy Cost of Work and Physical Activity

Being active promotes good health, strengthens muscles, helps maintain a good body weight, reduces risk factors for chronic disease, and makes us feel better. But the human body is amazingly efficient, such that in most people, the calories needed to support daily activities are considerably less than those needed for the BMR. To support a moderately active lifestyle, the calories for physical activity amount to about one third of total energy requirements for most individuals. The range, however, can be very large, with, for example, those engaged in heavy physical work needing many more calories than someone who sits at a desk all day.

Exercise physiologists have been able to measure the calorie cost of a huge array of human activities. Studies show that the calorie cost of a particular activity depends on its intensity—for example, how fast you run—and on body weight. It takes more calories to move a heavy body than it does a light one.

To put this in perspective, one 12-ounce (375 ml) soft drink contains about 150 calories. If you weigh about 130 pounds (59 kg), burning those calories requires that you walk for about 45 minutes at 3 miles (5 km) per hour. A 190-pound (86 kg) person would need to walk only 31 minutes at the same speed to burn 150 calories. As you can see, controlling how many calories one consumes might be a better strategy than relying on exercise to burn it off. Individuals also seem to differ in their spontaneous physical activity. Those who fidget may burn substantially more calories than their more relaxed counterparts—as much as 100 to 800 calories more per day.

All the recipes in this book provide the calorie content of the food along with the amount of brisk walking or jogging needed to burn the calories consumed. Remember, women have a slightly lower basal energy expenditure. Coupled with a lower body weight, this means that they may need to exercise longer and harder to burn the same number of calories a man burns.

UNDERSTANDING THE WORLD OF CALORIES

CONTROLLING BODY WEIGHT

If you habitually eat more calories than you use, you will gain weight, most of which will be in the form of fat. A pound of fatty tissue stores about 3,500 calories. From about 1960 to the early 2000s, the American population has been getting fatter. During this period, the average weight of adult men in the US went from 174 to 195 pounds (79 to 88 kg), while the average weight of women went from 145 to 165 pounds (66 to 75 kg). Remember that this 20-pound (9 kg) weight gain was the average; some did not change at all, while others gained much more than 20 pounds.

This weight gain resulted in substantial numbers of men and women becoming obese. Body weights are customarily classified by the relationship of body weight to height, termed the Body Mass Index (BMI). BMI is calculated by dividing body weight in kilograms by height in meters squared. A person who is 5 feet, 5 inches (165 cm) with a body weight of 129 pounds (58 kilograms) has a BMI of 21.5. The Appendix provides a handy chart for you to easily determine your own BMI.

Public health researchers have classified BMI into general categories relating to health; see the accompanying box.

BMI CLASSIFICATIONS

Underweight	<18.5
Normal weight	18.5–24.9
Overweight	25.0–29.9
Obese	>30
Extremely obese	>40

Based on this classification, about two-thirds of Americans are overweight or obese. Obesity is rapidly increasing in the rest of the world as well, even in countries where some of the population is undernourished. Keep in mind that these classifications are somewhat arbitrary, as a well-trained athlete, for example, could appear to be overweight but still be quite lean.

For children aged 2 to 19 years, the weight standard is based on national surveys of child growth carried out over the past fifty years. Children are considered overweight when their weight-for-height measurement is greater than the 85th percentile of children of the same age; they are obese if their weight for height exceeds that of 95th percentile of same-age children. As in the case of adults, the rates of overweight and obesity have nearly tripled from the period 1976 to 1980 to the present.

Concerns about obesity are not merely a matter of appearance: the risk of many health problems increases with obesity. The list is long and includes coronary heart disease, high blood pressure, type 2 diabetes, some cancers, risk of stroke, liver and gall bladder disease, sleep apnea, osteoarthritis, abnormal menses, and infertility. When several of these problems or conditions occur together—including high blood pressure, high blood triglycerides, high blood sugar, and excess abdominal fat—the condition is called *metabolic syndrome*.

In spite of this rise in overweight and obesity, we do have a remarkably efficient innate physiological system of maintaining our own body weight. Taking in 2,000 calories a day adds up to nearly one million calories a year, yet many adults remain at nearly the same weight throughout their lives without consciously doing anything to maintain it. The physiology of weight maintenance and control of calorie intake is complex and still not completely understood. Eating behavior is controlled by centers in the brain that respond to hormonal and neural signals originating in the mouth, intestinal tract, fatty tissues, and other organs. These centers in the brain mediate control of calorie intake, satiety, and body weight. It is also true that body weight regulation is controlled to a certain extent by genetic makeup. There are dozens of genes that influence eating behavior. The urge to eat is fundamental to life, and overlapping regulatory factors have evolved to maintain that urge and to prompt you to eat as much as you can at every opportunity. Exposure to highly palatable food in ways that increase your frequency and amount of consumption seems to be able to override the "stop eating" signals from our regulatory system.

Dieting to reduce body weight is difficult because the "eat-more" signals that come from reduced energy stores are difficult to ignore. This is why it is far better to prevent excessive weight gain rather than to undergo the rigors of dieting to reduce body weight to some desired level and then maintain it.

Why has the body weight of Americans increased in the past few decades, even though we do have efficient systems that help us control intake? Our present food environment has a great deal to do with it. The calories available in the US food supply from the early 1900s up to about 1980 amounted to about 3,200 calories per day. By the year 2000, there were 3,900 calories per day available in the food supply for every child and adult in the United States. This represents *available* calories and does not account for losses in processing and waste before the food is consumed. These changes were brought about by changes in agricultural policies that led farmers to increase production largely of the commodity crops corn and soybeans. The greater availability of these low-cost energy and protein sources resulted in inexpensive animal feeds, raw material for inexpensive packaged foods, and low-cost fast foods that made eating out less expensive. Competitive pressures to sell food have made food available just about everywhere. Food advertising is all-pervasive and contributes to our eat-more environment.

At the same time, large portion sizes became selling points for restaurants, food chains, and soft drink companies. Large portions encourage us to consume more calories than we need. All of this has resulted in an environment that severely challenges our ability to control our calorie intake. In food consumption surveys, men report consuming about 200 calories more per day now than in the period from 1971 to 1974, and women report consuming 300 calories more.

ARE DIETS EFFECTIVE, AND ARE ALL CALORIES ALIKE?

I often get asked if diets are effective and, if so, which is the best one to follow. There are thousands of diet books that advocate conflicting ways to lose weight, including low-carbohydrate, low-fat, and high-protein diet strategies. To the extent that any of these plans encourage consumption of fewer calories, they can work.

Is a calorie a calorie, or are those from carbohydrates different from those from protein or fat? There is little evidence that once calories are absorbed into the body, some are more readily burned off and lost as heat rather than stored as fat, other than the differences I've previously discussed in the thermic effects of the three primary food groups. Low-carbohydrate diets often show more rapid immediate weight loss as the body loses glycogen, the storage form of carbohydrate. When glycogen stores are depleted, the body loses considerable water, since the storage of glycogen is accompanied by about four times its weight of water. But longer studies comparing low-fat or low-carbohydrate diets show little advantage of one over the other in maintaining weight loss. The committee that advised the US government on the 2010 Dietary Guidelines for Americans concluded that "No optimal macronutrient (protein, fat, carbohydrate) proportion was identified for enhancing weight loss or weight maintenance. However, decreasing calorie intake led to increased weight loss and improved weight maintenance." In research on weight loss, study participants find that it is easier to gain weight than to lose it and easier to lose weight than to keep it off.

Sources of calories do differ in what they bring to the diet nutritionally. There is some evidence that the body has more difficulty in regulating the intake of calories from liquid sugars, such as those found in sodas or other sugary drinks, compared to calories from solid foods. High-protein diets have been reported to produce a greater feeling of satiety, at least in some individuals. Healthy sources of calories contribute more than just calories to a diet. They are accompanied by the macro- and micronutrients that we need for a balanced diet.

SO, HOW DO WE COPE WITH OUR CURRENT FOOD ENVIRONMENT?

In much of the United States today, food is readily available everywhere. Outlets that once never offered food to customers or patrons now often do, like bookstores and libraries. Candy is displayed at checkout counters in almost any store, drugstores have turned into mini supermarkets, and every city has dozens of fast-food restaurants where cheap, high-calorie food is available in ever-increasing portion sizes.

Food companies spend huge amounts of money to induce us to choose their products, which are often high-calorie processed foods with few nutrients.

In *Why Calories Count,* Marion Nestle and I provided suggestions for coping with this food environment. We encourage you to be clear about your objectives and motivation. Are you concerned about your health or appearance? Are your clothes starting to get tight? Do you want to please someone who is worried about your weight? Strong motivation helps you succeed. And managing weight and eating better make many people *feel* better—a very good reason to pay attention to your calories in and calories out.

That said, we encourage you to be aware of calories but not to be obsessive about them. Estimate how many calories you need each day. When you eat out, pay attention to the calorie counts now listed on many menus and food items. The best way to ensure you are in calorie balance is to monitor your weight. Weight varies from day to day because of water balance, but be aware of trends. If you're gaining weight, eat more carefully. If you wish to lose a substantial amount of weight, joining a weight-loss group can help you to maintain the discipline needed to reduce your food intake. Eat smaller portions, keep snacks to a minimum, and don't keep tempting treats in the house. Don't drink your calories in sugary drinks or excess alcohol, and eat a varied diet that follows dietary guidelines and includes plenty of fruits, vegetables, and whole grains. You might want to shop at farmers' markets for fresh healthy foods, while simultaneously helping local agriculture. I have gone back to my rural roots and taken up gardening; I find there is nothing like eating freshly picked vegetables that you have nurtured and watched grow.

Move more. Engage in moderately intense activities for more than two hours per week, and do muscle strengthening activity at least twice a week. Moderate activity can mean any brisk action—walking, dancing, gardening, bicycling, Pilates—something to get you moving and your heart rate up. I joined a local gym, which provides me with both motivation and opportunity. Be active in your day-to-day life. If yours is a sedentary occupation, get up and move around every once in a while.

Cooking at home is one of the best ways to control what you eat, how much you eat, and your calorie intake. That is why this book is so valuable: not only will you be able to make delicious food for you and your family, but you will be able to incorporate delicious eating into a weight-control program to keep you healthy.

Malden Nesheim, MS, PhD, *Professor of Nutrition Emeritus and Provost Emeritus of Cornell University, has had a long career as a teacher and researcher at Cornell University. He served as director of Cornell's Division of Nutritional Sciences for many years. He is a former president of the American Institute of Nutrition and a fellow of the American Society for Nutrition and of the American Academy of Arts and Sciences. He has served on many advisory committees dealing with nutrition at the National Institutes of Health and the US Department of Agriculture. He was also a member of the Food and Nutrition Board of the Institute of Medicine. His latest book, with Marion Nestle, is* Why Calories Count: From Science to Politics.

DETERMINING YOUR DAILY CALORIE AND EXERCISE NEEDS

NOW THAT YOU have been initiated into the world of calories, it's time to apply that knowledge to this book's recipes. Calorie counting is the main focus of this book, and to keep calorie counting as easy as possible, the recipes are divided into three color-coded sections: 0 to 199 calories, 200 to 299 calories, and 300 to 399 calories. Within each section, the recipes are categorized into chapters by type, such as Breakfasts, Soups, and Salads, and then, within each chapter, in increasing calorie order. Elaine and I both agree that if you, say, eat a big business lunch, when it comes time for dinner, you might aim for lighter-than-usual fare. Using the recipes and appendix you'll be able to design your perfect low-calorie meal.

The ultimate goal here is to make cooking and understanding your calorie intake easy for you, wherever you live. Each recipe provides both US and metric measurements, because in our highly interconnected global world, cooks are downloading cookbooks everywhere from New York and Toronto to London and Dubai.

Helpful at-a-glance conversion charts also appear in the Appendix on pages 355 to 396.

Elaine and I want *The Calories In, Calories Out Cookbook* to become the most useful calorie-focused cookbook you own—even your most trusted and useful cookbook, period. To that end, the recipes in this book, with few exceptions, include tons of calorie information that we designate as Calories In, Calories Out, Calorie Combos, and Calorie Cuts. Here's a brief orientation.

CALORIES IN

For each recipe, Calories In provides the following nutritional data: calories (cals), protein (grams), carbohydrates (grams), fat (grams), fiber (grams), sodium (milligrams), Carb Choices, and Diabetic Exchanges. Optional ingredients in the recipes were included in the breakdowns, while optional garnishes were not unless otherwise stated. Calorie values for optional garnishes are listed in the recipe's Calorie Combo section. When a range of a specific ingredient is called for, such as 2 to 3 tablespoons of canola oil, the lower amount was used in the nutritional calculations.

Special Note for Diabetics: Elaine calculated the Diabetic Exchanges based on the *Exchange List for Diabetes* guidelines from the American Diabetic Association and the Academy of Nutrition and Dietetics. She feels that personally reviewing a recipe is the most accurate way to determine the exchanges. The foods in the starch, fruit, and milk groups of the Exchange List for Diabetes each contain 15 grams of carbohydrate per serving and can be "exchanged" for one another. In the Carb Choices, one carbohydrate choice is based on 15 grams of carbohydrate, which is roughly equal to one slice of bread or ½ cup of cooked pasta. To calculate the Carb Choices of any food, simply divide the total carbohydrate grams by 15. A registered dietitian can help you determine how many grams of carbohydrates or Carb Choices you need each day in your meal plan. We do include recipes for alcoholic beverages, and we'd like to remind diabetics that alcohol can cause problems with blood sugar control; it should be consumed in moderation with meals or snacks. We hope this information will help you with all of your food decisions.

CALORIE COMBOS

The Calorie Combos feature that accompanies each recipe (except in the Desserts and Drinks sections) matches dishes and foods that you might expect to be served together. This info helps you quickly and easily count up calories as you plan your meals. I formulated the combinations based on how I would serve the dishes at my table, on culinary themes (such as Asian, Indian, Western, or Mediterranean), or how the various spices, herbs, and other flavors would complement each other. Some of the Calorie Combos include store-bought foods and prepared components of meals, when those dishes might typically accompany the recipe. Please note that metric conversions are not included in this section, but the conversion chart on page 389 will help if you need it. Also, all of the foods listed here, such as rice, pasta, and quinoa, are cooked without any added fat unless otherwise stated.

Each combo item comes with a calorie count for a single serving, and they are listed in ascending calorie order. *No single combo plus the featured dish exceeds 500 calories*. We chose 500 calories as the cutoff point so you can build your meal while factoring in other possible components including condiments, garnishes,

breads, and desserts, as well as beverages. For the recipes in the Sides sections, we limited the pairings to ten dishes, as any of those lists could go on forever. You will see how quickly things can add up. If you want to check on the calorie counts of popular foods not listed with the recipes, the list of Calorie Values in the Appendix is a terrific resource.

CALORIE CUTS

Calorie Cuts are designed to help those who need or want to cut back on their calorie and fat intakes. They offer ideas on how to reduce the calories and fat in each recipe by eliminating or altering the amounts of various ingredients, including optional garnishes, by substituting ingredients, or by cutting back on the serving size. Not every recipe includes this feature. We used a savings of about 25 calories per serving as our baseline. In other words, with a few exceptions, if a cut or a combination of cuts would save you at least 25 calories per serving, we listed it.

CALORIES OUT

Calories Out is the feature that instantly distinguishes this cookbook from virtually every other, but it's also the one that you might not be thrilled to see. It informs you how long you need to walk at a brisk pace or jog to burn off the calories in each recipe. It is broken down for women and men, but before we go any further, Elaine and I want to explain this concept, why we included it, and how the Calories Out numbers have been determined. We will also teach you how to determine your Total Daily Calorie Needs.

The idea to include the concept of Calories Out occurred to me one day as I was sweating buckets on the treadmill and had a flashback to my brother Mark's request for a cookbook that included the amount of work needed to burn off the calories for each recipe. Five minutes into my routine, and I felt as if I had been running forever. I kept my eyes on the red digital timer and calorie counter. This can't be right, I thought. I must be burning more than 100 calories in 12 minutes. Not fair, right?

It may not seem fair, but those treadmill numbers are probably accurate, particularly if you enter your age, height, and weight in the machine's database. Seeing that this cookbook cannot offer personalized databases, Elaine and I had to decide on two profiles, male and female, on which to base the Calories Out values. We chose to work with the 50th percentile of the *Anthropometric Reference Data for Children and Adults: US, 2007–2010 National Center for Health Statistics, CDC*. It provides recent and accurate height and weight values for Americans.

The characteristics of the "reference people" used to calculate the Calories Out values are as follows:

WOMAN

Age: 30 to 39 years old

Height: 5'4" (163 cm)

Weight: 160 lbs (73 kg)

MAN

Age: 30 to 39 years old

Height: 5'10" (178 cm)

Weight: 191 lbs (87 kg)

You may be nothing like this, but these profiles are simply reference points. You may be younger or older, shorter or taller, lighter or heavier, and you may have a super-fast or super-slow metabolism or even a medical condition that affects your weight and metabolism. *Just keep in mind that these reference people and the corresponding Calories Out values will inform you of the general amount of exercise, in the form of walking or jogging, it takes to burn off the calories in a particular recipe. Individual values will differ. Ultimately, these numbers are designed to empower you, not to freak you out, even though they can be sobering.*

By listing Calories Out values, we are not implying that every morsel you put in your mouth requires walking or jogging to burn it off. What it means is that once you have figured out how many calories you need per day, or your Total Daily Calorie Needs (see below), any calories you eat that exceed that limit will need to be burned off to keep you in energy balance. Admittedly, there is no way on earth you can keep track of every calorie you consume, so don't fret. The main goal here is calorie awareness. *The Calories In, Calories Out Cookbook* gives you the toolkit you need to make smart calorie decisions every day, whether you're contemplating that 450-calorie gooey maple-walnut twist with your coffee, wondering what to make for dinner, or deciding if you should go for a jog before breakfast or a walk after lunch or dinner.

Determining Your Total Daily Calorie Needs

When thinking about your daily calorie needs, energy balance, which depends on your dietary energy intake and energy expenditure, should be your goal. Many factors affect your energy expenditure, including your age, body composition, gender, physical activity level, nutritional status, genetics, and endocrine status (e.g., hypo- or hyperthyroidism). In Understanding the World of Calories, Malden pointed out that we all burn calories at different rates, which is why we provide different exercise values for women and men for each recipe. He also mentioned that our metabolism, often referred to as our metabolic rate or Basal Metabolic Rate (BMR), declines with age as we lose lean body mass. Since lean body mass is more metabolically active than fat tissue, the less lean body mass we have, the more our metabolic rate decreases. Women also naturally have less lean body mass than men, which explains why when couples attempt weight loss, the man almost always loses more weight than the woman.

To understand how many calories you need each day, it helps to step back and understand the components that make up our calorie needs. These needs are referred to as Estimated Energy Requirements (EER). EER is the average dietary energy intake you need to maintain energy balance and to sustain a stable body weight. Simply put, it is the number of calories you require every day to keep your body functioning and to maintain your ideal weight.

A significant majority of your body's energy expenditure goes toward your Basal Metabolic Rate, including metabolic activities such as blood circulation, respiration, and gastrointestinal and renal function. If you glance at the pie chart on page 6, you will remember that the BMR comprises about 70 percent of your total energy expenditure. Some people have a slightly higher BMR than others. These are generally the lucky folks who can eat all the time and stay thin. Some have a slightly lower BMR, so they tend to gain more weight than others who eat comparable amounts of food. Most of us have "predictable" metabolisms; hence, they can be calculated by prediction equations.

There are several prediction equations that scientists have developed, and they do a good job of estimating your daily calorie needs,

generally within about 10 percent of your precise needs. (To get an exact number for your body, you would need to visit a clinic or a research facility and undergo a calorimetry study.)

Typically the rates of Resting Energy Expenditure in adults—meaning at rest without movement—are 0.8 to 1.0 kcal per minute in women and 1.1 to 1.3 kcal per minute in men. This energy expenditure is about 10 to 20 percent higher than BMR, and it translates to:

CALORIES FOR RESTING ENERGY EXPENDITURE
1,150 to 1,440 kcal/day for women
1,580 to 1,870 kcal/day for men

So, now that you have a picture of how many calories you burn at rest, let's add movement to the equation. Here we will incorporate your weight (W), height (H) age (A), and gender. Using four simple steps, which include the Harris-Benedict equation, plus an Activity Factor (see chart below), you can calculate your Estimated Energy Requirements and your Total Daily Calorie Needs.

How to Calculate Your Total Daily Calorie Needs

Step 1. Calculate your BMR (using the Harris-Benedict equation)

BMR Using Pounds and Inches

Women: BMR (calories) = $655 + (4.35 \times W) + (4.7 \times H) - (4.7 \times A)$

Men: BMR (calories) = $66 + (6.23 \times W) + (12.7 \times H) - (6.8 \times A)$

where W = weight in pounds, H = height in inches, and A = age in years

---

or

Women: BMR (calories) = 655 + (9.56 x W)
+ (1.85 x H) − (4.7 x A)

Men: BMR (calories) = 66 + (13.75 x W)
+ (5.00 x H) − (6.8 x A)

where W = weight in kg, H = height in cm,
and A = age in years

Step 2. Determine your activity factor (AF) using the table below.

HOW TO DETERMINE YOUR ACTIVITY FACTOR (AF)

	SEDENTARY	LOW ACTIVE	ACTIVE	VERY ACTIVE
Women, 19 years and older	1.00	1.12	1.27	1.45
Men, 19 years and older	1.00	1.11	1.25	1.48
Girls, 3 to 18 years old	1.00	1.16	1.31	1.56
Boys, 3 to 18 years old	1.00	1.13	1.26	1.42
	Typical daily living activities (e.g., household tasks, walking to and from your car to the store)	Typical daily living activities plus 30 to 60 minutes of daily moderate activity (e.g., walking at 3 to 4 mph/ 5 to 7 km hour)	Typical daily living activities plus at least 60 minutes of daily moderate activity	Typical daily living activities plus at least 60 minutes of daily moderate activity plus an additional 60 minutes of vigorous activity, or 120 minutes of moderate activity

Source: Physical Activity Coefficients (PA Values) for Use in EER Equations, Dietary Reference Intakes, *The Essential Guide to Nutrient Requirements*. Washington, DC: The National Academies Press; 2006.

Step 3. Calculate your Total Daily Calorie Needs

Total Daily Calorie Needs (calories) =

_____ x _____
Your BMR   Your AF

Step 4. Congratulations! You now know your numbers. You are on your way to taking control of your energy balance. Knowing your numbers may not mean that you stay within them every day. You are going to have days where you are on target and others where you are not. But be assured, just the act of keeping track of your

calories will be rewarding and empowering, and you will be more successful with your goals.

So, now let's assess your goals. Do you simply want to maintain your weight? If so, you can stop here. Your Total Daily Calorie Needs for maintenance have been calculated. Remember, these are estimates, and the best way to keep in check is to step on the scale regularly and make sure you stay within one to two pounds of that weight.

If weight loss is your goal, though, your energy balance needs to be tipped in the direction of an energy deficit, which you can accomplish by eating fewer calories and/or by bumping up your physical activity level, preferably both. Cutting calories is the key factor in weight loss, even more so than exercise. Here's how to trim calories from your daily intake, a number we refer to Energy Needs for Weight Loss:

Energy Needs for Weight Loss =
_____ – (250 to 500 calories)
Your Total Calorie Needs

This 250- to 500-calorie cut is only a suggestion. Often a 500-calorie cut is used because at the end of a week, that adds up to 3,500 calories, and 3,500 calories equals one pound. So, in theory, by cutting 500 calories from your diet each day, you will have lost one pound by the end of a week. But keep in mind that our bodies are not mathematical machines and the numbers don't always add up. Initially you may lose one pound a week by cutting 500 calories a day, but over time, your metabolism will adjust to fewer calories and (brace yourself) it will slow down. So, with time, your weight loss slows down, too. Not to be discouraged though—slow weight loss is still weight loss, and slow weight loss is the kind that stays off! So, if a 500-calorie deficit is manageable for you, then go for it. Over time, even as little as 50 calories less per day will lead to weight loss.

Conversely, if weight gain is your goal, the balance will need to go in the other direction, which would mean an energy surplus: more calories, and/or less activity.

Energy Needs for Weight Gain =
_____+ (250 to 500 calories)
Your Total Calorie Needs

If this all seems a bit daunting, it is because our bodies are complex and there are a lot of factors that go into how we metabolize food and produce energy. No one has all the answers when it comes

to metabolism and energy balance. Based on what we do know, though, learning your calorie needs, journaling your calorie intake every day, controlling your calorie intake, and engaging in physical activity are all empowering approaches to achieving and maintaining an ideal weight and overall good health. Recording what you eat, using a computer program, an app, or a journal, will tell you how many calories you are consuming and expending. By knowing your Total Daily Calorie Needs, you have a baseline to compare this to, to gauge whether you are overconsuming and need to cut back. Studies have proven that people who keep food journals lose weight, and in some studies, people who kept journals lost twice as much weight as those who didn't.

EXERCISE GUIDELINES, BENEFITS, AND TIPS

In 2008, the federal government published the first-ever *Physical Activity Guidelines for Americans*. The report recommends that if you are a woman or man 18 to 64 years old, you should get at least 2½ hours each week of moderately intense aerobic physical activity. You need to do this activity for at least 10 minutes at a time; shorter intervals don't have the same health benefits. At least two days a week, you should also do strengthening activities, such as push-ups, sit-ups, and weight training.

For children and adolescents who are 6 to 17 years old, 60 minutes or more of physical activity daily is recommended. Most of that should be either moderate or vigorous aerobic physical activity, and it should also include vigorous physical activity at least three days a week. As part of the 60 or more minutes of daily physical activity, children and adolescents should include muscle- and bone-strengthening activity at least three days a week.

Approximate Calories Used in Physical Activity
(154 LB MAN)

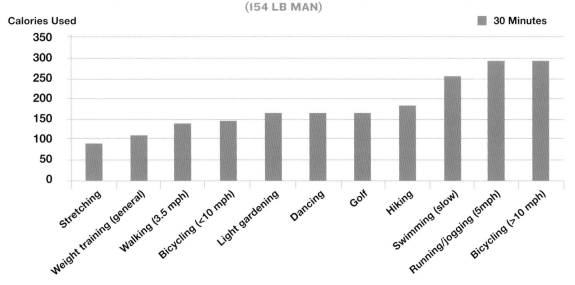

Calories Used

■ 30 Minutes

Activities (left to right): Stretching, Weight training (general), Walking (3.5 mph), Bicycling (<10 mph), Light gardening, Dancing, Golf, Hiking, Swimming (slow), Running/jogging (5mph), Bicycling (>10 mph)

Note: Those who weigh more will use more calories, and those who weigh less will use fewer.

Source: *Dietary Guidelines for Americans 2005*/MyPlate, http://www.choosemyplate.gov/food-groups/physicalactivity_calories_used_table.html

According to the *2008 Physical Activity Guidelines*, three kinds of exercise are essential to good health: 1) aerobic exercises, such as brisk walking at 3 mph (5 kph), jogging at 5 mph (8 kph), biking, rowing, swimming, or dancing; 2) muscle strengthening such as weight lifting, yoga postures, or Pilates, tai chi, or other forms of Eastern-style movement; and 3) bone-strengthening or weight-bearing activity, such as jumping jacks, running, brisk walking, and weight lifting. All are beneficial for burning fat and losing weight, the health of your heart and lungs, preventing osteoporosis, reducing stress, boosting energy, and revitalizing your body for optimal functioning. Although quite different, they complement each other. The great news about aerobic exercise is that your metabolism stays higher for many hours afterward. Exercise induces an additional small increase, about 15 percent, in expenditure for some time after activity completion (this could last for as long as 15 to 24 hours); the increase depends on the exercise intensity and duration. That's a reason to smile.

In *The Calories In, Calories Out Cookbook,* we focus on brisk walking—sometimes called walking for fitness—and jogging. Both move large muscle groups that cause you to breathe more deeply and your heart to work harder to pump blood. They are free, don't require a gym or class or any special equipment, and can be done anytime. Walking is safe for just about everyone; see the Note on page 18. With either, you should start with 3 to 5 minutes of stretching (the stretch-and-hold approach is recommended over stretching and bouncing to go deeper into the pose), then walk or jog briskly for 20 to 45 minutes. Cool down at a slower pace for 5 minutes, and stretch again. Stretching while your muscles are warm prevents stiffness and increases flexibility. Try a side stretch, forward bend, and calf, quadriceps, and hamstring stretches.

The pace of your walk should increase your heart rate gradually, which is most easily done by walking erect, talking full strides, and swinging your arms naturally. Jogging should be at your own comfortable pace. Your movement should be gentle but effective and not so rigorous as to harm the body. Breathe through your nose as much as possible. An extremely accurate way to indicate whether you are walking at a good pace is to measure your Target Heart Rate, or THR, which tells you how hard your heart is working. You can check your heart rate by counting your pulse for 15 seconds and multiplying that number by 4. The chart below lists different heart rates according to age. If you are new to exercise, aim for the lower Target Heart Rate at first and then, as your fitness improves, you can exercise harder to aim for the higher number.

AGE AND TARGET HEART RATE

AGE	TARGET HEART RATE (Beats per Minute)
20	120 to 170
25	117 to 166
30	114 to 157
35	111 to 157
40	108 to 153
45	105 to 149
50	102 to 145
55	99 to 140
60	96 to 136
65	93 to 132

Note: While walking is a safe and effective exercise for just about everyone, young or old, there are some people who should seek advice from a medical professional before engaging in any kind of exercise. This includes people with heart disease, diabetes, high blood pressure, arthritis, obesity issues, age-related issues, and other medical concerns, as well as pregnant women. If you find you are out of breath or you feel any pain, dizziness, or nausea while you are walking or jogging, stop and rest or seek medical help.

SAFETY TIPS FOR WALKERS AND JOGGERS

- Wear walking/jogging shoes with good arch support and a padded sole to protect your feet and legs and to ensure that your body gets the support it needs.
- Wear a watch with a second hand to measure your target heart rate if you need to.
- Layer your clothing so you can strip off layers as your body heats up.
- Walk/jog in a safe area, facing traffic, and on smooth surfaces, such as sidewalks or dirt paths. At night, use reflectors so drivers can see you and, ideally, walk/jog with a buddy, especially at night.
- If you wear headphones, keep the volume down or use just one earbud, so you can listen for traffic.
- Never use ankle weights—the added weight can hurt your back and joints. Very light hand weights can be used for gaining upper body strength, but be careful not to injure your shoulders, elbows, neck, or back.
- Ideally, get well hydrated before you walk or jog. Carry a water bottle to stay hydrated if needed, and drink more water after your routine.
- Carry ID and a cell phone, if possible.
- Protect yourself from the sun with SPF sunscreen and a hat.

Many of us are so gung ho about getting started with a new routine, we overdo it, and then stop doing it because we've injured ourselves or are turned off by the pain of pulled muscles and sore knees. The best advice is to ease into any form of exercise, especially if you are new to it or have not done it in a while. In order to attain the desired effects, it is critical that you exercise regularly, carefully, and in the correct manner. Going beyond your ability does more harm than good. Know your limits and don't push it, unless you feel it is the right thing to do. To prevent achy muscles and tight shoulders and calves, stretch before and after exercising. This is important for your muscles, circulation, and alignment.

CARDIO EXERCISE BENEFITS

- Improves cardiovascular functioning and circulation
- Decreases the risk of heart disease
- Helps control blood pressure
- Helps control blood sugar levels
- Aids with digestion and waste elimination
- Improves muscle tone and strength, and decreases the risk of osteroporosis
- Burns calories for weight management and weight loss
- Improves the body's response to stress
- Increases lung strength and capacity
- Improves circulation, as the network of blood vessels opens up to nourish and cleanse the body
- Reduces depression and anxiety
- Increases concentration and clarity
- Increases alertness and energy
- Improves sleep
- Improves creative thinking

STRETCHING AND STRENGTHENING EXERCISE BENEFITS

- Stretches and stimulates the muscles, ligaments, and joints
- Restores elasticity and tone to the body
- Improves spinal alignment and overall spinal health
- Stimulates circulation in all areas of the body
- Revitalizes the internal organs, the brain, and the nervous system
- Boosts the respiratory system
- Eliminates toxins, as more oxygen enters and leaves the body
- Massages and tones internal organs
- Improves digestion and bowel and kidney functions
- Stimulates the endocrine system and restores balance
- Relieves tension and reduces fatigue
- Reduces appetite
- Improves the complexion and hair vitality
- Improves mental clarity and balance and increases happiness
- Increases resistance to disease

Despite this litany of benefits, most of us need a little convincing to get moving. Inspiration can come from many different sources: a song that makes you want to move, an image that you admire, marking exercise time on your calendar or in your phone, or your family or friends. Motivation can also come from joining a walking or jogging club or fitness group, making exercise a regular family outing, taking a business walk instead of a business lunch, walking the dog, or exploring new places on foot. Perhaps the most important thing to remember is that not everyone responds to exercise in the same way. While some people lose weight when starting exercise programs, others, believe it or not, gain weight. Often they may be eating more calories to compensate for the calories burned. But don't look at exercise as an all-or-nothing proposition. Movement is an essential part of life. Once you start, you'll notice how much better you feel.

I'd like to end with a few words about stillness. We too often overlook our body's need for physical and mental stillness, and I'm not talking about lying in bed for a nap. After movement, be it cardiovascular exercise or yoga, a period of stillness can have a profound effect on mental clarity, awareness, creativity, and general happiness. Most yoga sessions end with the corpse pose (also known as *shavasina*), a restoring pose in which you lie on the floor in a comfortable position, legs slightly apart, arms slightly away from your sides, palms facing up, neck and shoulders relaxed, eyes closed. The aim is to simply let go, relax, and breathe. Your body melts into the ground and your breaths become rejuvenating.

Now, if you lie on the floor in the gym after a workout, people might think you're having a heart attack. But sit or stretch out on a mat, as you might in a yoga class, close your eyes, get comfortable, and connect with your breathing. Two to five minutes of this type of stillness, which some might call meditation, will make you happier and more productive for the rest of the day, and your mind and emotions will be more balanced. It's worth a try.

ABOUT THE RECIPES, PLUS SHOPPING AND COOKING TIPS

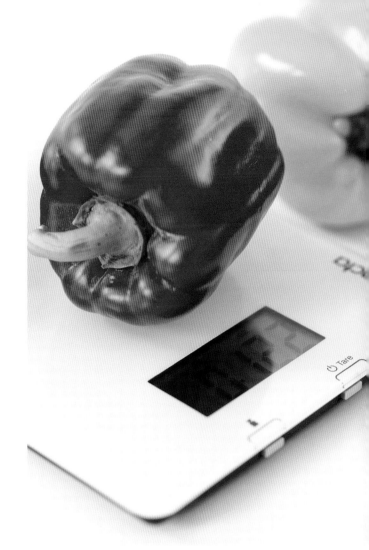

MY RECIPES

When I create a recipe, I think about *you*. I try to imagine you serving each dish at your table, to your family and friends. I try to gauge your joy, or possible frustration, when following the recipe. I try to anticipate your questions, and where you might be tempted to substitute an ingredient or adjust a quantity. And I picture the potential for a mess in your kitchen at the end of meal prep: how many dishes, pots, pans, bowls, whisks, spoons, and blenders you (or someone else) will have to clean. I try my best to look at the recipes from every one of these angles, simply because that's real life, and because I want you to succeed.

One thing to always bear in mind when you are in the kitchen is that you bring your own judgment, creativity, knowledge, experience, and taste buds to your cooking. Recipes don't come in one-size-fits-all packages. You may need to tweak them by substituting ingredients, adapting cooking times, or increasing or decreasing yields. Also, everyone's palate is unique. What appeals to me, or my husband, or children, or friends, might not appeal to you

or yours. I love Indian spices and tend to use them quite liberally. You may need to adjust or omit ingredients to suit your own tastes and those of the people you are feeding. But at the end of the day, if a recipe is structurally sound and delicious, it will become part of your life, and that is my goal here: to have my low-calorie recipes become yours.

As I mentioned earlier, feeding people can be complicated. There are times when I'm just plain tired of thinking about meals, food shopping, cooking, and, yes, even eating. During those moments I can't help but feel that food is overrated. Grossly overrated. But we can't do without it, and since we must fuel our bodies with food, we might as well get the most nutrients, flavor, and satisfaction we possibly can per calorie.

I am often asked where I get inspiration for my recipes. The answer: from everywhere and anywhere I find good food. This book's eclectic recipe lineup hails from around the globe. I've been on the global highway since birth (exactly five decades ago as I write this), and as it happens, my family and I have spent the past seven years in Southeast Asia, specifically the Philippines and Malaysia. While in Malaysia, I took numerous Indian cooking classes—hence the many wonderful Indian-inspired dishes you'll find throughout this book. I also squeezed in a few cooking lessons and classes while traveling in Thailand, Vietnam, and Vienna. I consider myself extremely lucky to have my food career and global lifestyle mesh together so perfectly, and I hope you'll enjoy the benefits as much as I do.

This book is a collection of the recipes I constantly come back to. They live in my kitchen. They are healthy and contain as few calories as I could manage without sacrificing taste or nutrition. I've cooked these recipes over and over again for weekday meals, family gatherings, formal dinners, casual lunches, working breakfasts, and brunches. No one ever seems to miss the excess calories and fat. Reviews are resoundingly positive. Clean plates, fellow diners going back for seconds, or being asked for a recipe are satisfying for me as the cook, and I hope that you will get the same responses when you make the recipes.

You don't need prior cooking experience to master my recipes. Some of them are quick to prepare, others may take more time. If you're a novice, I encourage you to follow each recipe exactly as written the first time you make it. After that, I invite you to play around. Have fun. Be creative. That is what cooking is all about.

MY RECIPE TESTERS

When it comes to testing recipes, I have always found that unpaid home cooks who volunteer as recipe testers are an essential part of preparing a cookbook for publication. I myself test each recipe that I develop at least three times and often many more times than that, since I'm not only developing recipes for this book but also constantly looking for new dishes to make for my family. It is only after I've made recipes at least three times that I farm them out for testing.

More than twenty friends, family, and acquaintances tested the recipes that appear here. All of my volunteers received a questionnaire along with the recipes, which helped ensure consistent feedback. In the questionnaire, I asked for input on serving sizes, the time it took to prepare the dish, the degree of difficulty, whether people liked it, what the cook did with the leftovers, and if he or she would serve it to guests. I took their praise, comments, recommendations, and criticisms into consideration as I tweaked the recipes and headnotes into their final form. One tester made my heart sing when she told me that she loved my food because she could *trust* it.

Why is this testing process so essential? One of my biggest pet peeves is complicated, expensive, time-consuming recipes that do not work. Actually, any recipe, simple or sophisticated, that fails to deliver on its promise drives me crazy. I've made my share of harebrained attempts at showstopping desserts that ended up total flops, worthy only of the garbage can. At first, just as you probably do, I blame myself, but that usually lasts only for a moment. Then I get mad at the wasted time, money, and energy. If you are investing in home cooking, cookbook authors and recipe developers should invest in you. I can assure you that I have.

SHOPPING TIPS

Start with Good-Quality Ingredients

A vital key to the success of any recipe is the quality of the ingredients. The better the quality, the better the outcome. Period. Even if things go wrong, which they sometimes do, if you started with something good, it usually still tastes good in the end. But this does not mean that you need to break the bank to eat well. Many of the tastiest and healthiest foods cost the least. As a general rule, buy the freshest, least-processed ingredients you can find. Farmers' markets and co-ops are wonderful places to purchase locally grown seasonal produce and homemade products, from heirloom tomatoes and straight-from-the-field corn to artisan cheeses and vinegars. You support your neighbors, the environment, and your own health. Win, win, win!

What about buying organic? By all means, do so. The benefits are clear. There is no question that foods free of chemicals, pesticides, antibiotics, and growth hormones, and neither genetically modified nor engineered, are better for you and the environment. If your budget has room for only a few organic products, choose the items that matter most to you. I tend to spend my extra dollars on organic, antibiotic-free, hormone-free meats, poultry, seafood, and dairy products. Then, whenever I can, I buy organic fruits and vegetables, greens, grains, and other staples.

Take the Time to Read Food Labels

When grocery shopping, please get in the habit of reading food labels. The section Understanding Nutrition Terms and Labels (page 356) explains what all of the numbers and percentage signs mean. I'm often surprised that the container I thought was enough for

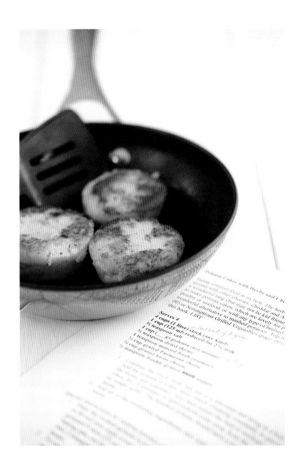

one person should, in fact, serve two or three, given the high calorie count per serving. Some expensive store-bought smoothies and health drinks are an example of this. Taking stock of nutritional information can save you unwanted calories, fat, and undesirable additives, such as artificial flavorings and colorings, gums, thickeners, preservatives, and MSG. As a rule of thumb, the shorter the ingredient list, the better. Also, try to shop more on the perimeters of the grocery store, where the whole foods tend to be, and less in the middle aisles, where most processed foods lurk.

Invest in Flavor

The dividends of a varied and extensive condiment collection are huge and will ultimately make cooking more fun. Invest in spices and condiments, fresh herbs, flavored vinegars and oils, Asian sauces, and anything else to excite your taste buds and olfactory senses. I have always found that the more flavorful my meal is, the less I tend to eat. Once you embrace spices, the creative possibilities are endless, in both Eastern and Western cuisines.

One of the best and cheapest places to purchase spices and other specialty items is an Indian or Asian grocery store. Turnover is usually high, so the spices tend to be fresher and more flavorful than what you find in a bottle from the grocery store. The downside to such markets is that often they are located off the beaten path, and many of the spices are sold only in bulk. But if you do buy in bulk, share your loot with friends who like to cook; it's a wonderful gift, believe me. Shopping online for spices is another convenient option; see Resources (page 393) for a list of websites for spices and other food items.

Admittedly, if you're new to cooking, or you haven't ventured much past Heinz ketchup and French's yellow mustard, buying Japanese, Thai, Indian, Mexican, or any other exotic products can be intimidating. The Ingredient Notes and Recommended Brands section (page 339) offers detailed descriptions of foods as well as brand recommendations. I think you'll find it helpful, so please take some time to read it before you shop or cook.

Time Savers

Some folks, like myself, love food shopping. Put me in a Whole Foods, gourmet or specialty food store, farmers' market, health food store, or a produce market on a distant shore, and I'm like a kid in a candy shop. I realize, though, that most people do not share this passion, and food shopping is a real chore for them. But whether you live alone or have a family, you will have to shop for food at some point, even if it's just venturing to the grocery store to buy coffee beans, cereal, and low-fat yogurt for breakfast. The following tips are designed to save you time, energy, and money.

Produce section: Look for washed and precut bagged or packaged vegetables and greens, including sliced or diced squash (summer and winter), stir-fry vegetables, baby carrots, broccoli and cauliflower florets, shucked corn, spinach, coleslaw, broccoli slaw, chopped or sliced onions, peeled shallots and garlic, cooked beets, cooked artichoke hearts, sliced mushrooms, and other ingredients. Some prepared vegetables come in a bag that you can just pop into the microwave oven. Fruits are often precut, which both saves time and allows you to purchase smaller amounts than, say, a whole watermelon or pineapple.

Salad bar: Many salad bars have precut vegetables and fruits that can save you prep time when cooking at home. Also, if you are cooking for only one or two people, you can pick up smaller amounts of foods such as chickpeas, beans, whole grains, lentils, olives, sun-dried tomatoes, and artichoke hearts. This way, you can avoid opening a can or jar and then wondering what to do with the portion you don't use. Some salad bars offer precooked foods that can save you loads of time, including hard-boiled eggs, cooked beets, cooked whole grains (particularly those with long cooking times, such as kamut or wheat berries), roasted peppers, blanched vegetables (such as peas and green beans), marinated mushrooms, and more. When putting together a salad, just be sure not to use too much dressing, and choose the healthiest offering possible, avoiding the creamy, fat-laden ones that can be tempting.

Freezer section: Frozen corn, peas, edamame (soybeans), French-style green beans, and artichoke hearts are all time savers. New products are constantly popping up on the shelves, and some of them are quite good. More and more of them cater to dietary restrictions: just look at the increasing number of gluten-free, vegan, vegetarian, and/or low-fat or diet products. Flavorful ethnic foods are usually my choice among frozen foods. Frozen breakfast foods are abundant, but be sure to read the labels so you can avoid high-calorie and fat-laden items.

Poultry, meat, and seafood sections: Meats, poultry, and seafood are sometimes sold seasoned with marinades or rubs. Some preseasoned raw meats and seafood can be found in the freezer section, too.

Emergency Meals

There are some days when cooking a homemade meal is simply not a reality. You can eat out, but that gets expensive, and you quickly lose track of your calories. Healthy choices at the prepared-foods sections of the grocery store can be a good option. And your freezer is an excellent standby. Mine bails me out at least twice a week. Also, I often double recipes, or components of recipes, to cook or heat later. The recipe headnotes offer freezing instructions wherever appropriate.

COOKING TIPS

Organize Your Kitchen

Being organized in the kitchen is absolutely essential. Take a moment to think about how you move around the kitchen. Ask yourself where you usually chop and mix things, roll out doughs, place hot pots and pans, then take those

answers and rearrange your kitchen accordingly. Make sure wooden spoons, spatulas, tongs, oven mitts, and other basic cooking utensils are in reach when you're at the stove or oven. Baking equipment ideally should be stored in one area. And you might want to keep canisters of flour, sugar, and other frequently used ingredients out on the countertop. You may find that making just a couple of minor adjustments makes a big difference.

Advance Prep

Advance prep is particularly helpful if you are juggling work and playing tag team with your husband or partner. Often you can prepare some of the ingredients of a recipe hours, or even days, before you cook or finish cooking the dish. Wash, chop, slice, or grate ingredients as appropriate. Nuts can be toasted in bulk and then frozen. Whole spices can be roasted and ground; they will keep for about a month. Instead of buying ground black pepper (which sometimes has little flavor), you can pregrind black peppercorns in a spice grinder and store the pepper in a spice jar. Sesame seeds can be toasted and stored; or buy them toasted. Many sauces, marinades, rubs, doughs, and batters can be prepped and then refrigerated or frozen. Be sure to label and date everything you freeze; those red sauces all look the same once frozen.

Advance prep also applies to the equipment you will be using for a recipe. When you're ready to cook, gather all the ingredients and tools you will need. This may seem obvious, but whenever I forget to do it, I inevitably regret it—especially when I'm baking and my hands are covered with dough. Also, you are less likely to forget an ingredient. Line up your tools alongside your prepped ingredients, and you are halfway there.

Freezing

Prep and freeze. Cook and freeze. Freeze, freeze, freeze! This advice is guaranteed to make you a happy camper in the kitchen. The key to fabulous Indian home cooking, for example, with its layers of intense flavors, is a freezer full of homemade sauces, curry bases, ginger-garlic paste, chutneys, spice mixes, and so much more. For those with different dietary predilections, the freezer may take on a different look, but the ease of adding flavors to a dish remains the same.

Planning Weekly Menus

If possible, take the time to plan menus for the week. Even if you don't stick with the plan exactly as written, it will at least give you a healthy starting point. Having menus set up for the week can relieve a lot of stress and prevent consuming unwanted calories. I know many people who cook on the weekends for the entire week. They are amazing, is all I can say. I often try to make leftovers roll into the next meal, or I double a recipe and freeze the extras.

Measuring Ingredients

Measuring ingredients is a good habit to get into for many reasons. First, of course, especially when baking, it could be critical for the success of your recipe. Second, it helps with portion control: the difference between 6 and 8 ounces (180 and 240 g) of raw salmon, for example, is almost 80 calories. Some folks weigh everything they eat, and I applaud them for that. They will see weight loss results for certain, and, more important, they will quickly learn to visually gauge portion sizes. Your eyes can play tricks on you, especially when you're hungry. Restaurant portions, which are usually large, will take on

an entirely new meaning when you are used to measuring everything and realize how much food is on your plate.

Snacking While Cooking

I admit that I'm guilty of snacking while cooking. It's torture to be hungry when you're surrounded by food. But now what I do is have a healthy snack before I begin to cook. It can be a piece of cheese with a few whole wheat crackers, nuts, or cut-up vegetables. A glass of water or unsweetened green tea might also take the edge off your hunger. I love to taste food as I cook. Apart from being vital to shaping the flavors of a dish, it's one of the real joys of cooking. But those spoonfuls, forkfuls, and mouthfuls can add up quickly, so I count them as part of the food that would go on my plate for the meal. If I've managed to taste my way through five spoonfuls of mashed potatoes, I serve myself that much less. It may sound crazy, but I'm keeping myself honest, and more important, I don't consider my smaller portion a punishment. If people ask why I am eating so little, I tell them that I ate the other half of my dinner while cooking it. They usually laugh.

Serving from the Kitchen

One easy way to control calories is to serve the meal in the kitchen and leave the rest of the food in the kitchen. That's right: leave that gorgeous stew on the stove-top, that lasagna dish or casserole on the counter. (The exceptions to this rule are salads, vegetable dishes, and healthy sides.) Fill the center of your table with a pretty arrangement of flowers and candles instead of food. You will quickly realize how keeping the extra food in the kitchen greatly reduces the temptation for second helpings, or mindless picking after you've finished your meal. Of course, if you have company, throw this suggestion out the window and bring your feast to the table.

Note: Some recipes call for ½ tablespoon of an ingredient; should you not have a ½ tablespoon measuring spoon, substitute 1½ teaspoons for the ingredient.

Note regarding recipe photographs:
If a recipe is featured in a photograph that does not appear right beside it, this 📷 following the recipe name directs you to the photograph in which a recipe is pictured.

HOW-TO . . .

Cooking is all about sharing. I've learned a few things from my years of professional and home cooking, and I want to share that knowledge with you, because often it's a subtle technique, or knowing how to choose the proper ingredient, that makes all the difference in the outcome of a dish. My "how-to" cooking tips are scattered throughout the book, and I've listed them here for easy reference.

HOW TO . . .

Slice Orange Segments (page 45)

Make Picture-Perfect Muffins Every Time (page 49)

Turn Milk into Buttermilk (page 52)

Freeze Bananas (page 53)

Make Homemade Croutons (page 62)

Roast Winter Squash (page 63)

Make Dashi (page 65)

Make Homemade Beef Stock (page 67)

Clean and Cook with Fresh Lemongrass (page 74)

Cook with Fresh Kaffir Lime Leaves (page 74)

Buy Seedless Cucumbers (page 75)

Make Perfect Coleslaw (page 79)

Clean Mushrooms (page 87)

Store and Clean Asparagus (page 88)

Cook Bok Choy (page 92)

Toast and Freeze Nuts and Seeds (page 93)

Trim Broccolini (page 96)

Wash Leeks (page 106)

Use Paneer (page 113)

Design a Makeshift Steamer (page 116)

Clean Shrimp (page 123)

Grill Skewered Food Evenly (page 129)

Soak Bamboo Skewers for Grilling (page 129)

Prevent an Avocado Half from Browning (page 157)

Keep Nuts Fresh (page 163)

Freeze Egg Whites (page 166)

Ripen Bananas Quickly (page 170)

Peel Ripe Mangoes (page 174)

Make Simple Syrup (page 175)

Take the Edge off Raw Onions (page 192)

Cook Beets (page 194)

Make a Basic Indian Tarka (page 210)

Clean Fresh Mung Bean Sprouts (page 215)

Cook Lentils (page 219)

Cook and Freeze Quinoa (page 219)

Make a Tandoori Yogurt Marinade (page 237)

Roast and Grind Spices (page 237)

Perfectly Roast a Chicken (page 245)

Score Bone-In Chicken Parts (page 245)

Mince Raw Chicken or Turkey (page 245)

Freeze Ginger and Garlic Paste (page 249)

Slice Flank and Skirt Steak or Brisket (page 260)

Make Homemade Applesauce (page 263)

Prevent Apples from Browning While Slicing (page 266)

Whip Perfect Egg Whites (page 272)

Make Perfect Hard-Boiled Eggs (page 290)

Slice Portobello Mushrooms (page 296)

Stir-Fry Rice (page 298)

Warm Tortillas Four Different Ways (page 330)

Clean Fresh Passion Fruit (page 332)

ESSENTIAL PANTRY

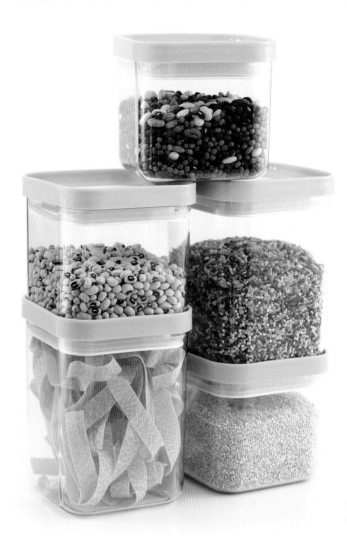

FOLLOWING IS A list of every ingredient used in this book, broken down into categories. Think of it as giant shopping list. Some of the items will be very familiar to you, others might not be. Foods marked with an asterisk indicate that more information is available in the Ingredient Notes and Recommended Brands section (page 339). In the Resources section (page 393) I've included some books and websites to help you learn more about spices, soy products, whole grains, and other items. I want you to have the confidence to try new things, so if you have any questions about the ingredients. please contact me through my website, www .caloriesinandcaloriesout.com.

CONDIMENTS, COMPONENTS, AND SAUCES

Anchovy fillets

Anchovy paste

Capers, medium

Dijon mustard, plain and whole-grain

Dill pickle relish

Dill pickles

Fish sauce*

French's yellow mustard

Green olives stuffed with pimientos

Green olives, pitted

Hoisin sauce*

Honey

Hot sauce

Japanese bonito flakes*

Japanese dashi*

Japanese seaweed products: kombu and wakame*

Jarred jalapeño peppers, whole or sliced

Kalamata olives, pitted

Ketchup

Lite soy sauce*

Maple syrup, Grade A or B

Mayonnaise, nonfat and light

Molasses

Oyster sauce*

Peperoncini

Prepared horseradish

Roasted red bell peppers

Sriracha hot sauce*

Sun-dried tomatoes in oil

Thai-style sweet red chili sauce*

Thousand Island dressing, reduced-fat

Tom Yam chili paste*

Worcestershire sauce

CANNED, JARRED, AND TETRA PAK FOODS

Artichoke hearts, in water

Canned black beans

Canned black-eyed peas

Canned cannellini beans

Canned chickpeas (garbanzo beans)

Canned great Northern beans

Canned green lentils

Canned kidney beans

Canned or jarred sliced red beets

Canned pineapple, in natural juice

Canned refried beans

Canned solid-pack pumpkin

Canned straw mushrooms, whole

Canned tomatoes, crushed, diced, puree, sauce

Canned yellow cling peaches, in light syrup

Coconut milk, regular and lite*

Low-sodium fat-free stock (any kind)*

Tomato paste

Unsweetened applesauce

V8 juice, low-sodium

OILS

Canola oil cooking spray

Canola oil

Extra virgin olive oil*

Toasted sesame oil

Vegetable oil (any kind)*

VINEGARS AND COOKING WINES

Balsamic vinegar, traditional or white*

Cider vinegar*

Distilled white vinegar

Red wine vinegar*

Seasoned rice vinegar*

Seasoned rice wine*

White wine vinegar*

HERBS, SPICES, AND EXTRACTS

Bay leaves

Black mustard seeds*

Black pepper, whole and freshly ground

Cayenne pepper*

Chili powder*

Chinese five-spice powder*

Chipotle chile powder

Cinnamon, ground and sticks *

Coriander, seeds and ground*

Cream of tartar

Cumin, seeds and ground*

Curry leaves, fresh or dried*

Curry powder, red and yellow*

Dried mint

Dried oregano

Dried tarragon

Dried thyme

Fennel seeds*

Garam masala*

Garlic powder*

Green cardamom, pods and ground*

Ground ginger

Ground nutmeg

Italian seasoning

Lemon extract

Old Bay Seasoning

Paprika, regular and smoked*

Red pepper flakes

Salt*

Sesame seeds, white, plain and toasted*

Star anise, pods and ground*

Tandoori spice mix*

Turmeric*

Vanilla extract

DRY GOODS FOR BAKING

All-Bran cereal

Baking powder, aluminum-free

Baking soda

Brown sugar, light or dark

Confectioners' sugar

Cornstarch

Dutch-processed unsweetened cocoa powder

Graham cracker crumbs

High-quality dark bittersweet chocolate

Instant coffee crystals

Low-fat granola

Oat flour*

Powdered gelatin

Semisweet chocolate chips

Sugar

Unbleached all-purpose flour

Whole wheat flour

NUTS AND DRIED FRUIT

Almonds, sliced

Cashews, roasted and salted

Dried cranberries

Dried mango

Dried pineapple

Peanuts, roasted and salted

Pecans

Pine nuts

Pumpkin seeds

Raisins, light or dark

Sunflower seeds

Walnuts

GRAINS, PASTAS, BREADS, AND LENTILS

Angel hair pasta

Arborio rice

Basmati rice, brown and white*

Corn tortillas, soft

Cornmeal, yellow*

Couscous*

Ditalini pasta

Dried lentils, green and red

Fusilli, bow-tie, or other bite-size pasta

No-boil lasagna noodles

Oats, rolled*

Orzo

Panko bread crumbs*

Polenta, instant*

Quinoa*

Rice, brown and white*

Rice noodles, for pad Thai* and thin (vermicelli)

Soba noodles*

Somen noodles*

Spaghetti, thin or regular

Udon noodles*

Whole grain bread

Whole wheat or white baguette

Whole wheat buns

Whole wheat pita or flatbread

Whole wheat tortillas

DAIRY AND SOY PRODUCTS

Alpine Lace, reduced-fat

Blue cheese, crumbled

Buttermilk, low-fat

Cheddar cheese, reduced-fat, shredded

Cream cheese, reduced-fat

Eggs, Grade A large

Feta cheese, reduced-fat

Goat cheese

Greek-style yogurt, plain nonfat or low-fat*

Milk, 2% fat and whole

Monterey Jack, reduced-fat, shredded

Mozzarella cheese, part-skim, low-moisture, shredded

Mozzarella mini balls

Paneer*

Parmesan cheese, grated

Provolone, reduced-fat

Ricotta cheese, part-skim

Sour cream, nonfat and reduced-fat

Swiss cheese, shredded

Tofu, extra-firm and soft*

Unsalted butter

Yellow miso*

FRESH VEGETABLES AND GREENS

Alfalfa sprouts

Arugula, regular and baby

Asparagus

Beets

Belgian endive

Bell peppers, red and green

Bok choy, regular and baby

Broccoli, spears and florets

Broccolini (also called broccolette)

Brussels sprouts

Butternut squash

Cabbage, green, red, and Napa

Carrots

Cauliflower florets

Celery

Cucumbers, seedless, unwaxed

Escarole

Fennel

Green beans, regular and French

Green chiles (hot or mild)*

Japanese eggplants (also called Asian eggplants)

Kale, regular and baby

Leeks

Mixed baby greens

Mung bean sprouts

Mushrooms, button, cremini (Baby Bella), shiitake, oyster, enoki, and portobello

Onions, yellow, sweet, and red*

Potatoes, new, russet, fingerling, and red

Radicchio

Red radishes

Romaine lettuce, regular and baby

Scallions

Snow peas

Spinach, regular and baby

Sweet potatoes

Swiss chard

Tomatillos

Tomatoes, plum, red, cherry, and grape

Watercress

Yellow summer squash

Zucchini

FRESH FRUITS

Apples, Granny Smith and others

Avocados

Bananas

Blackberries

Blueberries

Cantaloupe

Grapefruit

Grapes, green or red

Honeydew melon

Kiwis

Mangoes

Oranges

Papayas

Passion fruits

Peaches, white or yellow

Pears, Bosc

Pineapple

Plums, purple

Raspberries

Rhubarb

Strawberries

Watermelon

CITRUS AND JUICES

Lemons

Limes

Orange

Passion fruit juice

Pineapple juice

Pom (pomegranate) juice

FRESH HERBS AND AROMATICS

Basil

Chervil

Chives

Cilantro

Dill

Flat-leaf parsley

Garlic

Ginger

Kaffir lime leaves*

Lemongrass*

Mint

Rosemary

Tarragon

WHITE MEAT

Chicken tenderloins

Ground chicken

Ground pork, lean

Ground turkey

Pork shoulder

Pork tenderloin

Skinless bone-in chicken breasts, legs, and thighs

Skinless, boneless chicken breasts

Whole chicken

RED MEAT

Beef for stew, lean

Beef shank

Beef tenderloin steaks (filet mignon)

Flank steak

Ground beef, lean

Lamb chops, bone-in

Oxtail

Sirloin or top round steak

Skirt steak

SEAFOOD

Calamari, cleaned and sliced, frozen okay

Cod fillets

Center-cut salmon fillets

Mussels, cooked

Jumbo lump and/or backfin crabmeat

Sea scallops

Shrimp, raw, large and medium, peeled or unpeeled, frozen okay

Snapper fillets

Sole fillets

Tilapia fillets

Tuna steaks

Swordfish steaks

FROZEN

Blueberries

Corn

Edamame

Mangoes, sliced

Peaches, sliced

Peas

Raspberries

Spinach, whole leaves or chopped

ALCOHOL AND MIXERS

Agave syrup, light

Beer (any kind)

Blue agave tequila

Club soda

Cointreau

Frozen limeade

Peach liqueur

Pomegranate liquor

Prosecco

Red wine

Rum, dark or light

Stoli vodka, lemon and orange

Tequila, Cuervo Gold

Triple sec

Vodka

White wine

ESSENTIAL EQUIPMENT

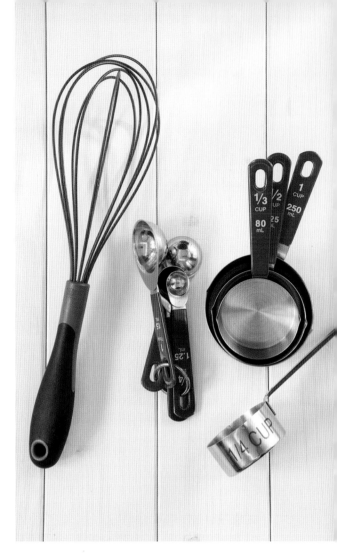

JUST ABOUT EVERY cookbook these days comes with a kitchen equipment section, and, truth be told, I always read them in the hopes of discovering a new gadget that will profoundly change my life in the kitchen. It's rare that that happens, and so my main message here is that you do not need a big fancy kitchen filled with gadgets to make healthy and delicious meals. I've listed all of my tools here, but I certainly don't expect you to have all of these as well. A small kitchen outfitted with the basics does just fine. What you do need are fresh, healthy ingredients, a bit of time, and, ideally, a sprinkle of passion.

Fresh flowers don't really count as essential equipment, but to me they are. They make my time spent in the kitchen a lot more pleasurable. Treat yourself and grab a bouquet of sunflowers, daffodils, roses, or hydrangeas on your next trip to the grocery store. A bowl or basket of colorful fresh fruits and vegetables, or a small potted herb garden by the window, can have an equally calming and joyful effect. Or light a candle before you cook, as Elaine does.

PREP AND HAND TOOLS

Bowls: An assortment of nesting bowls, metal, glass, or plastic, will serve you well. Buy at least one of each size: small, medium, and large. Ideally, at least one should be heatproof.

Chopping Boards: I highly recommend that you have a few plastic chopping boards: one for poultry, meats, and seafood; one for vegetables and fruits; and one for everything else. This is will help avoid potential cross-contamination with bacteria. Soft plastic boards (the hard plastic ones will destroy your knives) are excellent and cheap. They clean easily and effectively and can be bleached. I find a small board useful for slicing lemons and other quick jobs. I also love wooden boards, and I use them, but they can warp, are heavy, and can mold if not able to dry completely. Boos Block Board Cream, made from beeswax and mineral oil, is a good way to keep your wooden boards in top form.

Graters: Graters have come a long way since those rusted box graters of yesteryear. Remember those nasty finger scrapes? Ouch! I get shivers just thinking about it. Microplane graters, which come in many shapes and sizes, are razor sharp and super-efficient. (If you are really nervous about cutting yourself, Microplane even makes a kitchen cut-protection glove that might be worth a try.) I have Microplane's traditional four-sided box grater; the long thin one, for citrus zest, garlic, ginger, and cheese; and the fine spice grater for nutmeg.

Instant-read thermometer: Using a thermometer is best way to ensure the doneness of meats and poultry; if you want to take the second-guessing out of your cooking or grilling, invest in one. No need for an expensive one, though; a simple one from the grocery store will do.

Kitchen Scale: I have both an old-fashioned scale that I bought from Williams-Sonoma decades ago (it's a wonderful battery-free dinosaur) and a new digital Cuisinart scale that can measure in both ounces and grams, which is critical in recipe testing.

Kitchen Scissors: I use kitchen scissors all the time; in fact, I have them in three sizes. They're good for cutting fresh herbs, cutting

up hot quesadillas and pizzas, cutting baking paper to shape, and a thousand other things.

Knives: If you invest in a good set of knives, they should last you a lifetime. I'm partial to J. A. Henckels and Zwilling J. A. Henckels. There are also a number of excellent Japanese knives on the market, including Shun Kaju and Shun Hiro, though they tend to be very pricey. What draws me to Henckels is the feel of the handle in my hand. I suggest that you try holding knives before you buy them, especially bigger ones such as a chef's or santoku knife, or a cleaver. Handles vary in size, style, shape of the grip, texture, and how they balance the weight of the knife blade. You want knives that feel good in your hand when you chop or slice. The most important advice I can give you about knives is to keep them sharp. It's true that it's easier to cut yourself with a dull knife than a sharp one. Ideally knives should be professionally sharpened once a year, more if you cook a lot. Many hardware stores offer knife-sharpening services. A carbon steel is ideal for fine-tuning the blade every now and then.

Measuring Cups and Spoons: In the Pyrex category, which are used for measuring liquids, I would suggest having 1-, 2-, 4-, and 8-cup-capacity cups (in metrics, that would be 250-ml, 500-ml, 1-liter, and 2-liter capacities). For dry measuring, my set of cheap metal cups has served me well for years. The main problem with plastic ones is that sometimes the numbers on the handles fade, or they are so small you can't easily read them. I usually have at least three sets of measuring spoons in my kitchen (on some busy recipe testing days, I go through all of my cups and spoons numerous times).

Mortar and Pestle: Not essential, but people who use mortars and pestles tend to become attached to them. I have a number of them, which I use for different jobs: the gorgeous heavy brass one I picked up in Sri Lanka is perfect for grinding spices. My marble one is great for making garlic and ginger pastes. And my lava stone mortar and pestle works perfectly for pestos, guacamole, Thai-style curry paste, and herb oils (when I make these by hand; I admit the food processor saves time).

Pepper Mill: My recipes call for freshly ground pepper, and if you don't have a pepper mill, I urge you to buy one. It makes a huge difference. Get one that looks good on your table, too.

Ruler: As a cookbook author, I use rulers to make sure I have the correct size cake pan or skillet, or that I've rolled out the dough to the desired size. I keep a few in my kitchen, as they periodically disappear into my kids' bedrooms or backpacks.

Sieves and Colanders: I recommend having a medium-size stainless-steel mesh sieve with a handle for small jobs and a stainless-steel or plastic colander that can sit in the sink to drain pasta and other foods that require pouring off lots of hot water. I also keep a couple of small sieves on hand, for catching the pits when squeezing citrus fruits or for dusting baked goods with confectioners' sugar.

Small Bowls or Ramekins: I use small bowls and/or ramekins to hold my prepped ingredients. It makes cooking and baking much easier.

Spatulas for Cooking: I recommend investing in several spatulas in different sizes and shapes. A least a couple of them should be friendly for nonstick skillets. A long-handled grill spatula is another great investment. Heat-resistant silicone spatulas are good for stirring sauces and other hot mixtures.

Spatulas for Mixing: Spatulas have really evolved since the cheap white grocery-store varieties that often fell apart in the middle of mixing a batter, leaving you with the handle in your hand and the paddle buried somewhere deep in the bowl. Buy a few different sizes and widths: a thin one to get around the blade of a food processor or blender, a wider one for gently incorporating beaten egg whites into a batter, and something in between for everything else.

Tongs: Tongs are extremely useful for turning foods on the stove-top or in the oven. I like the inexpensive professional-kitchen metal ones. The thicker silicone-coated tongs can be difficult to slide under food, though they are gentle on nonstick skillets. Long-handled tongs are ideal for grilling.

Whisks: Whisks come in all different shapes and sizes, and depending on those factors, they perform differently (they really do). On my last trip to Williams-Sonoma, I noticed a variety of whisks on the shelves: ball-tip whisk, balloon whisk, standard French whisk, and a flat roux whisk. All very fancy. I suggest having three sizes: small (for dressings, sauces, and other small jobs), medium (for batters), and large (for large jobs such as incorporating whipped egg whites). The handle is important: it should be sturdy and comfortable. I do think you do get what you pay for in the whisk department: the cheaper ones tend to fall apart easily, so buy the best you can afford.

Wooden Spoons: I love my old, stained, heat-tempered wooden spoons, defined by their soft rounded edges and maybe a burn mark or two on the handle. The older they are, the better. I keep my wooden spoons for sweet and savory dishes separate. Wood does absorb flavor, and you don't want the taste of a curry in your raspberry jam. Ideally, get spoons in various shapes and sizes.

ELECTRICAL APPLIANCES

Blenders: If you have the money, Vitamix is the best. A Vitamix makes vegetable soups creamy without having to add any cream, it whips smoothies and other drinks in seconds, and it crushes ice beautifully for simple, instant fruit sorbets. Short of this gem, there are some excellent cheaper blenders on the market.

Food Processor: There are a number of fine brands, but I've used Cuisinart throughout my cooking career, and it's never let me down.

Handheld Blender: This is certainly one of my most-used gadgets. Also called immersion or stick blenders, handheld blenders are not expensive, and they are worth every penny; in fact, the cheaper ones seem to work just as well as the more expensive ones. (They are great for teaching your kids how to make smoothies.) Cuisinart is a good brand, and it is very easy to clean. Note that they don't last forever, especially if you use yours as much as I do mine.

Juicer: This cookbook includes some recipes that require a juicer, but it's not an essential piece of equipment unless you want to get into the juicing craze, which is certainly a healthy thing to do. Breville is one good brand.

Mini Food Processor: A gift to any cook, a mini processor does prep work, small mixing jobs, and grinding to perfection. It takes over the work of a mortar and pestle, though I do like to do things by hand when I have the time. Once again, Cuisinart is a trusted brand.

Mixers: A stand mixer is a worthwhile investment if you like to bake. KitchenAid, the king of the stand mixers, is one of my best friends in the kitchen. I also have a handheld mixer that I use for smaller jobs.

Spice Grinder/Coffee Grinder: If your budget allows, I highly recommend buying a spice grinder or a coffee grinder dedicated to grinding spices. Krups specializes in all things coffee and I have used their grinders for decades.

POTS AND PANS

6-Quart Heavy-Bottomed Stockpot: Think soups and stews. Le Creuset and Staub en France stockpots are beautiful and heat evenly, but they are very heavy, especially when they are full. (They are expensive, too!) One advantage is that they keep food warm for a long time, which is good if you are serving your dish directly from the pot. Other less expensive stainless-steel brands work well, too.

Cast-Iron Grill Pan: Not really essential, but if you cook a lot of chicken, meaty fish (such as tuna or swordfish steaks), or red meat, you might want to have one of these.

Nonstick Skillets: The price range for a set of nonstick skillets is astounding. The most important factor is how the pan conducts heat; a heavy base is essential. I prefer All-Clad skillets, which are expensive but will last. I have three sizes: 8-, 10-, and 12-inch (20, 25, and 30 cm). Store the pans with paper plates between them to protect them, and use the proper utensils to avoid scratching the surface.

Ovenproof Skillet: A 10- or 12-inch (25 or 30 cm) ovenproof skillet is essential for cooking certain dishes, such as my oven-baked breakfast pancake, frittatas, and some casseroles. My preference is cast iron.

Tiny Spice-Roasting Skillet: A 3- to 4-inch (8 to 10 cm) skillet is ideal for roasting spices, melting butter, cooking a single fried egg, and other small tasks.

BAKING EQUIPMENT

Baking Pans: Depending on how much you bake, your needs may vary. My essentials are 13 x 9 x 2-inch (33 x 23 x 5 cm) Pyrex and metal baking pans, a 3-quart (3-liter) Bundt pan, a 9-inch (23 cm) springform pan, 8- and 9-inch (20 and 23 cm) round cake pans, 9-inch (23 cm) Pyrex and metal pie dishes, and a 10-inch (25 cm) angel food cake pan. I invested in heavier, slightly more expensive pans, which have served me well over the years.

Baking Sheets and Cookie Sheets: The key here is to purchase heavy pans that will conduct heat evenly and are less likely to warp. A baking sheet is different from a cookie sheet in that it has four sides, whereas a cookie sheet has only one or two upturned edges.

Loaf Pans: I keep a range of sizes on hands, as I like to give smaller loaves as gifts. The ones I use most often are 8½ x 4½ x 2½-inch (21 x 12 x 7 cm) pans and 3¾ x 3 x 2⅛-inch (14.5 x 7.5 x 5 cm) pans.

Muffin Pans: I recommend 12-cup nonstick regular and mini size muffins pans. The minis are perfect for portion control. As with other baking pans, the heavier ones conduct heat better, and muffins will tend to rise more uniformly. In some of my recipes I call for muffin liners; in others, I specifically don't.

Oven Thermometer: An oven thermometer is a good idea, especially if your oven tends to heat unevenly. I always keep one in my oven to ensure dishes are cooking or baking at the correct temperature.

Pastry Brushes: I've been through many pastry brushes over the years, and I've come to rely on silicone brushes, which work well and clean easily.

Pie Dishes: I have 8- and 9-inch (20 and 23 cm) Pyrex and metal pie dishes, which I use interchangeably. I usually make no-bake pies in the Pyrex one and use the metal dish for baking, as the crusts tend to brown more evenly. Pie dishes are great for holding stir-fry ingredients; you simply slip them out of the dish and into the skillet as you go along. I also use pie dishes to hold partly cooked ingredients when the cooking process is staggered, or to hold portions of a dish that I am cooking in batches. As you can see, I'm a fan of pie dishes.

Silpat Baking Mats: A luxury worth investing in if you're a seasoned baker, or if you are new to baking. Not only do they keep cookies, crackers, tarts, and everything else from sticking, they make cleanup a dream. The mats come in different sizes, so choose the one best for you.

Timer: I have three timers in my kitchen, and I couldn't live without them. And, yes, I still manage to burn things sometimes.

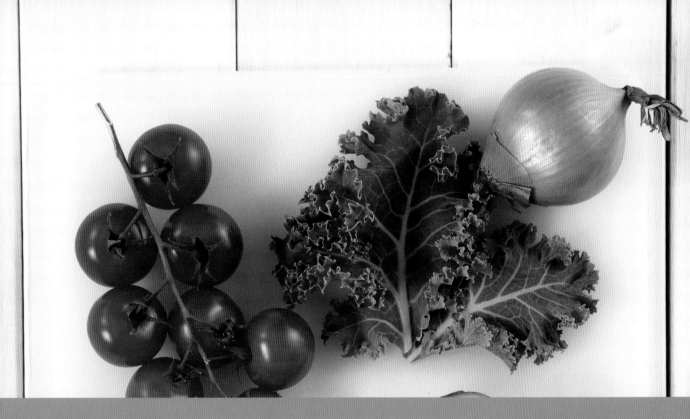

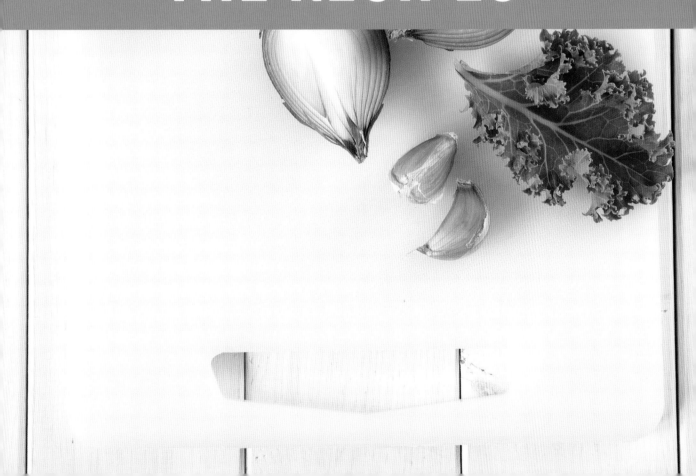

THE RECIPES

PART ONE

0 to 199

CALORIES PER SERVING

CUSTOMIZED FRUIT SALAD (📷 page xx)

I call this "customized" fruit salad because everyone likes different fruits and fruit combinations. My personal favorites are fresh mango, blueberries, and pineapple. Follow the suggestions below to make your own fruit salad according to your taste preferences and calorie needs. If you need to cut back, choose fruits low in calories, or use smaller amounts of the higher-calorie fruits. The optional garnishes are also a guideline. Note that 1 tablespoon of sugar is almost 50 calories (1 teaspoon is 16 calories); bear this in mind if you add sugar to your morning coffee or cereal. Calories Out values can be found on the opposite page. Note: ½ cup = 125 ml; the amount in grams will vary for each fruit.

Fresh Fruit Choices

Strawberries, rinsed, hulled, and quartered:
½ cup = 23 cals

Watermelon balls or cubes: ½ cup = 23 cals

Cantaloupe balls or cubes: ½ cup = 27 cals

Cubed papaya:
½ cup = 30 cals

Sliced peaches:
½ cup = 30 cals

Blackberries:
½ cup = 31 cals

Raspberries:
½ cup = 32 cals

Honeydew melon balls or cubes: ½ cup = 32 cals

Cubed pineapple:
½ cup = 40 cals

Blueberries:
½ cup = 41 cals

Orange segments:
½ cup = 42 cals

Diced apple:
½ cup = 47 cals

Sliced or cubed pears:
½ cup = 48 cals

Grapefruit:
½ cup = 48 cals

Cubed mango:
½ cup = 50 cals

Green or red grapes:
½ cup = 52 cals

Sliced peeled kiwi:
½ cup = 52 cals

Banana:
½ medium = 52 cals

Optional Additions

1 teaspoon sliced fresh mint leaves = 1 cal

¼ cup (60 ml) fresh orange juice = 28 cals

1 tablespoon sugar = 49 cals

Combine your choice of fruits and any optional additions and mix gently. If not serving immediately, cover and refrigerate. Fruit salad is best served on the same day it is made.

FOOD (½ CUP UNLESS OTHERWISE NOTED) | CALORIES IN	WOMEN WALKING (minutes)	WOMEN JOGGING (minutes)	MEN WALKING (minutes)	MEN JOGGING (minutes)
Strawberries 23	6	3	5	2
Watermelon 23	6	3	5	2
Cantaloupe 27	7	3	6	3
Papaya 30	7	3	6	3
Peaches 30	7	3	6	3
Blackberries 31	8	4	6	3
Raspberries 32	8	4	7	3
Honeydew 32	8	4	7	3
Pineapple 40	10	5	8	4
Blueberries 41	10	5	8	4
Orange 42	10	5	9	4
Apple 47	11	5	10	5
Pears 48	12	6	10	5
Grapefruit 48	12	6	10	5
Mango 50	12	6	10	5
Grapes 52	13	6	11	5
Kiwi 52	13	6	11	5
Banana (½ medium) 52	13	6	11	5
Fresh orange juice (¼ cup) 28	7	3	6	3
Sugar (1 tablespoon) 49	12	6	10	5

HOW TO SLICE ORANGE SEGMENTS

Cutting orange segments is easy once you get the hang of it. First, using a sharp paring knife, slice off the top and bottom of the orange to expose the flesh. Next, stand the orange upright. Working from top to bottom, and using your first slice as a guide to gauge the thickness of the peel, slice the peel off the orange in wide strips. Once it is peeled, working over a bowl, hold the orange in one hand and slice between the membranes on either side of each segment to release the segments, letting them drop into the bowl; set aside. Squeeze the juice from the membranes on top of your fruit salad to prevent fruits like apples, bananas, peaches, and pears from discoloring, or enjoy the juice as a drink (discard the membranes).

RHUBARB-RASPBERRY SAUCE (📷 page 281)

Rhubarb is wonderfully versatile—you can pair it with just about any fruit to make a delicious compote, pie, crisp, cobbler, or gorgeous deep-pink sauce like this one. My favorite way to eat the sauce is spooned over nonfat Greek-style yogurt, sprinkled with some Best-Ever Homemade Granola (page 184). One of my recipe testers noted that her family thought it was "excellent with pancakes." The sauce will keep for up to 1 week, covered and refrigerated, and it can be frozen for up to 1 month. Twelve ounces (360 g) of quick-frozen unsweetened raspberries can be used in place of the fresh ones: thaw the berries and omit the water called for in the recipe.

MAKES ABOUT 3 CUPS (750 ML)

8 ounces (240 g) rhubarb, any leaves trimmed, washed and cut into ½-inch (1.25 cm) pieces

½ cup (115 g) sugar, or to taste

12 ounces (360 g) fresh raspberries (about 3 cups, 75 0 ml)

2 tablespoons water

In a small saucepan, combine all of the ingredients and slowly bring to a boil, stirring to prevent sticking. Reduce the heat and gently simmer, stirring occasionally, for 15 to 20 minutes, until the rhubarb is soft and falling apart and the sauce is slightly thickened. (Note: The finished sauce should be the consistency of jam; it will thicken as it cools.) Serve warm, at room temperature, or chilled.

BLUEBERRY-PLUM SAUCE

Bursting with antioxidants, this is the ultimate sauce to pair with Greek-style yogurt, frozen yogurt, a bowl of oatmeal, waffles, pancakes, popovers, or anything else that begs for a hint of fruit. It is wonderful whipped into a luscious purple smoothie, which my kids sip as an after-school snack. Cover and refrigerate leftovers for up to 1 week, or freeze for up to 1 month.

MAKES ABOUT 2½ CUPS (625 ML)

1 pound (480 g) purple plums, pitted and cut into small cubes (about 3 cups, 750 ml)

1 cup (150 g) fresh blueberries

½ cup (115 g) sugar, or to taste

2 tablespoons water

1 cinnamon stick or ¼ teaspoon ground cinnamon

A few drops of vanilla extract, optional

In a small saucepan, combine all of the ingredients except the vanilla extract and slowly bring to a boil, stirring to prevent sticking. Reduce the heat and gently simmer, stirring occasionally, for 15 to 20 minutes, until the plums are soft and the sauce is slightly thickened. Smash some of the fruit against the sides of the pan to give the sauce extra body. Add the vanilla extract, if using. (Note: The finished sauce should be the consistency of jam; it will thicken as it cools.) Serve warm, at room temperature, or chilled.

57 CALORIES IN | 2 TABLESPOONS

Protein: 0 g; Carbohydrates: 14 g; Fat: 0 g; Fiber: 0 g; Sodium: 0 mg; Carb Choices: 1; Diabetic Exchange: 1 Fruit

57 CALORIES OUT

Women: Walk:
14 minutes | Jog: 7 minutes

Men: Walk:
12 minutes | Jog: 5 minutes

CALORIE COMBOS

4 ounces (120 g) nonfat plain yogurt: 72 cals

4 ounces (120 g) low-fat plain yogurt: 77 cals

4 ounces (120 g) nonfat frozen vanilla yogurt: 110 cals

Lemony Blueberry Corn Muffins (page 49): 120 cals

Mile-High Popovers (page 51): 143 cals

Carrot-Walnut Bran Muffins (page 52): 160 cals

8 ounces (240 g) instant oatmeal prepared with water: 166 cals

1 frozen waffle: 197 cals

Whole Wheat Pancakes (page 183): 216 cals

Best-Ever Homemade Granola (page 184): 286 cals

Oat Flour–Buttermilk Waffles (page 280): 303 cals

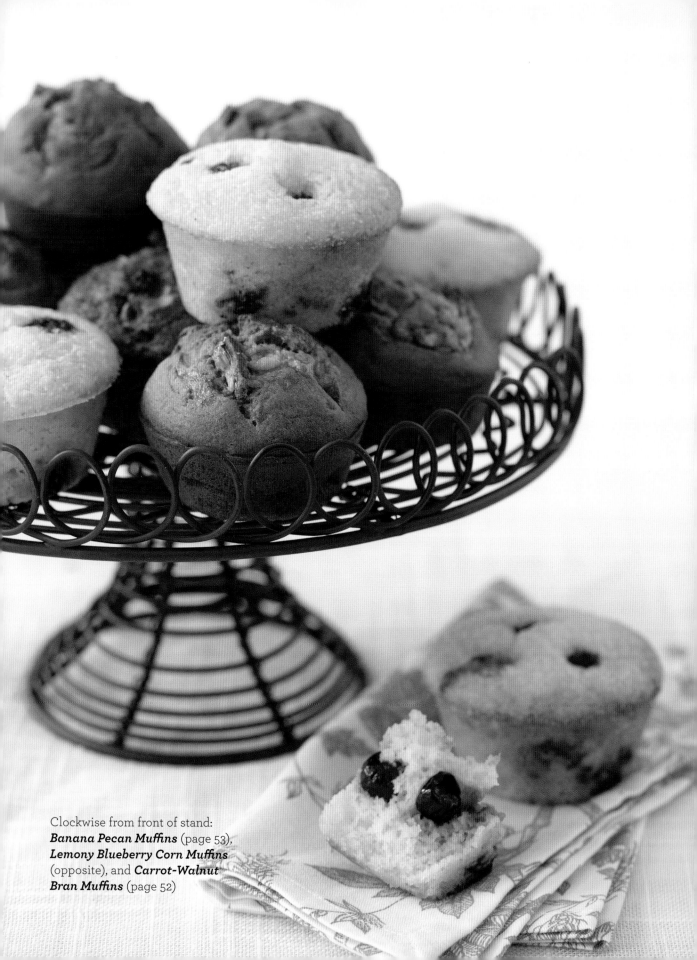

Clockwise from front of stand:
Banana Pecan Muffins (page 53),
Lemony Blueberry Corn Muffins
(opposite), and **Carrot-Walnut
Bran Muffins** (page 52)

LEMONY BLUEBERRY CORN MUFFINS

After they'd consumed many batches of these muffins, my family and friends unanimously decided that they are best made without muffin liners. Baking them directly in a greased muffin pan creates a crispy exterior, a wonderful foil to the fluffy, soft interior laced with juicy blueberries. Because blueberries have a tendency to sink, I roll them in a bit of flour before adding them to the batter, which helps keep them suspended. The muffins can be kept in an airtight container at room temperature for up to 3 days; they can be refrigerated for 5 days or frozen for up to 1 month. Muffins are best thawed at room temperature or in a conventional oven, not a microwave.

MAKES 12 MUFFINS

Canola oil cooking spray

1 cup (150 g) fresh blueberries

½ cup (65 g) plus 1 tablespoon unbleached all-purpose flour

½ cup (80 g) yellow cornmeal

1 teaspoon ground cinnamon

⅓ cup (70 g) sugar, plus a little extra for sprinkling

½ tablespoon baking powder

¼ teaspoon baking soda

¼ teaspoon salt

⅓ cup (80 ml) nonfat plain yogurt

¼ cup (60 ml) 2% milk

1 tablespoon grated lemon zest

2 tablespoons fresh lemon juice

¼ cup (60 ml) canola oil

1 large egg

1. Center an oven rack and preheat the oven to 375°F (190°C). Spray a 12-cup muffin pan with cooking spray; set aside. Roll the blueberries in 1 tablespoon of the flour and set aside.

2. In a large bowl, combine the remaining ½ cup (65 g) flour, the cornmeal, cinnamon, sugar, baking powder, baking soda, and salt and whisk until well combined. Set aside.

3. In a small bowl, combine the yogurt, milk, lemon zest, lemon juice, canola oil, and egg and whisk until blended. Add the wet ingredients to the dry ones, stirring until the flour is well incorporated. Fold in the reserved blueberries.

4. Divide the batter evenly among the muffin cups, filling each cup about three-quarters full. Sprinkle the top of each muffin with a little sugar. Bake for 20 minutes, or until a cake tester inserted in the center of a muffin comes out clean. Transfer the muffins to a rack and cool slightly before serving.

120 CALORIES IN I MUFFIN

Protein: 2 g; Carbohydrates: 16 g; Fat: 5 g; Fiber: 1 g; Sodium: 136 mg; Carb Choices: 1; Diabetic Exchange: 1 Starch, 1 Fat

120 CALORIES OUT

Women: Walk: 29 minutes | Jog: 14 minutes

Men: Walk: 24 minutes | Jog: 12 minutes

CALORIE COMBOS

Customized Fruit Salad (page 44): 23 to 57 cals

Rhubarb-Raspberry Sauce (page 46): 26 cals

½ cup (125 ml) orange juice: 56 cals

Blueberry-Plum Sauce (page 47): 57 cals

Three Delicious Fruit Smoothies (page 173): 62 to 89 cals

4 ounces (120 g) nonfat plain yogurt: 72 cals

4 ounces (120 g) low-fat plain yogurt: 77 cals

Five-a-Day Green Power Drink (page 176): 145 cals

Five-a-Day Pink Power Drink (page 177): 157 cals

HOW TO MAKE PICTURE-PERFECT MUFFINS EVERY TIME

When making fruit muffins, reserve some of the fruit before starting the recipe. For the Lemony Blueberry-Corn Muffins, reserve 1 to 2 blueberries per muffin. Do not roll these blueberries in flour. After you scoop the batter into the muffin cups, arrange the reserved fruit on top of the batter and then tuck it in, leaving it about halfway exposed, for a lovely presentation. You can also do this with nuts, banana chunks, berries, or dried fruits.

SPICED-UP HASH BROWNS (◎ page 55)

You would be hard-pressed to find a better friend for eggs than these spicy hash browns. My recipe testers loved the addition of smoked paprika; do try it. The high starch content of Yukon gold or russet potatoes will produce a soft, slightly mushy mix, while waxier potatoes will result in a bouncier texture. Sweet onions, such as Vidalia, are best. Also, think beyond breakfast: these potatoes make a great side dish for grilled foods (seafood, steak, chicken, sausages, pork chops, or veggie burgers) and are a lovely base on which to build a salad or soup. Any leftovers can be recycled in the Broccoli, Mushroom, and Cheddar Cheese Curry Frittata (page 216).

SERVES 5

133 CALORIES IN

Protein: 2 g; Carbohydrates: 19 g; Fat: 6 g; Fiber: 2 g; Sodium: 239 mg; Carb Choices: 1; Diabetic Exchange: 1 Starch, 1 Fat

133 CALORIES OUT

Women: Walk:
32 minutes | Jog: 15 minutes

Men: Walk:
27 minutes | Jog: 13 minutes

CALORIE COMBOS

1 tablespoon jarred salsa: 5 cals

1 tablespoon ketchup: 15 cals

½ cup (125 ml) orange juice: 56 cals

2 vegetarian breakfast links: 70 cals

1 whole wheat roll: 76 cals

1 poached egg: 78 cals

1 slice rye bread: 83 cals

2 bacon slices: 87 cals

1 fried egg: 90 cals

1 slice whole wheat bread: 120 cals

2 ounces (60 g) breakfast pork sausage: 180 cals

2 scrambled eggs, made with milk and butter: 182 cals

Spinach and Cheese Omelet (page 54): 193 cals

Broccoli, Mushroom, Cheddar, and Curry Frittata (page 216): 229 cals

½ teaspoon salt, or to taste, plus a pinch

4 cups (about 1 pound, 480 g) cubed peeled or unpeeled potatoes (see headnote above for potato varieties)

2 tablespoons vegetable oil

1 medium onion, chopped

1 garlic clove, minced

1 teaspoon regular or smoked paprika

Pinch of cayenne

1 teaspoon dried oregano or Italian seasoning

2 tablespoons chopped fresh flat-leaf parsley, optional

1. Bring a medium saucepan of water to a rolling boil and add the pinch of salt. Add the potatoes and cook for 5 to 7 minutes, or just until al dente. Do not overcook; the potatoes will be cooked again. Drain and set aside.

2. In a large nonstick skillet, heat the vegetable oil over medium-high heat. Add the onions and sauté, stirring occasionally, until light golden, 3 to 4 minutes. Add the garlic, paprika, cayenne, oregano, and potatoes, increase the heat to high, and cook until the potatoes are light golden, 10 to 15 minutes. If desired, smash some of the potatoes with a fork to break them up. Adjust the seasoning and garnish with the parsley, if using.

MILE-HIGH POPOVERS

My kids love these popovers; it's their #1 request for weekend breakfasts. I love them, too, piping hot from the oven with a spoonful of Rhubarb-Raspberry Sauce or Blueberry-Plum Sauce. They take 40 minutes to bake, so plan accordingly. You can play around with the ingredients, using different types of flour or adding millet, finely chopped nuts, or seeds for texture and protein. To freeze, cool almost completely, then place the popovers in a Ziploc bag and freeze. Reheat the popovers on a piece of foil in a preheated 350°F (180°C) oven for about 10 minutes. Do not microwave.

MAKES 6 POPOVERS

1 cup (130 g) unbleached all-purpose flour

1 cup (250 ml) 2% milk

2 large eggs plus 1 large egg white

1 tablespoon canola oil

Pinch of salt

Canola oil cooking spray

1. Center an oven rack and preheat the oven to 450°F (230°C). Have a six-cup nonstick popover pan ready.

2. In a large bowl, combine all of the ingredients and beat with an electric mixer on high speed for 30 seconds. Scrape down the sides of the bowl and beat 15 seconds more.

3. Preheat the popover pan for 2 minutes, then remove it from the oven and grease the cups with cooking spray. Divide the batter evenly among the cups.

4. Bake for 20 minutes, then reduce the heat to 350°F (180°C) and bake for 20 minutes longer, or until they are puffed and golden. Remove the popovers from the oven and serve immediately.

143 CALORIES IN | I POPOVER

Protein: 6 g; Carbohydrates: 18 g; Fat: 5 g; Fiber: 0 g; Sodium: 101 g; Carb Choices: 1; Diabetic Exchange: 1 Starch, ½ Low-Fat Milk

143 CALORIES OUT

Women: Walk:
35 minutes | Jog: 16 minutes

Men: Walk:
29 minutes | Jog: 14 minutes

CALORIE COMBOS

1 tablespoon diabetic-friendly, sugar-free strawberry jam (e.g., Polaner): 10 cals

Customized Fruit Salad (page 44): 23 to 57

Rhubarb-Raspberry Sauce (page 46): 26 cals

1 teaspoon unsalted butter: 34 cals

½ cup (125 ml) orange juice: 56 cals

Blueberry-Plum Sauce (page 47): 57 cals

4 ounces (120 g) nonfat plain yogurt: 72 cals

4 ounces (120 g) low-fat plain yogurt: 77 cals

CARROT-WALNUT BRAN MUFFINS (📷 page 48)

Quick, easy, tasty, and, best of all, super healthy. The more finely the carrots are grated, the better. I suggest All-Bran cereal because it is widely available, but you can certainly try other brands if you wish. I chuckled when I read one of my recipe tester's answers to the question "Would you make this again?" She wrote, "Yes, I've already made it three times." I call for using baking spray instead of muffin cup liners here, as the paper tends to stick to these muffins. The muffin batter can be made 1 day in advance; cover and refrigerate. Try to bring it to room temperate before baking, but if you can't, simply increase the baking time by a few minutes. Store muffins in an airtight container for up to 3 days; refrigerate for up to 5 days or freeze for up to 1 month. Frozen muffins are best thawed at room temperature or in a conventional oven, not a microwave.

MAKES 16 MUFFINS

160 CALORIES IN | 1 MUFFIN WITH WALNUTS AND CRANBERRIES

Protein: 4 g; Carbohydrates: 23g; Fat: 7 g; Fiber: 4 g; Sodium: 224 mg; Carb Choices: 1½; Diabetic Exchange: 1½ Starch, 1 Fat

160 CALORIES OUT

Women: Walk:
39 minutes | Jog: 18 minutes

Men: Walk:
33 minutes | Jog: 15 minutes

137 CALORIES IN | 1 MUFFIN WITHOUT WALNUTS AND CRANBERRIES

Protein: 3 g; Carbohydrates: 21 g; Fat: 6 g; Fiber: 3 g; Sodium: 224 mg; Carb Choices: 1½; Diabetic Exchange: 1 Starch, 1 Fat

137 CALORIES OUT

Women: Walk: 33 minutes | Jog: 16 minutes

Men: Walk:
28 minutes | Jog: 13 minutes

CALORIE COMBOS

Customized Fruit Salad (page 44): 23 to 57 cals

½ cup (125 ml) orange juice: 56 cals

Three Delicious Fruit Smoothies (page 173): 62 to 89 cals

4 ounces (120 g) nonfat plain yogurt: 72 cals

Five-a-Day Green Power Drink (page 176): 145 cals

Five-a-Day Pink Power Drink (page 177): 157 cals

Canola oil cooking spray

2 cups (130 g) All-Bran cereal

1 cup (250 ml) boiling water

⅓ cup (80 ml) canola oil

½ cup (115 g) sugar

2 tablespoons maple syrup

½ cup (125 ml) reduced-fat buttermilk

2 large eggs

1¼ cups (165 g) unbleached all-purpose flour

1½ teaspoons baking soda

1 teaspoon baking powder

¼ teaspoon salt

1½ teaspoons ground cinnamon

1½ cups (240 g) very finely shredded carrots

1 teaspoon vanilla extract

⅓ cup (40 g) chopped toasted walnuts, optional

⅓ cup (50 g) dried cranberries, optional

---

1. Center an oven rack and preheat the oven to 400°F (200°C). Grease 16 muffin cups with cooking spray; set aside.

2. Place the cereal in a small bowl and pour the boiling water over it; do not stir. Set aside.

3. Combine the canola oil, sugar, and maple syrup in a large bowl and whisk. Add the buttermilk and eggs and whisk again. Add the flour, baking soda, baking powder, salt, and cinnamon and whisk until combined. Add the All-Bran mixture and mix with a spoon, then add the carrots, vanilla, and walnuts and cranberries, if using, and mix until well incorporated. Let the batter sit at room temperature for 10 minutes.

4. Gently stir the batter, then divide it evenly among the muffin cups. Bake for 20 to 25 minutes, until a cake tester inserted in the center of a muffin comes out clean. Transfer the muffins to a rack and cool completely before serving.

HOW TO TURN MILK INTO BUTTERMILK

If you don't have buttermilk, no need to run out to the grocery store. Pour the specified amount of milk (whole or reduced-fat) into a Pyrex measuring cup. Add 1 tablespoon distilled white or cider vinegar per each 1 cup (250 ml) milk and heat in a microwave oven until warm to the touch, about 20 seconds. Let sit at room temperature for 10 minutes. When you see the milk beginning to curdle, you're good to go.

BANANA PECAN MUFFINS (📷 page 48)

Who doesn't love a deliciously moist and nutty banana muffin? This no-fuss recipe does not require a mixer, which greatly reduces cleanup. The key here, and with other recipes calling for ripe bananas, is to use bananas that are seriously overripe (see How to Ripen Bananas Quickly, page 170). You can substitute another ¾ cup (105 g) all-purpose flour for the whole wheat flour. The muffins keep well in an airtight container at room temperature for up to 3 days; they can be refrigerated for up to 5 days or frozen for up to 1 month. The muffins are best thawed at room temperature or in a conventional oven, not the microwave.

MAKE 12 MUFFINS

Canola oil cooking spray for greasing the muffin pan, or use muffin cup liners

¾ cup (105 g) whole wheat flour

¾ cup (105 g) unbleached all-purpose flour

1½ teaspoons baking soda

¼ teaspoon salt

⅓ cup (40 g) chopped toasted pecans or walnuts

⅓ cup (60 g) packed brown sugar

⅓ cup (80 ml) canola oil

1 teaspoon vanilla extract

1 large egg

¼ cup plus 2 tablespoons (60 ml plus 2 tablespoons) 2% milk

1¼ cups (330 g) coarsely mashed ripe bananas (3 to 4 large bananas)

1. Center an oven rack and preheat the oven to 375°F (190°C). Grease a 12-cup muffin pan with cooking spray or line with muffin cup liners.

2. In a large bowl, whisk together the flours, baking soda, salt, and pecans until well combined.

3. In a small bowl, combine the brown sugar, canola oil, vanilla, egg, and milk and whisk until well blended. Add the bananas and mix well, then add the wet ingredients and mix until well blended.

4. Divide the batter evenly among the muffin cups. Bake for 25 to 30 minutes, until a cake tester inserted into the center of a muffin comes out clean. Transfer the muffins to a rack and cool slightly before serving.

188 CALORIES IN | I MUFFIN WITH PECANS

Protein: 3 g; Carbohydrates: 25 g; Fat: 9 g; Fiber: 2 g; Sodium: 215 mg; Carb Choice: 1½; Diabetic Exchange: 2 Starch

188 CALORIES OUT

Women: Walk:
46 minutes | Jog: 22 minutes

Men: Walk:
38 minutes | Jog: 18 minutes

167 CALORIES IN |I MUFFIN WITHOUT PECANS

Protein: 3 g; Carbohydrates: 25 g; Fat: 7 g; Fiber: 2 g; Sodium: 215 mg; Carb Choices: 1½; Diabetic Exchange: 2 Starch

167 CALORIES OUT

Women: Walk: 4
1 minutes | Jog: 19 minutes

Men: Walk:
34 minutes | Jog: 16 minutes

CALORIE COMBOS

Customized Fruit Salad (page 44): 23 to 57 cals

½ cup (125 ml) orange juice: 56 cals

Three Delicious Fruit Smoothies (page 173): 62 to 89 cals

4 ounces (120 g) nonfat plain yogurt: 72 cals

Five-a-Day Green Power Drink (page 176): 145 cals

Five-a-Day Pink Power Drink (page 177): 157 cals

HOW TO FREEZE BANANAS

Ripe and overly ripe bananas can be frozen peeled or unpeeled. To freeze *peeled* bananas, place the banana pulp in a Ziploc freezer bag and mark it with a label indicating the number of bananas or the volume measurement. The frozen pulp can be thawed at room temperature or in a microwave oven for a minute or two. You can also freeze whole *unpeeled* bananas in a freezer bag; the skin will turn completely brown. To facilitate peeling frozen bananas, after thawing, use a paring knife and start at the bottom of the banana versus the top stem end. The bananas will be soft and very juicy, so work over a bowl.

193 CALORIES IN

Protein: 15 g; Carbohydrates: 2 g; Fat: 14 g; Fiber: 0; Sodium: 194 mg; Carb Choices: 0; Diabetic Exchange: 2 High-Fat Meats

193 CALORIES OUT

Women: Walk: 47 minutes | Jog: 22 minutes

Men: Walk:
39 minutes | Jog: 19 minutes

CALORIE COMBOS

1 tablespoon jarred salsa: 5 cals

1 tablespoon ketchup: 15 cals

Customized Fruit Salad (page 44): 23 to 57 cals

½ cup (125 ml) orange juice: 56 cals

2 vegetarian breakfast links: 70 cals

2 bacon slices: 87 cals

1 slice whole wheat bread: 120 cals

Spiced-Up Hash Browns (page 50): 133 cals

2 ounces (60 g) breakfast pork sausage: 180 cals

SPINACH AND CHEESE OMELET

Some chefs assert that one of the hardest things to make is a perfect omelet, and there is definitely some truth to that. The heat of the pan is critical. The omelet needs to set without the outer surface overbrowning. You can always remove the skillet from the stove if the eggs are cooking too quickly. Apart from spinach, tomatoes, and cheese, other filling possibilities include sautéed thinly sliced mushrooms, sautéed diced onions, diced jarred red bell peppers, chopped blanched broccoli florets, diced ham, thinly sliced chives or chopped fresh herbs, and dried herbs. Sautéing vegetables reduces their water content, thereby preventing a watery omelet, but if you're in a hurry, you can skip that. I always use butter when I cook eggs because it gives them a rich flavor and creamy texture. You can substitute a teaspoon of vegetable oil or use cooking oil spray. If you like ketchup with your eggs, consider switching to salsa, which has about 5 calories per tablespoon compared to ketchup's 15 calories.

SERVES 1

2 large eggs

Sprinkle of salt and freshly ground pepper

½ teaspoon unsalted butter

1 tablespoon diced ripe tomatoes

2 tablespoons thawed frozen spinach, patted dry, or ⅓ cup (10 g) fresh baby spinach

1 tablespoon grated reduced-fat cheddar cheese

1. Whisk the eggs, salt, and pepper in a bowl until very light and frothy. The more you whip the eggs, the lighter the omelet will be; set aside.

2. Melt the butter in a small nonstick skillet over medium heat. Add the tomatoes and spinach and cook for 1 minute, stirring, just until hot. Transfer to a small plate or bowl and set aside. (Do not rinse the skillet.)

3. Return the skillet to medium-low heat, add the eggs, and cook for about 20 seconds. Then, while tilting the skillet, use a spatula to push the cooked egg toward the center of the pan, allowing the raw eggs to hit the skillet. Distribute the cheese on top, followed by the reserved tomato-spinach mixture. Reduce the heat to low and cook for 1 to 2 minutes, until the eggs are set.

4. Fold the omelet in half, tuck in the sides if necessary, and cook for 10 to 30 seconds longer, until the omelet is the way you like it. Serve immediately.

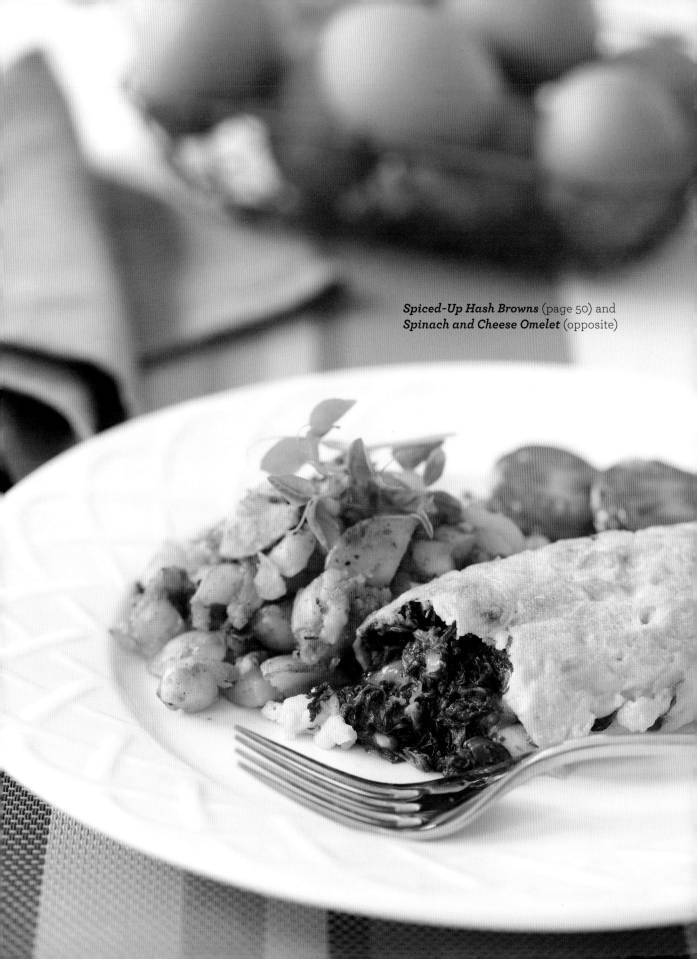

Spiced-Up Hash Browns (page 50) and
Spinach and Cheese Omelet (opposite)

SOUPS

HOMEMADE ROASTED VEGETABLE STOCK

20 CALORIES IN | I CUP

Protein: 0 g; Carbohydrates: 5 g; Fat: 0 g; Fiber: 0 g; Sodium: 330 mg; Carb Choices: 0; Diabetic Exchange: 1 Vegetable

NOTE: Because the cooked vegetables are not part of this recipe, low-sodium fat-free vegetable stock was used to calculate the nutritional information.

20 CALORIES OUT

Women: Walk:
5 minutes; Jog: 2 minutes

Men: Walk:
4 minutes; Jog: 2 minutes

This stock is a great base for the vegetarian soup recipes in this book, or any other recipes that call for the addition of stock. Oregano and thyme are used here, but feel free to change the flavors to jibe with whatever you are cooking. A wonderful Asian nuance can be achieved with a few fresh cilantro sprigs, a couple of stalks of lemongrass, and a handful of kaffir lime leaves, added in Step 3. The stock keeps for up to 3 days refrigerated and can be frozen for up to 3 months. Freeze it in small containers so you can thaw only what you need. Chipping away at an ice block of stock is no fun.

MAKES ABOUT 6 CUPS (I.5 LITERS)

1½ tablespoons extra virgin olive oil or vegetable oil

1 medium onion, quartered

2 carrots, coarsely chopped

½ red or green bell pepper, cored, seeded, and coarsely chopped

2 large garlic cloves, crushed

8 ounces (200 g) mushrooms (any kind), rinsed, stems trimmed, and quartered

1 teaspoon dried oregano

1 teaspoon dried thyme

1 cup (125 ml) boiling water

8 cups (2 liters) cold water

One 14.5-ounce (411 g) can diced tomatoes, with their juices, or 1½ cups (375 ml) diced fresh tomatoes, with their juices

1 teaspoon salt, or to taste

1. Preheat the oven to 450°F (230°C). Place the olive oil in a large baking dish and add the onions, carrots, red bell peppers, garlic, and mushrooms. Sprinkle with the oregano and thyme and stir to lightly coat the vegetables. Roast, stirring once, for 30 to 40 minutes, until the vegetables are nicely browned.

2. Transfer the roasted vegetables to a stockpot. Add the boiling water to the baking dish and scrape up as much of the roasted bits as possible. Add the liquid and any bits to the stockpot.

3. Add the remaining ingredients and bring to a boil, then reduce the heat and gently simmer for 1 hour, or until the stock is slightly reduced and the flavors have had a chance to develop. Strain the stock into a heatproof bowl; use the back of a ladle to press the juices and some of the pulp through the strainer (this is an important step as your stock will be more flavorful). If not using immediately, let cool and refrigerate or freeze.

HOMEMADE CHICKEN STOCK

There is nothing quite like the soul-warming smell of chicken stock simmering on the stove. Use this recipe as a blueprint, then spring off into any direction you wish. While I was living in Malaysia, my fabulous Chinese cook, Luan, always rubbed the raw chicken with salt before rinsing it. Luan believes this helps remove impurities and also flavors the meat. It's an extra step, admittedly, but I've adopted it and you can too, if you wish. I also learned not to boil the chicken too long; 45 minutes to 1 hour is about right, depending on the size of the bird. Too long, and the meat dries out. Luan used only ginger, no other vegetables or herbs, to flavor the broth. I've gone the traditional Western route with the flavors in this recipe. This stock keeps for up to 3 days refrigerated and can be frozen for up to 3 months.

MAKES ABOUT 10 CUPS (2.5 LITERS)

One 3- to 3½-pound (1.5 to 1.7 g) whole chicken or 3 pounds (1.5 kg) skinless bone-in chicken parts, rinsed and any visible fat removed

1 onion, quartered

1 carrot, quartered

1 celery stalk, quartered

3 fresh parsley sprigs

2 bay leaves

2 teaspoons salt, or to taste

½ teaspoon black peppercorns

10 to 12 cups (2.5 to 3 liters) water, or enough to completely cover all of the ingredients

1. In a stockpot, combine all of the ingredients and bring to a boil. Reduce the heat and simmer, uncovered, for about 1 hour, or until the chicken is completely cooked.

2. Remove the chicken and strain the stock into a heatproof bowl. Allow the stock to cool to room temperature, then refrigerate until chilled. Meanwhile, when the chicken is cool enough to handle, remove the meat from the bone. (Note: This is more easily done while the chicken is still warm.) Cover the meat and refrigerate it if not using promptly.

3. Once the stock has chilled, remove it from the refrigerator and, using a large spoon, scrape off as much fat from the surface as possible. If not using immediately, refrigerate or freeze.

Note: The cooked chicken from this stock can be used in the Lemony Turkish-Style Chicken Salad (page 195) and the Asian-Style Chicken Noodle Salad (page 285). It can also be added to the Caesar Salad with a Light Touch (page 83), substituted for the tuna in the Salad Niçoise with Roasted Potatoes, Green Beans, and Tuna Steak (page 289), or tossed into any of the grain-based or green salads. More ideas include substituting it for the shrimp in the Thai-Style Hot-and-Sour Shrimp Soup (page 59), using it in the Thai-Style Chicken Soup with Coconut Milk (page 73), or adding it to the Easy Black Bean Soup with Fixins (page 191).

22 CALORIES IN | 1 CUP

Protein: 2 g; Carbohydrates: 3 g; Fat: 0; Fiber: 0; Sodium: 538 mg; Carb Choices: 0; Diabetic Exchange: 1 Vegetable

NOTE: Because the cooked chicken is not part of this recipe, low-sodium fat-free chicken stock was used to calculate the nutritional information.

22 CALORIES OUT

Women: Walk: 5 minutes; Jog: 3 minutes

Men: Walk: 4 minutes; Jog: 2 minutes

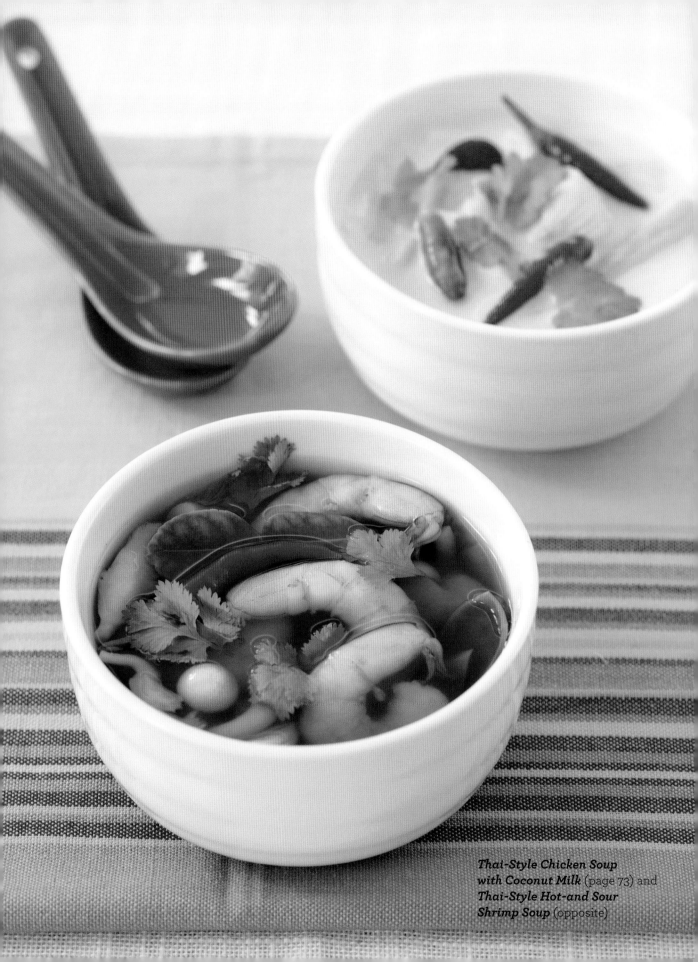

*Thai-Style Chicken Soup
with Coconut Milk* (page 73) and
*Thai-Style Hot-and Sour
Shrimp Soup* (opposite)

THAI-STYLE HOT-AND-SOUR SHRIMP SOUP

I first learned how to make this at a cooking class in northern Thailand. It's just amazing how much flavor this low-calorie soup packs. You allow the broth to infuse with the aromatic lemongrass, kaffir lime leaves (see How to Cook with Fresh Kaffir Lime Leaves, page 74), and cilantro, then add the mushrooms and shrimp. To save a little time, use frozen cooked shrimp thawed, rinsed, and drained. You can also replace the shrimp with an equal amount of diced chicken or tofu. This soup does not freeze well; it is best eaten the same day it is made. Final word: if you like heat, add lots of chili paste.

SERVES 4

5 cups (750 ml) low-sodium fat-free stock

3 fresh lemongrass stalks, bottom 3 inches (8 cm) only, crushed to release the juices (see How to Clean and Cook with Fresh Lemongrass, page 74)

6 thin slices peeled fresh ginger

8 to 10 fresh kaffir lime leaves, torn into 4 pieces each

Root ends of 2 cilantro stalks, trimmed and thoroughly rinsed, plus 3 tablespoons chopped fresh cilantro

2 bird's-eye chiles or other hot chiles, left whole, or sliced for more heat

4 ounces (120 g) shiitake or oyster mushrooms, rinsed, stems trimmed and thinly sliced, or ¾ cup (3 ounces/90 g) canned straw mushrooms, rinsed and halved or quartered

6 ounces (180 g) medium shrimp, peeled and deveined

2 tablespoons fish sauce, or to taste

1 tablespoon fresh lime juice, or to taste

1 teaspoon Tom Yam red chili paste, or to taste, optional

3 tablespoons sliced scallions

1. Place the stock in a medium saucepan and bring to a boil. Add the lemongrass, ginger, kaffir lime leaves, cilantro stalks, and chiles and bring to a boil. Reduce the heat and gently simmer for 10 minutes.

2. Add the mushrooms and return the soup to a boil, then reduce the heat to a gentle simmer and cook for 5 minutes. (Note: To increase the flavor, at this point, turn the heat off and allow the soup to infuse for 15 to 20 minutes before adding the shrimp.)

3. Add the shrimp, increase the heat to medium, and simmer until the shrimp are cooked and opaque throughout, about 7 minutes. Add the fish sauce, lime juice, and chili paste, if using, and let the flavors infuse for a few minutes before serving. Serve garnished with the scallions and chopped cilantro.

Note: I like to serve this soup with all of the Asian aromatics (such as the lemongrass stalks and kaffir lime leaves) in the bowl, even though they are not meant to be eaten in this particular dish. Most Thai restaurants do it this way, too. However, if you prefer a cleaner look or are worried about someone choking, you can pick them out before serving.

83 CALORIES IN

Protein: 11 g; Carbohydrates: 8 g; Fat: 1 g; Fiber: 0 g; Sodium: 965 mg; Carb Choices: ½; Diabetic Exchange: 1 Lean Meat, 1 Vegetable

83 CALORIES OUT

Women: Walk: 20 minutes; Jog: 10 minutes

Men: Walk: 17 minutes; Jog: 8 minutes

CALORIE COMBOS

½ cup (80 g) plain white rice: 103 cals

½ cup (90 g) plain brown rice: 108 cals

Sweet-and-Spicy Fried Tofu (page 114): 151 cals

Tofu and Bok Choy with Chili Sauce (page 116): 174 cals

Stir-Fried Tofu, Shiitakes, and Bean Sprouts (page 214): 226 cals

Quinoa, Paneer, and Cabbage Patties (page 220): 235 cals

Old Bay and Dill Salmon Patties (page 231): 283 cals

Vegetarian Stir-Fried Rice (page 297): 367 cals

Shrimp Pad Thai (page 312): 391 cals

GENTLY COOKED GAZPACHO

Gazpacho is one of the best low-calorie soups out there, but sometimes the raw onion, garlic, and vegetables can leave you with unpleasant breath and gas in your tummy. To prevent this, I gently cook my gazpacho. I lightly brown the onions and garlic, then I add the rest of the vegetables and bring the soup just to a boil; be sure not to overcook it. Jarred or fresh jalapeños and sun-dried tomatoes add a wonderful layer of flavor. Ideally gazpacho should be eaten the same day it's made; it does not freeze well.

SERVES 4

1 tablespoon extra virgin olive oil

1 sweet onion, chopped

1 garlic clove, minced

2 tablespoons thinly sliced jalapeños, or to taste

¼ cup (35 g) sun-dried tomatoes in oil, drained (about 3 pieces)

1¼ pounds (600 g) ripe tomatoes, diced (4 cups, 1 liter)

1 cup (150 g) diced seedless cucumber

1 cup (250 ml) water or low-sodium fat-free vegetable stock

¼ teaspoon salt, or to taste

Freshly ground pepper or hot sauce, to taste

2 tablespoons chopped fresh cilantro, dill, or chervil

1. In a medium saucepan, heat the olive oil over medium heat. Add the onions and cook, stirring occasionally, until they turn light golden brown, about 5 minutes. Add the garlic, jalapeños, and sun-dried tomatoes and sauté for 1 minute. Add the remaining ingredients except the fresh herbs, stir, and bring to the point just before boiling. Remove from the heat and let cool.

2. In a blender or food processor or using a handheld immersion blender, puree the gazpacho to the desired consistency. Adjust the seasoning, and refrigerate until well chilled. Garnish with the fresh herbs before serving.

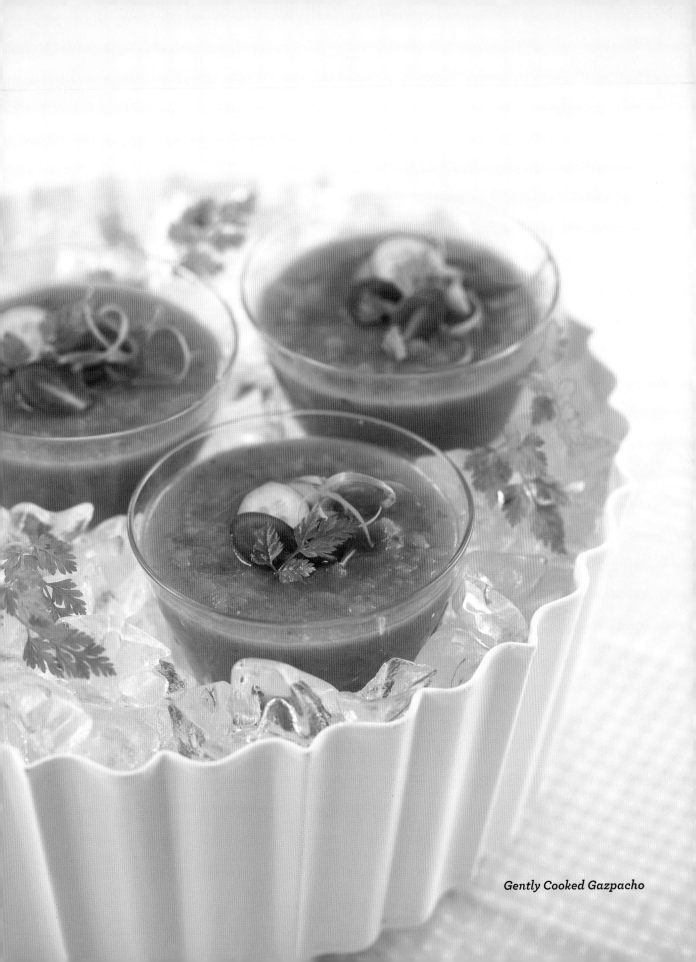

Gently Cooked Gazpacho

QUICK ZUCCHINI-BASIL SOUP

99 CALORIES IN

Protein: 4 g; Carbohydrates: 10 g;
Fat: 6 g; Fiber: 2 g; Sodium: 213
mg; Carb Choices: ½; Diabetic
Exchange: 1 Starch

99 CALORIES OUT

Women: Walk:
24 minutes; Jog: 11 minutes

Men: Walk:
20 minutes; Jog: 10 minutes

CALORIE COMBOS

1 whole wheat roll: 76 cals

Savory Corn Cakes (page 111):
98 cals

Caesar Salad with a Light Touch
(page 83): 163 cals

Allie's Bruschetta (page 71):
172 cals

Cheese Toasts with Tomatoes,
Cucumbers, and Greens (page 72):
175 cals

Everyone's Favorite Veggie Burgers
(page 212): 223 cals

Broccoli, Mushroom, Cheddar, and
Curry Frittata (page 216): 229 cals

Quinoa, Paneer, and Cabbage
Patties (page 220): 235 cals

CALORIE CUTS

Reduce the vegetable oil to ½
tablespoon and save 15 calories
and about 2 grams of fat per
serving. Use the fresh basil rather
than the pesto, which has 25
calories and 2.5 grams of fat per
teaspoon.

If you like zucchini, or you find it growing with abandon in your garden during the summer months, this super-easy soup is for you. The potato is cooked first, then the zucchini is added, and the basil comes at the end for the perfect smack. To keep the basil flavor fresh, I make the soup in small quantities. No garnish is necessary, but feel free to embellish it with grated cheese, croutons (see How to Make Homemade Croutons, below), sprouts, toasted pine nuts or pumpkin seeds, or diced tomatoes. Also, you can substitute an equal amount of broccoli or any other vegetable for the zucchini. (Note: After a few hours, the zucchini and basil will oxidize, causing the bright green soup to turn a muted green. This color change does not affect the flavor, but my advice is to serve it promptly.) The soup freezes well.

SERVES 4

1½ tablespoons vegetable oil

1 onion, chopped

1 small garlic clove, chopped

2 teaspoons Italian seasoning

1 medium potato, diced

4 cups (1 liter) low-sodium fat-free stock, or as needed

1 large zucchini (about 12 ounces/360 g), cut lengthwise in half and diced

⅓ cup (10 g) chopped fresh basil or 2 teaspoons Reduced-Fat Basil Walnut Pesto (page 156)

Salt and freshly ground pepper, to taste

1. In a large saucepan, heat the vegetable oil over medium-high heat. Add the onions, garlic, and Italian seasoning and sauté for 2 minutes. Add the potatoes and stock and bring to a boil. Cook, uncovered, for 7 minutes.

2. Add the zucchini and cook for 5 minutes, or until the potatoes and zucchini are tender. Remove from the heat and let cool slightly.

3. Add the basil and puree the soup, thinning it with a small amount of additional stock or water if necessary. Season with salt and pepper and serve immediately.

HOW TO MAKE HOMEMADE CROUTONS

Homemade croutons are infinitely better than their store-bought counterparts, and they are easy to make. Using day-old bread is ideal, but you can start with fresh, too. Any kind of bread will do, from a white or whole wheat baguette to a rustic country loaf laced with olives and sun-dried tomatoes. Preheat the oven to 300°F (150°C). Slice the bread into small squares or rectangles and arrange them in a single layer on a baking sheet with sides. Bake until dry, about 30 minutes, flipping them once. I don't use oil or seasonings, because croutons usually end up in salads, where they soak up the oil and flavors in the dressing. If you'd like, spray the croutons with extra virgin olive oil or canola oil cooking spray before baking and sprinkle them with dried herbs such as Italian seasoning or oregano, or garlic powder.

GINGERY SQUASH SOUP (📷 page 70)

The perfect companion to a salad or a half sandwich. If I'm entertaining, I like to jazz up this soup with some of the optional garnishes. Peeled and cut fresh butternut squash, found in the refrigerated produce section of many grocery stores, is a big timesaver. Or, if I buy a whole butternut squash, I sometimes roast it to avoid having to peel and cut it, which can be time-consuming (see How to Roast Winter Squash, below). For more Indian flavor, in addition to the spices listed, I add ½ teaspoon each roasted ground cumin and cardamom in Step 1. It you're serving this soup to kids, though, you might want to cut back on the spices, although some kids love the intense flavors. The soup, without the garnishes, freezes well.

SERVES 6

2 tablespoons vegetable oil

1 large onion, chopped

1½ tablespoons minced peeled fresh ginger

1 large garlic clove, minced

½ teaspoon ground ginger

¼ teaspoon ground cinnamon

1½ teaspoons garam masala or mild curry powder

1 cup (100 g) diced carrots

1¼ pounds (600 g) peeled, seeded, and diced butternut squash (about 5 cups, 1.25 liters)

6 to 7 cups (about 1.5 liters) low-sodium fat-free stock

1 teaspoon salt, or to taste

Optional Garnishes

¼ cup (20 g) toasted pumpkin seeds or sunflower seeds

3 tablespoons chopped fresh cilantro

½ cup (15 g) cup fresh alfalfa sprouts

1. Heat the vegetable oil in a large saucepan over medium heat. Add the onions, ginger, and garlic and sauté for 3 minutes. Add the ground ginger, cinnamon, garam masala, carrots, butternut squash, stock, and salt and bring to a boil, then reduce the heat and simmer for 15 to 20 minutes, until the squash and carrots are tender.

2. Remove the soup from the heat and allow to cool slightly, then puree in batches. Return the soup to the rinsed-out saucepan.

3. Just before serving, bring the soup to a boil over medium-high heat. Thin it with water, if necessary. Garnish with any of the optional garnishes and serve promptly.

118 CALORIES IN | 1 SERVING WITHOUT GARNISHES

Protein: 4 g; Carbohydrates: 16 g; Fat: 5 g; Fiber: 3 g; Sodium: 477 mg; Carb Choices: 1; Diabetic Exchange: 1 Starch, 1 Fat

118 CALORIES OUT

Women: Walk: 29 minutes; Jog: 14 minutes

Men: Walk: 24 minutes; Jog: 11 minutes

CALORIE COMBOS

1 tablespoon chopped fresh cilantro: 0 cals

1 tablespoon fresh alfalfa sprouts: 0 cals

1 tablespoon sunflower seeds: 47 cals

2 cups (500 ml) salad greens with 1 tablespoon Balsamic Vinaigrette (page 150): 73 cals

1 whole wheat roll: 76 cals

1 tablespoon pumpkin seeds: 82 cals

Caesar Salad with a Light Touch (page 83): 163 cals

Allie's Bruschetta (page 71): 172 cals

Cheese Toasts with Tomatoes, Cucumbers, and Greens (page 72): 175 cals

Broccoli, Mushroom, Cheddar, and Curry Frittata (page 216): 229 cals

Quinoa, Paneer, and Cabbage Patties (page 220): 235 cals

CALORIE CUTS

Reduce the vegetable oil to ½ tablespoon and save 15 calories and about 2 grams of fat per serving. Skip the optional seed garnishes; use only the fresh herbs and sprouts.

HOW TO ROAST WINTER SQUASH

To roast a butternut squash (or any variety of winter squash), preheat the oven to 375°F (190°C). Using a sharp knife, cut the squash lengthwise in half. Scoop out the seeds, then find a baking dish large enough to accommodate the squash. Line the baking dish with foil and grease it with canola oil or cooking spray. Season the flesh of the squash with salt and pepper and place it cut side down in the baking dish. Bake for 35 to 40 minutes, until the flesh is tender. Check it by piercing with a bamboo skewer or knife. Allow the squash to cool slightly, then scoop out the flesh and proceed with your recipe.

MISO SOUP WITH TOFU, SHIITAKES, NOODLES, AND BABY SPINACH

I'd like to dedicate this recipe to Yukiko Jacques, who patiently taught me the nuances of Japanese miso soup, which she eats for breakfast every day. You don't need to go to a Japanese restaurant for a good bowl of miso soup. In fact, homemade soup is best because you can tailor it to your taste. See page 340 for information on the different types of miso pastes, good brands, and how they can be used. This recipe calls for yellow miso, called *shinshu*, which is the most popular one for soup. Traditional Japanese miso soup is made with a dashi, a stock using kelp (*kombu*), bonito flakes (*katsuo-bushi*), and seaweed (*wakame*), which are all boiled together and strained. Many Japanese cooks make a large batch of dashi and freeze it for the week (see How to Make Dashi, opposite.) For non-Japanese kitchens, any kind of low-sodium fat-free stock, or even water, can be used as the soup base.

Some traditional additions to miso soup include tofu noodles, daikon, mushrooms (such as fresh shiitake, enoki, or oyster, or canned straw mushrooms), clams or other small shellfish, onions, spinach, potatoes, and seaweed. Ideally the soup should be made just before serving. See page 348 for more information on udon and soba noodles, and page 342 for notes on tofu.

SERVES 4

4 cups (1 liter) dashi (see headnote above)

2 ounces (60 g) thin soba noodles, udon, or other Asian-style noodles

4 ounces (120 g) enoki mushrooms, rinsed, stems trimmed, or shiitake mushrooms, stems removed, thinly sliced

7 ounces (210 g) firm or silken tofu, drained and cut into ½-inch (1.25 cm) dice

2 tablespoons thinly sliced scallions

3 cups (90 g) baby spinach or 1½ ounces (45 g) wakame (soak the seaweed for 15 minutes to soften it before using)

Tiny pinch of sugar

¼ cup (70 g) yellow miso, or to taste

1. In a medium saucepan, bring the dashi to a boil. Add the noodles and return to a boil, then reduce the heat and gently simmer for 3 minutes. Add the enoki, tofu, scallions, baby spinach, and sugar and simmer until the noodles are tender, 4 to 5 minutes. Turn off the heat.

2. Add the miso and gently stir. (Note: Do not boil the soup after you add the miso, or it will kill the enzymes and mute the flavor.) Adjust the seasoning and serve.

HOW TO MAKE DASHI

To make this recipe, you will need to get your hands on some specialty ingredients, such as kelp, fish flakes, and seaweed. All of these are available at Whole Foods; see pages 339 and 341 for more information on them.

SERVES 4

A 4-inch (10 cm) piece of dried kelp (*kombu*)
4 cups (1 liter) water
1 ounce (30 g) bonito flakes (*katsuo-bushi*)

Wipe both sides of the kelp with a wet cloth. Place the water and kelp in a saucepan and let sit for 20 minutes at room temperature. Then place the saucepan over high heat and bring to a boil; just before the water boils, remove the seaweed and discard it. Once the water is boiling, reduce the heat to low, add the bonito flakes, and simmer very gently for 4 minutes. Turn off the heat and allow the stock to sit for 15 minutes. Strain, and it's ready to use or refrigerate.

HEARTY BEET SOUP

147 CALORIES IN | 1 SERVING WITHOUT SOUR CREAM

Protein: 5 g; Carbohydrates: 21 g; Fat: 5 g; Fiber: 5 g; Sodium: 454 mg; Carb Choices: 1½; Diabetic Exchange: 1 Starch, 1 Vegetable, 1 Fat

CALORIES OUT

Women: Walk: 36 minutes; Jog: 17 minutes

Men: Walk: 30 minutes; Jog: 14 minutes

CALORIE COMBOS

1 teaspoon fat-free sour cream: 4 cals

Spinach, Feta, and Dill Dip (page 154): 65 cals

1 whole wheat roll: 76 cals

Savory Corn Cakes (page 111): 98 cals

7 whole wheat crackers: 120 cals

Tomato, Artichoke Heart, Feta, and White Bean Salad (page 84): 168 cals

Cheese Toasts with Tomatoes, Cucumbers, and Greens (page 72): 175 cals

Broccoli, Mushroom, Cheddar, and Curry Frittata (page 216): 229 cals

Couscous Salad with Harissa Dressing (page 198): 241 cals

My Russian roots are evident in this rich, ruby-colored, vitamin-packed soup, which I adapted from my Russian mother's delicious recipe. She makes homemade beef stock (see How to Make Homemade Beef Stock, opposite), which she simmers for hours until it develops a deep flavor and the meat falls off the bone. Because I am usually crunched for time, I use a good-quality store-bought stock. A Microplane grater (a good workout for your arms) or a food processor fitted with a grater attachment is ideal for grating the root vegetables. Because grating or slicing all the vegetables does take time, you might want to pick up as many as you can from a salad bar, or look for packaged bags in the salad section of the produce department. If you are using store-bought stock, there will not be any meat in the soup. If you'd like meat, you will have to make the homemade beef stock. Without the garnishes, the soup freezes well.

SERVES 8

3 tablespoons vegetable oil

1 large onion, chopped

1 pound (500 g) red beets, coarsely grated (about 4 cups, 1 liter)

2 large carrots, coarsely grated

3 tablespoons cider vinegar or red wine vinegar

12 ounces (360 g) white cabbage, tough outer leaves and core removed, quartered, and very thinly sliced (about 5 cups, 750 ml)

2 medium potatoes, coarsely grated

1 cup (140 g) finely chopped green bell pepper

8 cups (2 liters) low-sodium fat-free stock

1½ cups (375 ml) tomato juice or V8 juice

Squeeze of fresh lemon juice, or to taste

3 tablespoons chopped fresh dill, plus additional for serving

3 tablespoons chopped fresh flat-leaf parsley, plus additional for serving

½ teaspoon salt, or to taste

Freshly ground pepper, to taste

Fat-free sour cream, for serving

1. Heat the vegetable oil in a large saucepan over medium-high heat. Add the onions and sauté until light golden, about 3 minutes. Add the beets, carrots, and vinegar and sauté, stirring occasionally, for 3 minutes. Add the cabbage and sauté for 5 minutes more. Add the potatoes and green bell peppers and sauté for 2 minutes longer.

2. Add the stock and tomato juice and bring to a boil. Reduce the heat and gently simmer, uncovered, for 1 hour, stirring occasionally.

3. Add the lemon juice, dill, and parsley. Season with salt and pepper and serve. Pass the sour cream and additional herbs at the table.

HOW TO MAKE HOMEMADE BEEF STOCK

Beef stock is used less often than chicken or vegetable stock (see pages 57 and 56), but it's still worth learning to make your own. For this stock, allow about 3 hours for the meat to get tender and the flavors to meld into a wonderful broth.

MAKES ABOUT 9 CUPS, JUST OVER 2 LITERS

1½ to 2 pounds (720 g to 1 kg) cross-cut beef shank or oxtails

1 carrot, quartered

1 celery stalk, quartered

1 large onion, quartered

3 bay leaves

7 black peppercorns

2 teaspoons salt

4 quarts (4 liters) water

1. Place the beef in a stockpot and add just enough water to cover it. Bring to a boil and cook for 5 minutes. Drain the meat, rinse it well, and return it to the stockpot.

2. Add all of the remaining ingredients to the stockpot, cover, and bring to a boil. Reduce the heat and simmer for about 3 hours, skimming as needed, until the meat is very tender. Remove from the heat and strain the stock into a large heatproof bowl or clean stockpot. Discard the vegetables and save the meat.

3. When the beef is cool enough to handle, remove the meat from the bones and shred or cut it into small pieces. (This is most easily done when the meat is still warm.) Proceed with your recipe, or let cool down, then refrigerate for 3 days or freeze for up to 1 month.

ROASTED CARROT AND FENNEL SOUP

I love the deep, robust, sweet flavors of roasted vegetables, so transforming them into a soup seemed logical. When entertaining, I often serve this soup as a first course, as it goes well with just about any menu. For a smooth finish, I strain the soup after pureeing it; the fennel tends to be a bit stringy otherwise. The fennel seeds heighten the natural licorice flavor of the fennel bulb, but if you don't have them, no worries. The soup, without the garnishes, freezes well.

SERVES 6

3 tablespoons vegetable oil

1 medium onion, quartered, or 1 large leek, sliced (see How to Wash Leeks, page 106)

3 carrots, sliced

1 large fennel bulb (8 ounces/240 g), trimmed and sliced

2 medium potatoes, diced

1 garlic clove, smashed and peeled

1 teaspoon fennel seeds, optional

1 teaspoon garam masala

1 teaspoon brown sugar

½ teaspoon salt, or to taste

Freshly ground pepper, to taste

6 cups (1.5 liters) low-sodium fat-free stock

Optional Garnishes

Squeeze of fresh lemon juice

¼ cup (20 g) roasted pumpkin or other seeds

3 tablespoons chopped fresh flat-leaf parsley or fennel fronds

1. Center an oven rack and preheat the oven to 450°F (230°C). Place the vegetable oil in a large roasting pan. Add all of the remaining soup ingredients except the stock and toss until the vegetables are well coated with the oil and seasonings. Spread them out in a single layer so they roast evenly.

2. Roast for 15 minutes. Using a spatula, turn the vegetables over and roast for another 15 minutes, or until they feel soft when pierced with a fork.

3. Remove the roasting pan from the oven. Add ½ cup (125 ml) of the stock to deglaze the pan. Using a spatula, scrape up all the caramelized bits. Carefully transfer half of the contents of the pan to a blender. Add half of the remaining stock and puree to a smooth consistency. Strain the soup through a strainer into a saucepan. Repeat this process with the remaining vegetables, and remaining stock. Thin with additional stock or water if necessary.

4. Reheat the soup and adjust the seasoning, and top with any of the optional garnishes.

CAULIFLOWER, WATERCRESS, AND PARMESAN SOUP (page 70)

A natural combination of flavors delivers a lovely green soup bursting with vitamins. So it retains its color, the watercress is added at the end of the cooking process. For a chunkier soup, puree all but 2 cups (500 ml) of the soup. The Parmesan cheese can be replaced with Monterey Jack, sharp cheddar, or your favorite cheese. For a wonderful finishing touch, garnish with some reserved watercress sprigs, chopped parsley, or the Parsley Drizzle. You can freeze the soup before adding the milk, cheese, and parsley. One of my recipe testers mentioned that she likes this soup both hot and chilled.

SERVES 6

2 tablespoons vegetable oil

1 medium onion, chopped

⅓ cup (80 ml) white wine, optional

4 cups small cauliflower florets (about 12 ounces/360 g)

1 medium potato, diced

½ teaspoon salt, or to taste

Freshly ground pepper, to taste

4 cups (1 liter) low-sodium fat-free stock

6 cups (5 ounces/150 g) watercress leaves, plus extra leaves for garnish, if desired

1 cup (250 ml) whole milk

½ cup (40 g) grated Parmesan cheese

¼ cup (10 g) chopped fresh flat-leaf parsley or a couple of drops of Parsley Drizzle (page 144)

1. In a large saucepan, heat the vegetable oil over medium-high heat. Add the onions and sauté for 2 minutes. Add the wine, if using, and cook for 1 minute. Add the cauliflower florets, potatoes, salt, pepper, and stock and bring to a boil, then reduce the heat and simmer for 15 to 20 minutes, until the potatoes and cauliflower are tender. Remove the soup from the heat and stir in the watercress. The soup will be rather thick at this point.

2. Allow the soup to cool slightly, then puree it using an immersion or regular blender (in batches if necessary); return the soup to the saucepan if you used a regular blender.

3. Add the milk to the soup, then reheat over medium-high heat. Add the cheese, reduce the heat to low, and stir until the cheese is melted; do not boil the soup after adding the cheese. Adjust the seasoning, garnish with watercress, if using, parsley, or the Parsley Drizzle, and serve.

159 CALORIES IN

Protein: 8 g; Carbohydrates: 12 g; Fat: 8 g; Fiber: 2 g; Sodium: 391 mg; Carb Choices: 1; Diabetic Exchange: 1 Whole Milk

159 CALORIES OUT

Women: Walk: 39 minutes; Jog: 18 minutes

Men: Walk: 32 minutes; Jog: 15 minutes

CALORIE COMBOS

2 cups (40 g) salad greens with 1 tablespoon Balsamic Vinaigrette (page 150): 73 cals

1 whole wheat roll: 76 cals

Savory Corn Cakes (page 111): 98 cals

Caesar Salad with a Light Touch (page 83): 163 cals

Allie's Bruschetta (page 71): 172 cals

Cheese Toasts with Tomatoes, Cucumbers, and Greens (page 72): 175 cals

Everyone's Favorite Veggie Burgers (page 212): 223 cals

Quinoa, Paneer, and Cabbage Patties (page 220): 235 cals

Spinach Salad with Mushrooms, Fennel, and Avocado (page 201): 251 cals

Pasta Salad with Sun-Dried Tomato Pesto and Mozzarella Cheese (page 202): 264 cals

CALORIE CUTS

Reduce the vegetable oil to 1 tablespoon and save 20 calories and 2 grams of fat per serving. Omit the white wine and save about 10 calories per serving. Omit the Parmesan cheese and save 28 calories and about 2 grams of fat per serving. Use chopped parsley or watercress instead of the Parsley Drizzle.

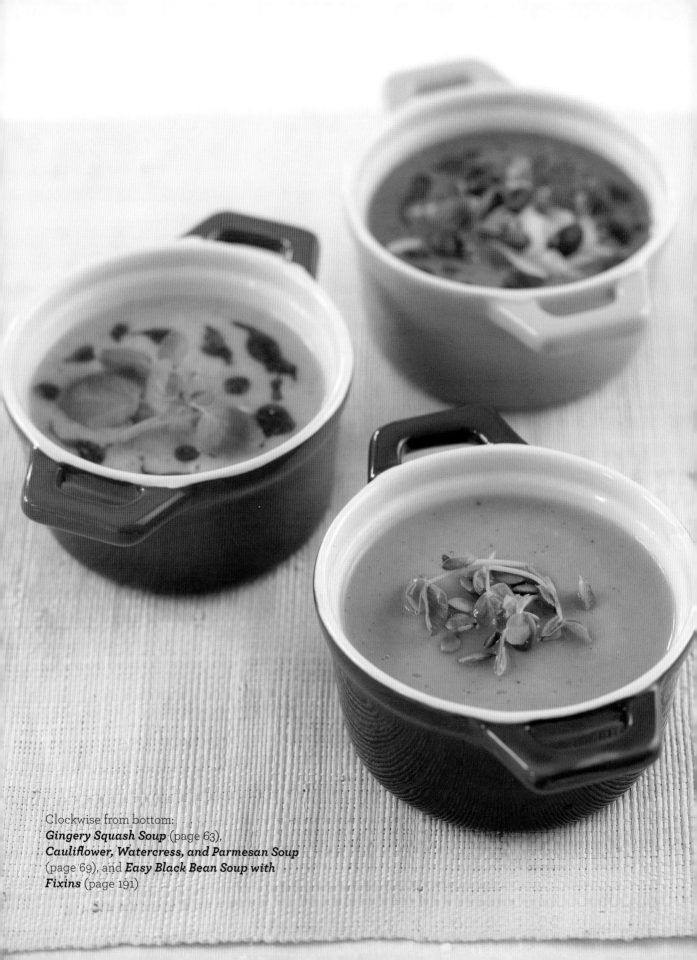

Clockwise from bottom:
Gingery Squash Soup (page 63),
Cauliflower, Watercress, and Parmesan Soup
(page 69), and *Easy Black Bean Soup with
Fixins* (page 191)

ALLIE'S BRUSCHETTA

My daughter Allie and I both like the bread on the crisp side, so before adding the topping, she toasts it on both sides. Then she adds a thin layer of Parmesan cheese, melts it under the broiler, and finishes with the fresh tomato-basil topping. I sometimes add chopped olives, marinated artichoke hearts, or jarred roasted red bell peppers. The Parmesan cheese not only tastes delicious, but also forms a barrier to prevent the juicy tomatoes from soaking the bread. Yummy is all I can say.

MAKES 8 SLICES

Topping

8 ounces (240 g) ripe tomatoes, finely diced and drained in a sieve

1 teaspoon balsamic vinegar, or to taste

½ teaspoon crushed garlic or a sprinkle of garlic powder

Sprinkle of Italian seasoning

A couple of fresh basil leaves, sliced

Salt and freshly ground pepper, to taste

8 slices whole-grain bread, preferably from a baguette or small country-style loaf, or your favorite bread

About ¼ cup (20 g) grated Parmesan cheese

1. To make the topping, combine all of the ingredients in a bowl and gently mix. Adjust the seasoning and set aside.

2. Preheat the broiler or toaster oven to high. Lightly toast the bread on both sides. Distribute the grated Parmesan cheese evenly over the bread slices and then place them under the broiler again until the cheese melts and begins to bubble.

3. Transfer to a serving plate and top with the topping. Serve promptly.

---

172 CALORIES IN | 2 SLICES

Protein: 9 g; Carbohydrates: 25 g; Fat: 4 g; Fiber: 5 g; Sodium: 298 mg; Carb Choices: 1½; Diabetic Exchange: 2 Starch

172 CALORIES OUT

Women: Walk: 42 minutes; Jog: 20 minutes

Men: Walk: 35 minutes; Jog: 17 minutes

CALORIE COMBOS

Gently Cooked Gazpacho (page 60): 87 cals

Grilled Vegetables (page 108): 89 cals

Quick Zucchini-Basil Soup (page 62): 99 cals

Gingery Squash Soup (page 63): 118 cals

3 cups (60 g) salad greens with 2 tablespoons Sublime Parmesan-Lime Dressing (page 151): 137 cals

Cauliflower, Watercress, and Parmesan Soup (page 69): 159 cals

Roasted Carrot and Fennel Soup (page 68): 159 cals

Caesar Salad with a Light Touch (page 83): 163 cals

Mediterranean Vegetable Soup (page 186): 205 cals

Italian Meatball and Noodle Soup with Greens (page 189): 221 cals

Spinach Salad with Mushrooms, Fennel, and Avocado (page 201): 251 cals

CALORIE CUTS

The bread has the most calories in this recipe, so to cut back, use a small loaf and slice the bread as thin as possible. The Parmesan cheese has about 11 calories and 0.5 gram of fat per ½ tablespoon.

175 CALORIES IN | I SERVING MADE WITH LOW-FAT ALPINE LACE CHEESE

Protein: 12 g; Carbohydrates: 16 g; Fat: 7 g; Fiber: 2 g; Sodium: 322 mg; Carb Choices: 1; Diabetic Exchange: 1 Starch, 1 High-Fat Meat

175 CALORIES OUT

Women: Walk:
43 minutes; Jog: 20 minutes

Men: Walk:
36 minutes; Jog: 17 minutes

CALORIE COMBOS

Gently Cooked Gazpacho (page 60): 87 cals

Grilled Vegetables (page 108): 89 cals

Quick Zucchini-Basil Soup (page 62): 99 cals

3 cups (60 g) salad greens with 2 tablespoons Classic Red Wine Vinaigrette (page 146): 105 cals

Gingery Squash Soup (page 63): 118 cals

Cauliflower, Watercress, and Parmesan Soup (page 69): 159 cals

Roasted Carrot and Fennel Soup (page 68): 159 cals

Caesar Salad with a Light Touch (page 83): 163 cals

CALORIE CUTS

The bread has the highest amount of calories in this recipe, so to cut back, use a small loaf and slice the bread as thin as possible. Choose a reduced-fat or low-fat cheese.

CHEESE TOASTS WITH TOMATOES, CUCUMBERS, AND GREENS

Cheese toasts are simply open-faced grilled cheese sandwiches, nothing fancy, just plain good. You can use any type of bread or cheese. I like my bread crisp, so I always toast the slices on both sides. Depending on what I am serving, I might sprinkle the toasts with chopped fresh basil, dried Italian seasoning, or a dash of paprika. One of my recipe testers suggested placing tomatoes, cucumbers, and greens on top of the melted cheese for a fresh crunch—an excellent idea that I incorporated.

SERVES I

1 slice country-style whole-grain bread

Dijon mustard, optional

1 slice (about 1 ounce/30 g) reduced-fat cheese, such as Alpine Lace, Swiss, cheddar, Provolone, or Monterey Jack (see calorie counts below)

1 tomato slice

3 cucumber slices

¼ cup (10 g) baby greens or other greens or sprouts

Preheat the broiler or toaster oven to high. Lightly toast the bread on both sides. Spread a bit of Dijon on the bread, if using, then add the cheese and place under the broiler just until the cheese melts and bubbles. Top with the tomato and cucumber slices and baby greens.

CALORIE COUNTS FOR CHEESES

1 slice (30 g) low-fat Swiss = 49 cals

1 slice (30 g) reduced-fat (50%) Cheddar = 70 cals

1 slice (30 g) low-fat Monterey Jack = 88 cals

1 slice (30 g) low-fat Alpine Lace = 91 cals

1 slice (30 g) provolone = 100 cal

1 slice (30 g) Monterey Jack = 106 cals

1 slice (30 g) Swiss = 108 cals

THAI-STYLE CHICKEN SOUP WITH COCONUT MILK (page 58)

Called *tom ka gai*, this is one of my all-time favorite soups, and, surprisingly, one of the easiest to make. Unless you live in Asia, assembling the ingredients will likely be the hardest part. If you've never experienced the flavors of fresh lemongrass and kaffir lime leaves, you're in for a treat. See How to Clean and Cook with Fresh Lemongrass and How to Cook with Fresh Kaffir Lime Leaves (page 74). Lime zest can be used in place of the kaffir lime leaves, but I urge to you try to find the fresh leaves. Coconut milk adds a silky texture; see page 340 for brand recommendations. Shrimp or tofu can be substituted for the chicken. This soup is best on the same day it is made; it cannot be frozen.

SERVES 4

4 cups (1 liter) low-sodium fat-free chicken stock

3 fresh lemongrass stalks, bottom 3 inches (8 cm) only, crushed to release the juices (see page 74)

6 thin slices peeled fresh ginger

8 to 10 fresh kaffir lime leaves, torn into 2 or 3 pieces each

Root ends of 2 cilantro stalks, trimmed and thoroughly washed, plus 3 tablespoons chopped fresh cilantro

1 to 2 bird's-eye or other hot chiles, left whole or sliced, depending on the heat you want (leaving them whole is less hot)

4 ounces (120 g) fresh shiitake or oyster mushrooms, rinsed, stemmed, and thinly sliced, or ¾ cup (90 g) canned straw mushrooms, rinsed and halved or quartered

8 ounces (240 g) chicken tenderloins, sliced into very thin strips

¾ cup (200 ml) lite coconut milk

2 to 3 tablespoons fish sauce, to taste

2 tablespoons fresh lime juice, or to taste

2 to 3 teaspoons Thai red chili paste, to taste, optional

3 tablespoons sliced scallions

1. Place the chicken stock in a medium saucepan and bring to a boil over high heat. Add the lemongrass, ginger, kaffir lime leaves, cilantro stalks, and chiles, reduce the heat, and gently simmer for 10 minutes.

2. Add the mushrooms and chicken and return the soup to a boil, then reduce the heat to a gentle simmer and cook for 7 minutes, or until the chicken is fully cooked.

3. Add the coconut milk, fish sauce, lime juice, and chili paste, if using. Allow the the flavors infuse for 10 to 15 minutes off the heat before serving. Serve hot, garnished with the scallions and chopped cilantro.

Note: I like to serve this soup with all of the Asian aromatics (such as the lemongrass stalks and kaffir lime leaves) in the bowl, even though they are not meant to be eaten in this particular dish. Most Thai restaurants do it this way, too. However, if you prefer a cleaner look or are worried about someone choking, you can pick them out before serving.

178 CALORIES IN

Protein: 17 g; Carbohydrates: 9 g; Fat: 8 g; Fiber: 2 g; Sodium: 958 mg; Carb Choices: ½; Diabetic Exchange: 1 Medium-Fat Meat, 1 Vegetable

178 CALORIES OUT

Women: Walk: 43 minutes; Jog: 20 minutes

Men: Walk: 36 minutes; Jog: 17 minutes

CALORIE COMBOS

½ cup (80 g) plain white rice: 103 cals

½ cup (90 g) plain brown rice: 108 cals

Sweet-and-Spicy Fried Tofu (page 114): 151 cals

Tofu and Bok Choy with Chili Sauce (page 116): 174 cals

Stir-Fried Tofu, Shiitakes, and Bean Sprouts (page 214): 226 cals

Quinoa, Paneer, and Cabbage Patties (page 220): 235 cals

Old Bay and Dill Salmon Patties (page 231): 283 cals

Vegetarian Stir-Fried Rice (page 297): 367 cals

Shrimp Pad Thai (page 312): 391 cals

HOW TO CLEAN AND COOK WITH FRESH LEMONGRASS

Fresh lemongrass is a joy to cook with, but there are a few steps you should follow to release the maximum amount of flavor from it. To start, when shopping, look for stalks that are not dried out, moldy, or blemished. After rinsing, cut off the woody green tops and discard, unless you plan to use them in a soup or curry. Then cut off the bottom tip of the root end and discard. You should have a piece that is about 3 inches (8 cm) long. Remove any tough outer layers, then slice the lemongrass very thin. The areas with the purple lines (you will see them as you slice) are the most flavorful. Pulse the slices in a mini food processor to release more flavor and to break up the fibers. Lemongrass prepared this way is entirely edible. If you want to use lemongrass stalks as an aromatic in soups or curries, simply wash them and crush the lower part of the stalks using a blunt object, such as a pestle, to release the juices.

HOW TO COOK WITH FRESH KAFFIR LIME LEAVES

Fresh kaffir lime leaves add a wonderful citrusy flavor to Asian dishes. Be sure to use only fresh leaves, not dried, as they contain the flavorful essential oils. In Thai soups like the one on page 73, the leaves are torn into pieces to release their oils. They are not intended to be eaten, but they are usually served in the soup as a garnish. For many Asian salads and other savory dishes, the leaves are very finely sliced and eaten; see Asian-Style Chicken Noodle Salad (page 285). See page 345 for more information on fresh kaffir lime leaves.

INDIAN-STYLE CUCUMBER YOGURT SALAD

This refreshingly light yogurt-based salad includes the classic additions of cucumbers, tomatoes, yogurt, and cumin. Indian yogurt-based salads come in endless varieties, from yogurt and spices mixed with cooked spinach and eggplant, which are totally sublime, to salads made with fresh fruits. They are best made no more than about 2 hours before serving, but if you want to get a head start, you can prepare the yogurt base a day in advance, then add the tomatoes and cucumbers before serving. For more spice, consider adding about ½ teaspoon minced fresh green or red chile, to taste. Serve with just about anything, from curries to grilled foods, or serve as a dip with Indian breads, pita crisps, or cut-up fresh vegetables. I like to use roasted cumin seeds, cayenne, and chopped cilantro as garnishes.

MAKES ABOUT 4 CUPS (I LITER)

1½ cups (405 g) nonfat plain Greek-style yogurt

1½ teaspoons roasted ground cumin, or to taste

1 teaspoon fresh lemon juice, or to taste

2 tablespoons minced onion

2 tablespoons chopped fresh mint

2 tablespoons chopped fresh cilantro

Salt and freshly ground pepper, to taste

1 cup (160 g) finely diced ripe tomatoes

¾ cup (130 g) well-washed and finely diced or grated seedless unwaxed cucumber

Combine all of the ingredients in a bowl and mix well. Adjust the seasoning and serve.

45 CALORIES IN | GENEROUS ¼ CUP (60 ML)

Protein: 4 g; Carbohydrates: 7 g; Fat: 0 g; Fiber: 1 g; Sodium: 50 mg; Carb Choices: ½; Diabetic Exchange: ½ Skim Milk

45 CALORIES OUT

Women: Walk:
11 minutes | Jog: 5 minutes

Men: Walk:
9 minutes | Jog: 4 minutes

CALORIE COMBOS

1 whole wheat chapati (Indian flatbread): 137 cals

Paneer with Spinach, Tomatoes, and Spices (page 312): 143 cals

Dieter's Chicken Skewers (page 124): 154 cals

Grilled Lemony Lamb Chops (page 130): 177 cals

Beans and Rice Indian-Style (page 118): 189 cals

Grilled Chicken Tandoori (page 236): 212 cals

Classic Dal (page 217): 232 cals

1 naan (Indian bread): 234 cals

Indian-Spiced Broiled Salmon (page 226): 262 cals

Classic Chicken Curry with Coconut Milk (page 248): 266 cals

Chicken Curry Stir-Fry (page 317): 352 cals

HOW TO BUY SEEDLESS CUCUMBERS

The word "seedless" here is something of a misnomer, as no cucumber is entirely seedless, but certain varieties have been cultivated to have underdeveloped seeds. These include Japanese, English (also called burpless), Mediterranean, and Persian or Lebanese. Cucumbers with lots of seeds include regular American cucumbers and Kirbys, which are good for pickling or juicing. Seedless cucumbers have thin unwaxed skin and are often sold sealed in plastic; they can be eaten unpeeled. My advice is to opt for smaller cucumbers, usually 6 to 8 inches (15 to 20 cm), which tend to be juicier and sweeter than larger ones. If you can't find seedless cucumbers, no worries—simply remove the seeds of a regular cucumber by running a teaspoon down the seedy core in the middle of the cucumber.

TOMATO, CUCUMBER, AND RADISH SALAD

This simple salad is a great side for just about any main dish. I also like to serve it on a bed of cooked whole grains, such as bulgur or couscous, lightly seasoned with lemon and olive oil. See opposite for information on varieties of seedless cucumbers. Other possible additions include diced avocado, sliced fennel, alfalfa sprouts, sprouted legumes, and fresh dill or chervil.

SERVES 4

1½ cups (240 g) diced tomatoes (3 to 4 ripe tomatoes), drained in a sieve

1½ cups (225 g) diced seedless cucumber, half peeled in alternating strips

½ cup (60 g) sliced red radishes

2 tablespoons extra virgin olive oil

1 tablespoon fresh lemon juice, or to taste

2 tablespoons minced red onion or thinly sliced scallions

2 tablespoons chopped fresh mint

½ teaspoon dried mint

Pinch of sugar

Salt and freshly ground pepper, to taste

Combine all of the ingredients in a bowl and mix gently. Adjust the seasoning and serve promptly.

HOT-AND-SWEET CUCUMBER, CARROT, AND RED BELL PEPPER SALAD (📷 page 125)

Colorful, fresh, tasty, and low-cal. What more could you want? This salad is best made no more than 20 minutes before serving. The vegetables tend get weepy if made too far in advance. See page 75 for information on seedless cucumbers; and if you don't have a seedless cucumber, just scoop out the seeds. One of my recipe testers added sautéed spicy tofu to turn this salad into a main course.

SERVES 4

1 medium seedless cucumber (4 ounces/120 g), halved lengthwise and thinly sliced

½ small red onion, thinly sliced

1 small red bell pepper, cored, seeded, quartered, and sliced crosswise

1 carrot, shaved into thin strips or coarsely grated

2 tablespoons chopped fresh cilantro

3 tablespoons seasoned rice vinegar, or to taste

2 tablespoons sugar, or to taste

½ teaspoon toasted sesame oil, or to taste

Pinch of red pepper flakes, optional

Salt, to taste

Combine all of the ingredients in a bowl and mix gently. Serve promptly.

---

61 CALORIES IN

Protein: 1 g; Carbohydrates: 13 g; Fat: 1 g; Fiber: 2 g; Sodium: 53 mg; Carb Choices: 1; Diabetic Exchange: 2 Vegetable

61 CALORIES OUT

Women: Walk: 15 minutes | Jog: 7 minutes

Men: Walk: 12 minutes | Jog: 6 minutes

CALORIE COMBOS

Savory Corn Cakes (page 111): 98 cals

Crab Cakes with Super-Easy Tartar Sauce (page 119): 145 cals

Sweet-and-Spicy Fried Tofu (page 114): 151 cals

Dieter's Chicken Skewers (page 124): 154 cals

Grilled Chicken Tandoori (page 236): 212 cals

Indian-Spiced Broiled Salmon (page 226): 262 cals

Old Bay and Dill Salmon Patties (page 231): 283 cals

Aussie-Style BBQ Chicken (page 252): 279 cals

Swordfish with Cilantro-Mint Sauce (page 233): 284 cals

Chicken Curry Stir-Fry (page 317): 352 cals

Sesame-Coated Salmon with Soy Sauce–Lime Drizzle (page 310): 363 cals

LEMONY DILL CABBAGE SLAW (📷 page 232)

A lemony twist on coleslaw that is sure to please. I like to mix white and red cabbage for a beautiful presentation. The dressing can be made up to 3 days in advance, covered, and refrigerated, but don't dress the salad until just before serving: cabbage wilts quickly, especially when it comes in contact with salt. It may not look as if you have enough dressing at first, but keep tossing, and you'll find it is plenty. One of my recipe testers used tarragon instead of dill and said it was a very nice switch. Another mentioned that she was tempted to throw in some diced green mango. See the box opposite for making perfect slaw every time.

SERVES 6

Lemony Dressing

2 tablespoons fresh lemon juice, or to taste

2 tablespoons extra virgin olive oil

1 tablespoon nonfat mayonnaise

1½ teaspoons grated lemon zest, or to taste

Salt and freshly ground pepper, to taste

Pinch of sugar

Cabbage Slaw

About 5 cups (12 ounces/ 360 g) thinly sliced white or red cabbage, or a mix of both, or packaged coleslaw

½ cup (50 g) grated carrots

¼ cup (40 g) sliced celery

2 tablespoons chopped fresh dill

1. To make the dressing, combine all of the ingredients in a small bowl and whisk until emulsified. Cover and refrigerate until ready to use.
2. Combine the cabbage, carrots, celery, and dill in a large bowl and toss gently.
3. Just before serving, dress the slaw and adjust the seasoning.

HOW TO MAKE PERFECT COLESLAW

- Keep the dressing light, and preferably a bit acidic, with vinegar or lemon. Go easy on the oil, which will weigh down the slaw.
- A little sugar brings out the natural sweetness of cabbage (and other greens) and offsets any bitterness.
- Never put too much dressing on slaw. Remember, less is always more.
- Cabbage "weeps" when it comes in contact with salt or a dressing, so the liquid content will naturally increase. Some people toss their cabbage with salt in advance of dressing. This breaks down the cell walls. If you do this, rinse the cabbage, drain thoroughly, and pat dry before dressing.
- Always dress slaw at the last minute to prevent it from turning soggy and limp. Add a little dressing at first, mix, and then add more as needed.
- Add crunch to your slaw with carrots, celery, jicama, and/or broccoli.

CREAMY ALL-AMERICAN POTATO SALAD

Creamy potato salad conjures up summer BBQs with friends and family. I call it all-American because the dressing is made from three quintessentially American products: Hellman's mayonnaise (or any other high-quality light mayonnaise), French's yellow mustard (the kind served on hot dogs at the ballpark—it's the best mustard for this dressing), and Thousand Island dressing. The celery adds a welcome crunch, while the dill pickles give it a kick and the eggs some creaminess. Allow the salad to sit in the refrigerator for at least 4 hours before serving to give the potatoes a chance to absorb the other flavors. If you want a moister potato salad without more fat, add 1 tablespoon of nonfat plain Greek-style yogurt. Two of my recipe testers mentioned that they would love the crispness of bacon here. It's up to you: 1 slice of regular bacon has 43 calories and 3 grams of fat.

SERVES 6

1½ pounds (720 g) red or white new potatoes, scrubbed

⅓ cup (40 g) minced red onion, or to taste

1 hard-boiled egg, diced

⅓ cup (50 g) sliced celery

⅓ cup (50 g) diced dill pickles or dill pickle relish

2 tablespoons light or nonfat mayonnaise

1 teaspoon French's yellow mustard, or to taste

3 tablespoons reduced-fat or nonfat Thousand Island dressing

Salt and freshly ground pepper, to taste

2 tablespoons chopped fresh flat-leaf parsley, for garnish

1. Bring a large pot of salted water to a boil and cook the potatoes until they are tender but not mushy. There is a fine line here, check them after about 15 minutes. Drain and let cool slightly.

2. When the potatoes are cool enough to handle, peel and cut into ½-inch (1.25 cm) cubes. Mix the potatoes with the red onions, eggs, celery, and dill pickles in a bowl.

3. In a small bowl, whisk together the mayonnaise, mustard, and Thousand Island dressing. Add to the potatoes and gently mix until well combined. Cover and refrigerate for at least 4 hours and up to 12 hours before serving to allow the flavors to meld.

4. Garnish the salad with the parsley and serve.

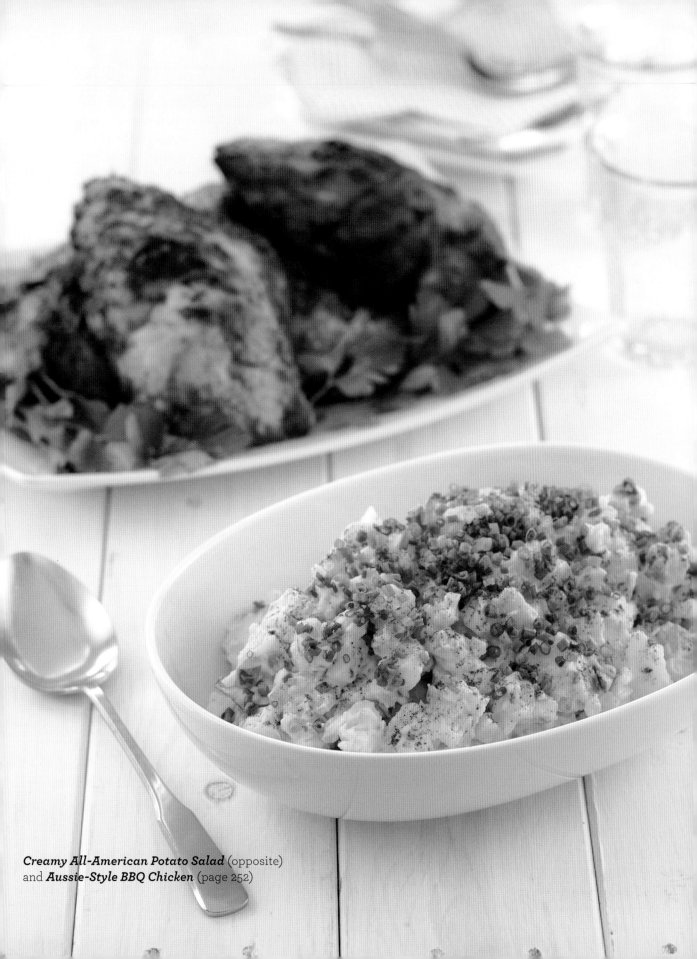

Creamy All-American Potato Salad (opposite)
and *Aussie-Style BBQ Chicken* (page 252)

AUSTRIAN-STYLE POTATO SALAD

The addition of stock to the potatoes is what makes this salad typically Austrian. The stock gets absorbed by the warm potatoes and helps make them wonderfully creamy without much oil. The type of potato is critical here: they should be a long, thin, waxy variety, such as Austrian Crescent, Russian or French fingerling, or banana potatoes. Austrians typically don't add fresh herbs, but I do.

SERVES 6

2 pounds (1 kg) fingerling or other small, thin waxy potatoes

3 tablespoons minced red onion or shallots

⅓ cup (80 ml) low-sodium fat-free stock

1 tablespoon canola oil or very mild extra virgin olive oil

3 tablespoons white wine vinegar, or to taste

Salt and freshly ground pepper, to taste

3 tablespoons chopped fresh dill

3 tablespoons finely sliced fresh chives

1. Cook the potatoes in boiling salted water until tender, about 15 minutes. The cooking time will depend on the size, so test frequently with the tip of a knife; you may want to remove any small potatoes first. Drain and let cool slightly.

2. Using a sharp paring knife, peel the potatoes (this is a bit time-consuming because they are so small); or leave the skin on if you prefer. Slice the potatoes into ¼-inch (6 mm) slices and put them in a bowl.

3. Add the onions and stock to the potatoes and mix gently, then add the oil, vinegar, salt, pepper, dill, and chives and mix again. Adjust the seasoning, and allow the salad to sit for 30 minutes at room temperature before serving. (It can be made up to 6 hours ahead, covered, and refrigerated.) Serve at room temperature or chilled.

CAESAR SALAD WITH A LIGHT TOUCH

With this recipe, you can have your Caesar and eat it, too. To turn this salad into a meal, add grilled chicken or shrimp or sautéed tofu. The croutons are optional, but homemade are always healthier than their store-bought counterparts, which are usually high in fat (see How to Make Homemade Croutons, page 62). In a hurry? Use bagged baby romaine lettuce. Use the dressing with any greens, not just romaine. I like the anchovy paste, but you can skip it if you want. There are separate breakdowns for the dressing and salad; the total for both is 163 calories and 10 grams of fat. By the way, the average restaurant Caesar salad clocks in at close to 400 calories, with 25 grams of fat.

SERVES 4

Caesar Dressing
(makes about ½ cup, (125 ml)

¼ cup (60 g) nonfat plain Greek-style yogurt

¼ to ½ teaspoon anchovy paste, to taste, optional

1 small garlic clove, halved

2 tablespoons fresh lemon juice, or to taste

1 teaspoon Dijon mustard

2 teaspoons Worcestershire sauce

2 tablespoons extra virgin olive oil

¼ cup (20 g) grated Parmesan cheese

Salt and freshly ground pepper, to taste

Salad

About 7 cups (about 350 g) romaine lettuce sliced into bite-size pieces or bagged baby romaine, washed and dried

¼ cup (20 g) grated or shaved Parmesan cheese

1 cup (40 g) homemade croutons (see box, page 62), optional

Freshly ground pepper, to taste

1. For the Caesar dressing, combine all of the ingredients in a mini food processor or place them in the cup of an immersion blender, and process until emulsified. Adjust the seasoning.

2. Combine all of the salad ingredients in a large bowl, add half of the dressing, and toss gently to mix. Add a bit more dressing, a little at a time, tossing gently, until the salad is dressed to your liking. (Note: You'll have some extra dressing that is good on any greens; cover and refrigerate.) Adjust the seasoning and serve promptly.

97 CALORIES IN | CAESAR DRESSING ONLY

Protein: 3 g; Carbohydrates: 2 g; Fat: 8 g; Fiber: 0 g; Sodium: 160 mg; Carb Choices: ½; Diabetic Exchange: 2 Fat

97 CALORIES OUT

Women: Walk: 24 minutes | Jog: 11 minutes

Men: Walk: 20 minutes | Jog: 9 minutes

66 CALORIES IN | CAESAR SALAD ONLY, NO DRESSING

Protein: 4 g; Carbohydrates: 8 g; Fat: 2 g; Fiber: 2 g; Sodium: 135 mg; Carb Choices: ½; Diabetic Exchange: 1 Starch

66 CALORIES OUT

Women: Walk: 16 minutes | Jog: 8 minutes

Men: Walk: 13 minutes | Jog: 6 minutes

CALORIE COMBOS

2 ounces (60 g) cooked shrimp: 67 cals

Gently Cooked Gazpacho (page 60): 87 cals

2 ounces (60 g) cooked chicken breast: 94 cals

Crab Cakes with Super-Easy Tartar Sauce (page 119): 145 cals

Grilled Lemony Lamb Chops (page 130): 177 cals

Roasted Chicken with Rosemary-Lemon-Garlic Rub (page 244): 244 cals

Aussie-Style BBQ Chicken (page 252): 279 cals

Old Bay and Dill Salmon Patties (page 231): 283 cals

Filet Mignon with Zesty Black Pepper Sauce (page 327): 307 cals

CALORIE CUTS

Omit the croutons and save 31 calories per serving. (Store-bought croutons range in calories from 30 to 70 calories with up to 3 grams of fat per ¼ cup/60 ml.) You can also reduce the Parmesan cheese in both the dressing and salad: 1 tablespoon grated Parmesan cheese has 22 calories and 1 gram of fat.

TOMATO, ARTICHOKE HEART, FETA, AND WHITE BEAN SALAD

This protein- and vitamin-packed salad is lovely on a bed of baby greens or on top of toasted slices of whole wheat baguette, similar to Allie's Bruschetta (page 71). I also love it served over cooked whole grains. You can use any canned beans, from chickpeas to black-eyed peas. Sliced canned hearts of palm can be substituted for the artichoke hearts. Cherry tomatoes tend to be a bit juicier than grape tomatoes (they are famous for squirting), and some say they are sweeter; grape tomatoes have thicker skins. The dressing can be made up to 3 days in advance, covered, and refrigerated.

SERVES 6

Lemony Dressing

1 small garlic clove, crushed and peeled

1 teaspoon Dijon mustard

1 to 2 teaspoons grated lemon zest

2 tablespoons fresh lemon juice, or to taste

3 tablespoons extra virgin olive oil

Salt and freshly ground pepper, to taste

Pinch of sugar

Salad

2 cups (340 g) halved cherry or grape tomatoes

One 15.5-ounce (439 g) can white beans, such as great Northern or cannellini, rinsed and well drained (1½ cups, 375 ml)

One 13.75-ounce (390 g) can artichoke hearts, drained and cut into quarters

2 tablespoons sliced fresh basil leaves

2 tablespoons thinly sliced scallions

⅓ cup (60 g) pitted Kalamata or green olives, or a mix

½ cup (80 g) crumbled reduced-fat feta cheese

1. To make the dressing, combine all of the ingredients in a small bowl and whisk until emulsified.
2. Combine the salad ingredients in a large bowl and pat with paper towels to remove as much of the water as possible. (This will prevent any excess juices from watering down the dressing.) Add the dressing and toss gently. Adjust the seasoning and serve promptly.

ORZO WITH SNOW PEAS, FENNEL, AND BENIHANA-STYLE DRESSING

Orzo gone Asian is how I describe this dish. The bright fresh flavors go especially well with grilled foods. Feel free to substitute the orzo with any other small pasta, or any whole grain, from quinoa to farro. If you'd like more veggies, add sliced cooked asparagus or green beans, edamame, or small broccoli florets. Note that the green vegetables will lose their bright green color soon after they come in contact with the dressing, but the taste will not be affected. Ideally, dress the orzo just before serving.

SERVES 6

4 ounces (120 g) snow peas, ends trimmed and sliced lengthwise into thin strips

6 ounces (180 g) fennel, trimmed and cut into small pieces

1 cup (180 g) uncooked orzo

⅓ cup (80 ml) Benihana-Style Ginger-Sesame Dressing (page 155), or to taste

3 tablespoons chopped fresh cilantro

¼ cup sliced scallions

Salt, to taste

1. In a medium saucepan of boiling salted water, cook the snow peas and fennel for 3 minutes. Remove them with a slotted spoon and transfer to a large bowl. Keep the water boiling.
2. Add the orzo to the boiling water and cook until done (follow the package directions). Drain and add to the bowl with the snow peas and fennel. Add the dressing and toss, then add the remaining ingredients. Adjust the seasoning, using more dressing (1 tablespoon at a time) if needed, and serve.

179 CALORIES IN

Protein: 5 g; Carbohydrates: 26 g; Fat: 6 g; Fiber: 3 g; Sodium: 105 mg; Carb Choices: 2; Diabetic Exchange: 1½ Starch, 1 Fat

179 CALORIES OUT

Women: Walk:
44 minutes | Jog: 21 minutes

Men: Walk:
37 minutes | Jog: 17 minutes

CALORIE COMBOS

Thai-Style Hot-and-Sour Shrimp Soup (page 59): 83 cals

Japanese Eggplant in Sweet Chili Sauce (page 94): 86 cals

Miso Soup with Tofu, Shiitakes, Noodles, and Baby Spinach (page 64): 139 cals

Crab Cakes with Super-Easy Tartar Sauce (page 119): 145 cals

Sweet-and-Spicy Fried Tofu (page 114): 151 cals

Easy Lime-Cilantro Grilled Chicken (page 238): 215 cals

Quinoa, Paneer, and Cabbage Patties (page 220): 235 cals

Chicken-Zucchini Burgers with Ricotta and Sun-Dried Tomatoes (page 247): 261 cals

Old Bay and Dill Salmon Patties (page 231): 283 cals

Beef and Vegetable Kebabs with Cilantro–Green Olive Drizzle (page 325): 304 cals

CALORIE CUTS

Apart from the orzo, which has 105 calories per serving, the other major source of calories is the dressing. The ⅓ cup (80 ml) dressing used for this recipe has about 52 calories and 6 grams of fat). You can cut back on both the orzo and the dressing, adding more vegetables in place of some of the orzo.

SIDES

BROILED PORTOBELLO MUSHROOMS WITH HERBS

There are few things more satisfying than a perfectly grilled or broiled portobello mushroom infused with sweet balsamic vinegar, mixed herbs, and a hint of garlic. These meaty delights are perfect alongside just about anything. They can also be sliced and added to salads, or dice them for veggie burgers, omelets, or quesadillas. For a fantastic dinner, toss the sliced mushrooms with pasta and top with a generous dusting of Parmesan cheese and fresh herbs. Feel free to play around with the marinade ingredients: dried oregano, tarragon, basil, or, if you've got some growing in your garden or a pot, a bit of chopped fresh rosemary (dried rosemary does not work here). One of my recipe testers suggested spraying the mushrooms with cooking oil instead of drizzling olive oil over them—a very good idea that saves on fat.

MAKES 6 MUSHROOM CAPS

6 portobello mushrooms (about 14 ounces/420 g total), stems removed and caps wiped clean (see How to Clean Mushrooms, opposite)

Canola or olive oil cooking spray

1 tablespoon balsamic vinegar

1 tablespoon minced garlic or ½ teaspoon garlic powder

2 teaspoons Italian seasoning, or to taste

Salt and freshly ground pepper, to taste

1. Place the mushrooms on a foil-lined baking sheet, gill side down, and spray with cooking, spray. Then turn the mushrooms over and spray the gills. Sprinkle with the balsamic vinegar, followed by the garlic (gently press it between the gills a bit, or sprinkle with garlic powder, if using), Italian seasoning, salt, and pepper.

2. To broil: Preheat the broiler to high and position a rack on the second rung down from the heating element. Turn the mushrooms gill side up on the baking sheet. Broil for 5 minutes, then flip and broil the other side for 2 to 3 minutes. The timing will depend on the thickness of the mushrooms and your broiler. Check

doneness by inserting the tip of a knife into the thickest part of the mushroom—it should give slightly but not be too soft. Save the juices on the baking sheet and spoon over the mushrooms before serving.

3. To grill: Heat the grill to medium heat. For a charcoal grill: Light a chimney starter filled with charcoal briquettes. When the coals are hot, spread them evenly over the bottom of the grill and set the cooking grate in place. Cover and heat until hot, about 5 minutes. For a gas grill: Turn all the burners to medium, cover, and heat until hot, about 10 minutes.

4. Oil the grill grate. Add the mushroom caps, gill side up, and grill for 4 to 5 minutes, then flip and grill the gill side for 2 to 3 minutes. (You will lose some of the juices by grilling instead of broiling, but don't worry, lots of flavor will remain.) Serve the mushrooms warm or at room temperature.

HOW TO CLEAN MUSHROOMS

There are many different opinions on how to clean mushrooms without having them absorb oodles of water, turning them into organic sponges. What works best for me with capped mushrooms, such as button and portobello, is to trim the stems and then hold the cap side, not the gills, under cold running water while I rub off any dirt. If the underside of the mushroom is dirty, run it under water briefly. Pat the mushrooms dry with paper towels and proceed. Some folks avoid water and use a mushroom brush or damp paper towel for cleaning. The main objective is get the mushrooms clean without submerging them in water.

ROASTED ASPARAGUS WITH DILL AND LEMON ZEST (📷 page 223)

Boiling or steaming asparagus the traditional way is great, but if you want an earthier flavor, try roasting it. A tiny bit of sugar helps caramelize the stalks. I call for fresh dill here, but parsley, chervil, mint, or just about any other fresh herb will work. Leftovers can be sliced and tossed into a salad, used in a frittata (see page 216) or an omelet (see page 54), or added to a quesadilla (see page 301). One of my recipe testers suggested a sprinkle of lemon juice and finely grated Parmesan cheese as a garnish.

SERVES 4

12 ounces (360 g) medium or thin asparagus, bottom ends trimmed

1 to 2 tablespoons extra virgin olive oil, as needed

Salt and freshly ground pepper, to taste

Pinch of sugar

1 teaspoon grated lemon zest, or to taste

2 tablespoons chopped fresh dill

1. Center an oven rack and preheat the oven to 400°F (200°C). Line a baking sheet with foil.
2. Place the asparagus spears on the baking sheet and toss with the olive oil, salt, and pepper until well coated. Roast for about 10 minutes, or until the spears are crisp-tender (the time will depend on the thickness of the spears).
3. Add the lemon zest and dill, gently toss, and transfer to a serving dish. Serve warm or at room temperature.

HOW TO STORE AND CLEAN ASPARAGUS

You may have noticed that many grocery stores display fresh asparagus with the spears standing in a shallow basin of water. This helps keeps the asparagus at its prime, firm from the base to the tips, without any shriveled spots. If you are not using asparagus the day you purchase it, you might want to trim the stems and stand the stalks in a bowl of water. To prevent possible freezer burn, keep the asparagus in the front of the fridge, not the back. If your asparagus is thin and tender, cleaning it will involve only a quick rinse with cold water and trimming the stem ends. Thicker asparagus should be washed and trimmed, and then the tough lower ends of the stalks peeled with a vegetable peeler.

NAPA CABBAGE WITH GINGER AND OYSTER SAUCE

Quick and simple, this is a good side dish for any Asian-style main course. Look for oyster sauce that does not contain MSG; see page 341 for suggested brands. If you are vegetarian, hoisin sauce (which is sweet, not salty) can be substituted for the oyster sauce; use about ½ tablespoon and omit the pinch of sugar. Keep a good supply of minced ginger in your freezer so you can make this dish in a flash; see How to Freeze Ginger and Garlic Paste (page 249).

SERVES 4

2 teaspoons vegetable oil

1 teaspoon toasted sesame oil

1 tablespoon minced peeled fresh ginger

Sprinkle of red pepper flakes, optional

12 ounces (360 g) Napa cabbage, large leaves halved lengthwise, all leaves cut into 1-inch (1.25 cm) strips (about 8 cups, 2 liters)

Pinch of sugar

1 tablespoon oyster sauce

1 tablespoon water

1. In a large nonstick skillet, heat the vegetable and sesame oils over medium-low heat. Add the ginger and red pepper flakes, if using, and cook, stirring, just until the ginger is light golden, about 1 minute. Add the Napa cabbage and pinch of sugar, increase the heat to medium, and sauté, stirring, for 1 minute, or until the cabbage begins to wilt.

2. Combine the oyster sauce and water in a small bowl, add it to the cabbage, and cook for 3 minutes. Adjust the seasoning and serve promptly.

48 CALORIES IN

Protein: 1 g; Carbohydrates: 4 g; Fat: 4 g; Fiber: 1 g; Sodium: 117 mg; Carb Choices: 0; Diabetic Exchange: 1 Vegetable

48 CALORIES OUT

Women: Walk: 12 minutes; Jog: 6 minutes

Men: Walk: 10 minutes; Jog: 5 minutes

CALORIE COMBOS

Sweet-and-Spicy Fried Tofu (page 114): 151 cals

Tofu and Bok Choy with Chili Sauce: 174 cals (page 116)

Shrimp with Broccoli and Red Bell Peppers (page 121): 198 cals

Easy Lime-Cilantro Grilled Chicken (page 238): 215 cals

Stir-Fried Tofu, Shiitakes, and Bean Sprouts (page 214): 226 cals

Chicken with Zucchini, Mushrooms, Celery, and Cashews (page 246): 254 cals

Fish Sticks for Hale (page 230): 280 cals

Soba Noodles with Tofu, Kale, and Miso Dressing (page 291): 349 cals

Sesame-Coated Salmon with Soy Sauce–Lime Drizzle (page 310): 363 cals

Vegetarian Stir-Fried Rice (page 297): 367 cals

BROILED ZUCCHINI WITH PARMESAN

49 CALORIES IN

Protein: 3 g; Carbohydrates: 4 g; Fat: 3 g; Fiber: 1 g; Sodium: 84 mg; Carb Choices: 0; Diabetic Exchange: 1 Vegetable

49 CALORIES OUT

Women: Walk:
12 minutes; Jog: 6 minutes

Men: Walk:
10 minutes; Jog: 5 minutes

CALORIE COMBOS

Dieter's Chicken Skewers (page 124): 154 cals

Vegetarian Chili (page 115): 156 cals

Grilled Lemony Lamb Chops (page 130): 177 cals

Roasted Pork Tenderloin with Mustard-Tarragon Marinade (page 127): 198 cals

Snapper with Olive-Artichoke-Tomato Tapenade (page 228): 279 cals

Old Bay and Dill Salmon Patties (page 231): 283 cals

Grilled Chicken Tandoori (page 236): 212 cals

Roasted Chicken with Rosemary-Lemon-Garlic Rub (page 244): 244 cals

Swordfish with Cilantro-Mint Sauce (page 233): 284 cals

Spaghetti with Bolognese Sauce (page 328): 339 cals

So simple and so delicious. I think the Parmesan cheese is perfect, but you may modify with other cheeses and herbs. One of my recipe testers did not stop with zucchini; she added red bell peppers, eggplant, and mushrooms and reported that it was really good.

SERVES 4

2 medium zucchini, cut lengthwise in half, flesh scored in a crisscross pattern about ¼ inch (6 mm) deep

Extra virgin olive oil for brushing, or canola or olive oil cooking spray

Salt and freshly ground pepper, to taste

1 teaspoon dried oregano or Italian seasoning

¼ cup (20 g) finely grated Parmesan cheese

1. Preheat the broiler to high and position a rack on the second rung down from the heating element. Place the zucchini halves on a baking sheet lined with foil. Brush with olive oil (or spray with cooking spray) and season with salt, pepper, and the oregano. Broil the zucchini until crisp-tender, about 5 to 7 minutes, turning once. The time will depend on the size of the zucchini; do not overcook.

2. Remove the baking sheet; leave the broiler on. Sprinkle the flesh side of the zucchini with the Parmesan cheese and return them to the broiler just until the cheese melts and bubbles. Serve promptly.

GREEK-STYLE BROCCOLI

A lovely and simple way to serve cooked broccoli or cauliflower, or other vegetables such as green beans and zucchini, or a mix of vegetables. Lemon and olive oil are quintessential Greek flavorings, and anyone who has dined in a Greek taverna will have had vegetables prepared this way—though most Greek restaurants serve whole broccoli spears, not just the florets, which you are welcome to do. Use a vegetable peeler to remove the tough skin from the lower stalks. It is important to add the olive oil before the lemon juice; this will coat the florets to prevent discoloration from the acid in the lemon. Finish with a sprinkle of fresh herbs, if desired.

SERVES 4

1 pound (480 g) broccoli florets

1 to 2 tablespoons extra virgin olive oil, to taste

1 to 2 tablespoons fresh lemon juice, to taste

Salt and freshly ground pepper, to taste

2 to 3 tablespoons chopped fresh parsley, dill, or your favorite fresh herb

1. Boil or steam the broccoli florets until crisp-tender. Drain well and blot dry with paper towels. (This is important, as extra water will dilute the dressing.)

2. Place the broccoli in a bowl, add the olive oil, and gently mix. Add the remaining ingredients and mix again. Adjust the seasoning and serve warm or at room temperature.

71 CALORIES IN

Protein: 3 g; Carbohydrates: 8 g; Fat: 4 g; Fiber: 3 g; Sodium: 39 mg; Carb Choices: ½; Diabetic Exchange: 1 Vegetable, 1 Fat

71 CALORIES OUT

Women: Walk: 17 minutes; Jog: 8 minutes

Men: Walk: 14 minutes; Jog: 7 minutes

CALORIE COMBOS

Crab Cakes with Super-Easy Tartar Sauce (page 119): 145 cals

Vegetarian Chili (page 115): 156 cals

Quick Herb-Coated Tilapia (page 120): 196 cals

Everyone's Favorite Veggie Burgers (page 212): 223 cals

Memorable Meat Loaf (page 253): 233 cals

Grilled Chicken with Fresh Mango Salsa (page 243): 234 cals

Quinoa, Paneer, and Cabbage Patties (page 220): 235 cals

Fish Sticks for Hale (page 230): 280 cals

Filet Mignon with Zesty Black Pepper Sauce (page 327): 307 cals

Baked Marinated Salmon with Mustard-Dill Sauce (page 308): 324 cals

79 CALORIES IN

Protein: 3 g; Carbohydrates: 6 g; Fat: 5 g; Fiber: 2 g; Sodium: 219 mg; Carb Choices: ½; Diabetic Exchange: 1 Vegetable, 1 Fat

79 CALORIES OUT

Women: Walk: 19 minutes; Jog: 9 minutes

Men: Walk: 16 minutes; Jog: 8 minutes

CALORIE COMBOS

Sweet-and-Spicy Fried Tofu (page 114): 151 cals

Tofu and Bok Choy with Chili Sauce (page 116): 174 cals

Easy Lime-Cilantro Grilled Chicken (page 238): 215 cals

Roasted Chicken with Rosemary-Lemon-Garlic Rub (page 244): 244 cals

Chicken with Zucchini, Mushrooms, Celery, and Cashews (page 246): 254 cals

Soba Noodles with Tofu, Kale, and Miso Dressing (page 291): 349 cals

Sesame-Coated Salmon with Soy Sauce–Lime Drizzle (page 310): 363 cals

Vegetarian Stir-Fried Rice (page 297): 367 cals

SAUTÉED BABY BOK CHOY AND RED BELL PEPPERS

The simple trick to this dish is cooking the garlic over medium-low heat until it turns a light golden brown and develops a sweet taste. The heat must be low, or the garlic will burn and become bitter. Once the garlic is cooked, you add the bok choy and red bell peppers and sauté briefly before adding the soy sauce and water, which provide moisture to finish the cooking process.

SERVES 4

½ tablespoon vegetable oil

2 teaspoons toasted sesame oil

1 tablespoon minced garlic

1 pound (480 g) baby bok choy, stalks trimmed and halved or quartered lengthwise, depending on size

1 red bell pepper, cored, seeded, quartered, and thinly sliced crosswise

Pinch of sugar

1 tablespoon lite soy sauce

1 tablespoon water

1 tablespoon toasted sesame seeds

1. In a large nonstick skillet, heat the vegetable and sesame oils over medium-low heat. Add the garlic and cook, stirring, just until light golden, about 30 seconds. Add the baby bok choy and red bell peppers, increase the heat to medium-high, and sauté, stirring, for 1 minute. Add the sugar, soy sauce, and water and cook for 3 to 4 minutes, until the vegetables are crisp-tender.

2. Adjust the seasoning, sprinkle with the sesame seeds, and serve promptly.

HOW TO COOK BOK CHOY

The great thing about bok choy, also called Chinese cabbage, is not only how tasty it can be, but how easy it is to cook. While there are many kinds of Chinese cabbages available throughout Asia, only two, bok choy and Napa, are widely available in the West. Within the bok choy category, the three most common varieties here are: bok choy, with ivory stalks and dark green leaves; Shanghai bok choy, with jade stalks and more delicate light green leaves; and bok choy sum, which looks like Shanghai bok choy and has small edible yellow flowers. All three can be used interchangeably in recipes. For large mature bok choy, with big heads that can weigh up to 2 pounds, the stems and leaves are often cooked separately to avoid overcooked leaves or tough stems. Baby bok choy varieties weigh just a few ounces and can be cooked whole, halved, or quartered. When cooking bok choy, there are three things to remember: keep it simple, cook it fast, and serve it promptly.

ROASTED CAULIFLOWER AND MUSHROOMS WITH PINE NUTS

To keep things easy, I use only two common Indian spices, cumin and coriander, but branch out by adding turmeric, fennel seeds, or other fragrant spices that you may have in your collection. Add red pepper flakes for a dash of heat and color, if desired.

SERVES 4

1 tablespoon vegetable oil

12 ounces (360 g) cauliflower florets

8 ounces (240 g) shiitake mushrooms, rinsed, stems removed, and quartered

1 onion, thinly sliced

½ teaspoon roasted ground coriander

½ teaspoon roasted ground cumin

¼ teaspoon sugar

Pinch of red pepper flakes, optional

Salt, to taste

2 tablespoons toasted pine nuts

2 tablespoons chopped fresh cilantro or flat-leaf parsley, or a mix of both

Small squeeze of fresh lemon juice, or to taste, optional

1. Center an oven rack and preheat the oven to 450°F (230°C). Line a baking sheet with sides with aluminum foil or baking paper; set aside.

2. In a bowl, combine all of the ingredients except the pine nuts, herbs, and lemon juice and toss to coat the cauliflower and shiitakes. Transfer the vegetables to the prepared baking sheet, spread them out in a single layer, and roast for 20 to 30 minutes, until the cauliflower is light golden and crisp-tender.

3. Adjust the seasoning, transfer to a serving bowl, and garnish with the pine nuts, cilantro, and the lemon juice, if using. Serve promptly.

85 CALORIES IN

Protein: 6 g; Carbohydrates: 9 g; Fat: 4 g; Fiber: 1 g; Sodium: 13 mg; Carb Choice: ½; Diabetic Exchange: 2 Vegetable, 1 Fat

85 CALORIES OUT

Women: Walk: 21 minutes; Jog: 10 minutes

Men: Walk: 17 minutes; Jog: 8 minutes

CALORIE COMBOS

Grilled Lemony Lamb Chops (page 130): 177 cals

Quick Herb-Coated Tilapia (page 120): 196 cals

Roasted Pork Tenderloin with Mustard-Tarragon Marinade (page 127): 198 cals

Classic Dal (page 217): 232 cals

Roasted Chicken with Rosemary-Lemon-Garlic Rub (page 244): 244 cals

Chicken Thighs with Capers and Parsley (page 250): 273 cals

Beef and Vegetable Kebabs with Cilantro–Green Olive Drizzle (page 325): 304 cals

Sesame-Coated Salmon with Soy Sauce–Lime Drizzle (page 310): 363 cals

CALORIE CUTS

Skip the pine nuts and save 29 calories and 3 grams of fat per serving.

HOW TO TOAST AND FREEZE NUTS AND SEEDS

Having pretoasted nuts and seeds in the freezer is a real bonus, especially when you're in a hurry. They are great tossed into salads, used in baked goods, and added to breakfast cereals or almost anything else. There are a couple of ways to toast nuts and seeds. Preheat the oven to 300°F (150°C). Spread them in a single layer (it's okay if they overlap a bit) on a baking sheet and bake for 10 minutes. Stir and bake for 10 minutes more, or until they give off a nutty smell and are light golden. Watch carefully to prevent burning; some nuts and seeds may take less than 20 minutes. Transfer to a plate to cool. You can also toast nuts or seeds in a dry skillet on the stove-top over low to medium heat. Stir them every now and then to prevent overbrowning, and keep a close eye on them. The timing will depend on how high your heat is. Once they are completely cooled, store in an airtight container in the freezer.

JAPANESE EGGPLANT IN SWEET CHILI SAUCE

You've undoubtedly seen this dish on the menu at your local Chinese restaurant. It's easy to make at home, but be sure to use the right type of eggplant and chili sauce. Look for unblemished small- to medium-size, deep purple, long, thin Asian eggplants. They are usually called Japanese or Chinese eggplants. When cooked, these eggplants tend to have creamy, mild-tasting, tender flesh. See page 342 for information on Thai-style chili sauces. The eggplant is cooked in batches in oil, and then the sauce is made in the same skillet. If you want more heat, use fresh red chiles instead of green.

SERVES 6

Sweet Chili Sauce

1½ tablespoons ketchup

2 tablespoons Thai-style sweet chili sauce

1 tablespoon yellow miso

½ tablespoon lite soy sauce, or to taste

½ teaspoon cornstarch, dissolved in ¼ cup plus 1 tablespoon water

Eggplant

2 tablespoons plus 1 teaspoon vegetable oil, or as needed

1 pound (480 g) Japanese eggplants, cut into matchsticks about 2 inches (5 cm) long by ½-inch (1.25 cm) thick

1 cup (40 g) sliced scallions (1-inch/1.25 cm pieces)

1 tablespoon minced garlic

1 tablespoon minced green chile

1. To make the sauce, in a small bowl, combine the ingredients and stir until well blended; set aside.

2. In a large nonstick skillet or wok, heat 1 tablespoon of the vegetable oil over medium heat. Add half of the eggplant and sauté, stirring occasionally, for 3 to 5 minutes, until the flesh starts to get soft. (Note: The eggplant may seem dry due to the small amount of oil, but don't worry, it will be moistened later with the sauce; however, if it seems too dry, you can add a little more oil.) Transfer to a heatproof serving bowl or platter. Heat another 1 tablespoon vegetable oil in the skillet. Add the remaining eggplant and sauté for 3 to 5 minutes, or just until soft. Transfer to the serving bowl or platter.

3. Add the remaining 1 teaspoon vegetable oil to the pan, then add the scallions, garlic, and green chile and sauté, stirring occasionally, for 2 minutes. Add the sautéed eggplant, then make an empty space in the middle of the skillet and add the reserved sauce. Bring it to a boil, stirring constantly, and boil, stirring, just until it begins to thicken, 1 to 2 minutes. If it gets too thick, thin with a couple of tablespoons of water. Stir the eggplant into the sauce, adjust the seasoning, transfer to a serving dish, and serve.

MAPLE-GLAZED CARROTS

Carrots come to life with a simple drizzle of golden maple syrup and a dash of spices. These might even tempt your kids, who, like most, probably prefer raw carrot sticks. The technique of stove-top braising is a typical French method (although in France, the liquid is added little by little, and a finishing touch would normally include a dollop of crème fraîche).

SERVES 4

½ tablespoon unsalted butter

5 large carrots (a little over 1 pound, 500 g), sliced into ¼-inch (6 mm) rounds

Salt and freshly ground pepper, to taste

¼ teaspoon ground star anise, cardamom, or cinnamon, or a mix of spices, to taste

½ cup (125 ml) water or low-sodium fat-free stock

2 tablespoons maple syrup, or to taste (you may need less if your carrots are really sweet)

1. In a medium skillet, melt the butter over medium heat. Add the carrots, salt, pepper, and star anise and sauté for 2 minutes, or just until the carrots begin to give off their juices. Add the water and bring to a boil, then reduce the heat to a strong simmer and cook, covered, for 7 to 10 minutes, until the carrots are tender and almost all of the water has evaporated.

2. Add the maple syrup and stir to coat, adjust the seasoning, and serve.

98 CALORIES IN

Protein: 1 g; Carbohydrates: 17 g; Fat: 3 g; Fiber: 3 g; Sodium: 432 mg; Carb Choices: 1; Diabetic Exchange: 4 Vegetables

98 CALORIES OUT

Women: Walk: 24 minutes; Jog: 11 minutes

Men: Walk: 20 minutes; Jog: 9 minutes

CALORIE COMBOS

Crab Cakes with Super-Easy Tartar Sauce (page 119): 145 cals

Dieter's Chicken Skewers (page 124): 154 cals

Grilled Lemony Lamb Chops (page 130): 177 cals

Roasted Pork Tenderloin with Mustard-Tarragon Marinade (page 127): 198 cals

Memorable Meat Loaf (page 253): 233 cals

Roasted Chicken with Rosemary-Lemon-Garlic Rub (page 244: 244 cals

Butter Chicken Made Easy (page 251): 276 cals

French-Style Beef Stew (page 261): 286 cals

Slow-Cooker Pulled Pork with Whole Wheat Buns (page 318): 360 cals

Sesame-Coated Salmon with Soy Sauce–Lime Drizzle (page 310): 363 cals

BROCCOLINI WITH SESAME AND SPICE (📷 page 299)

Versatility is thy name: this spicy sesame sauce, which can be made up to 2 days in advance, can be used with just about any vegetable, or drizzle it over grilled seafood or poultry for a quick and easy flavor boost. It's sublime on sautéed or steamed bok choy, steamed spinach, grilled eggplant, or regular broccoli. Adjust the amounts of soy sauce and other ingredients to suit your taste. The pinch of sugar in the boiling water helps to keep the broccolini bright green.

SERVES 5

Sesame-Spice Sauce

1 tablespoon vegetable oil

1 tablespoon toasted sesame oil

2 garlic cloves, minced

2 tablespoons sesame seeds, white or black, or a mix of both

Pinch of red pepper flakes, or to taste, optional

2 tablespoons lite soy sauce, or to taste

½ teaspoon sugar

Broccolini

Pinch of sugar

Pinch of salt

12 ounces (360 g) broccolini, stems trimmed (see below)

1. To make the sauce, in a very small skillet, heat the vegetable and sesame oils over medium-low heat until hot. Add the garlic, sesame seeds, and red pepper flakes, if using, and cook for 30 seconds. (Be careful not to burn the garlic and sesame seeds, or they will develop a bitter taste.) Add the soy sauce and sugar, stir, and cook for 30 seconds. Set aside.

2. To cook the broccolini, bring a medium pot of water to a boil and add the sugar and salt. Add the broccolini and cook for 2 to 3 minutes, until crisp-tender; do not overcook. Drain well, pat dry with paper towels, and transfer to a serving bowl.

3. Pour the sauce over the broccolini and mix gently. Adjust the seasoning and serve warm or at room temperature.

HOW TO TRIM BROCCOLINI

The stems of broccolini, sometimes called broccolette, should be about 4 inches (10 cm) long, with green florets emerging at the top. Avoid those with yellow flowers as they tend to be past their prime. After rinsing, trim the bottoms of the stems. If the stems are thick, more than ½ inch (1.25 cm) in diameter, you will probably need to peel them. Use a paring knife, grab a little piece of the skin's bottom edge, and pull it off in an upward motion. It will stop automatically at the florets and then you can simply twist or slice it off. The upward peeling motion is key here.

SAUTÉED KALE WITH BEANS AND BALSAMIC VINEGAR

Balsamic vinegar is the perfect dressing for these hearty, nutrient-packed greens and meaty beans. It simultaneously adds a welcome sweetness and tartness. Feel free to substitute the kale with mustard greens, Swiss chard, or bok choy. If the kale leaves are large, cut them in half vertically before you slice into thin strips. Play around with different bean varieties as well. Chickpeas, cannellini beans, and lentils are all delicious. Everything in this recipe can be adjusted to your taste. Slice the kale into small strips that will meld together with the beans more easily.

SERVES 6

- 2 tablespoons vegetable oil
- 1 medium onion, chopped
- 1 garlic clove, minced
- 10 ounces (300 g) kale, tough stems trimmed, leaves sliced into thin strips
- Salt and freshly ground pepper, to taste
- One 15-ounce (425 g) can black-eyed peas, cannellini, or your favorite beans, rinsed and drained
- 1 to 2 tablespoons balsamic vinegar, to taste

1. In a large nonstick skillet, heat the vegetable oil over medium heat. Add the onions and garlic and sauté, stirring, just until light golden, about 3 minutes. Add the kale, salt, and pepper and sauté for 2 to 3 minutes, moving the kale around as it wilts. If you need more moisture, sprinkle 2 tablespoons of water over the kale and continue cooking.

2. Once the kale is wilted, add the black-eyed peas and cook until heated through. Add the balsamic vinegar, adjust the seasoning, and serve promptly.

116 CALORIES IN

Protein: 4 g; Carbohydrates: 14 g; Fat: 5 g; Fiber: 3 g; Sodium: 123 mg; Carb Choices: 1; Diabetic Exchange: 3 Vegetable, 1 Fat

116 CALORIES OUT

Women: Walk: 28 minutes; Jog: 13 minutes

Men: Walk: 24 minutes; Jog: 11 minutes

CALORIE COMBOS

Savory Corn Cakes (page 111): 98 cals

Grilled Lemony Lamb Chops (page 130): 177 cals

Aromatic Brown Basmati Rice (page 107): 184 cals

Quick Herb-Coated Tilapia (page 120): 196 cals

Roasted Pork Tenderloin with Mustard-Tarragon Marinade (page 127): 198 cals

Chicken, Mushroom, Red Bell Pepper, and Pineapple Kebabs (page 239): 224 cals

Memorable Meat Loaf (page 253): 233 cals

Roasted Chicken with Rosemary-Lemon-Garlic Rub (page 244): 244 cals

Chicken-Zucchini Burgers with Ricotta and Sun-Dried Tomatoes (page 247): 261 cals

Slow-Cooker Pulled Pork with Whole Wheat Buns (page 318): 360 cals

ROASTED NEW POTATOES (📷 page 223)

There is no way to go wrong with the classic combination of fresh rosemary, Italian seasoning, and potatoes. The caramelized brown bits of potato have the best flavor, so be sure to scrape them off the roasting pan at the end. If you don't have fresh rosemary, use a bit more Italian seasoning or oregano. Minced garlic (one large clove, or to taste) can be mixed into the potatoes in Step 2. You can peel the potatoes or leave the skin on. Leftovers make wonderful hash browns for breakfast or any meal.

Cooking Note: In this recipe I call for putting the potatoes directly in the oven. If I have the time, though, I boil them first for 5 minutes, and then I drain and roast them in step 2. It adds a step, but it shaves off a bit of the oven time. It's a great do-ahead step for entertaining.

SERVES 6

2 pounds (1 kg) new potatoes, cut in half or into quarters, depending on size

½ teaspoon salt

Freshly ground pepper, to taste

1 tablespoon chopped fresh rosemary, or to taste

1 teaspoon Italian seasoning

Olive oil or canola oil cooking spray

1. Center an oven rack and preheat the oven to 450°F (230°C). Line a large baking sheet with sides with baking paper or aluminum foil and set aside.

2. In a large bowl, combine the potatoes, salt, pepper, rosemary, and Italian seasoning. Spray with cooking spray, then toss until well combined. Transfer the potatoes to the baking sheet and arrange them so that they are evenly spaced in a single layer. Roast for 15 to 20 minutes, until light golden brown and tender.

3. Transfer to a serving dish, adjust the seasoning, and serve.

BRUSSELS SPROUTS WITH PARMESAN AND PINE NUTS

Some folks resist cooking Brussels sprouts because they claim that they make their kitchen and often the entire house stink. But I find that this is only true if you overcook the sprouts. The key to this recipe is to boil the sprouts just until crisp-tender, then sauté them until golden. To save on cleanup, I use the same large skillet for boiling and sautéing them. Butter browns the sprouts more than oil and gives them a nutty flavor. The Parmesan cheese melts upon contact with the hot sprouts.

SERVES 6

1¼ pounds (600 g) Brussels sprouts, bottoms trimmed, loose or damaged outer leaves removed, and halved if small, quartered if large

2 tablespoons unsalted butter

1 teaspoon sugar

Salt and freshly ground pepper, to taste

⅓ cup (30 g) finely grated Parmesan cheese

¼ cup (30 g) toasted pine nuts

1. Fill a large skillet about half-full with water and bring to a boil. Add the Brussels sprouts and cook for 4 minutes. (Note: Do not overcook them at this stage; they will be sautéed in Step 2.) Drain the sprouts and pat dry with a paper towel; set aside. (Do not rinse the skillet.)

2. Heat the butter in the same skillet over medium-high heat. Just when the butter is turning golden brown (be careful it does not burn), add the sprouts, sugar, salt, and pepper and sauté until the sprouts are golden brown, about 5 minutes, or to the desired tenderness (lower the heat if the sprouts are browning too quickly). Adjust the seasoning, transfer to a serving dish, and immediately sprinkle the hot sprouts with the Parmesan cheese. Top with the pine nuts and serve hot.

118 CALORIES IN

Protein: 6 g; Carbohydrates: 10 g; Fat: 7 g; Fiber: 4 g; Sodium: 479 mg; Carb Choices: ½; Diabetic Exchange: 2 Vegetable, 1 Fat

118 CALORIES OUT

Women: Walk: 29 minutes; Jog: 14 minutes

Men: Walk: 24 minutes; Jog: 11 minutes

CALORIE COMBOS

Grilled Lemony Lamb Chops (page 130): 177 cals

Roasted Pork Tenderloin with Mustard-Tarragon Marinade (page 127): 198 cals

Rosemary-and-Smoked-Paprika Chicken Kebabs (page 128): 199 cals

Grilled Chicken Tandoori (page 236): 212 cals

Memorable Meat Loaf (page 253): 233 cals

Roasted Chicken with Rosemary-Lemon-Garlic Rub (page 244): 244 cals

Glazed Flank Steak with Honey-Dijon Onions (page 259): 282 cals

Swordfish with Cilantro-Mint Sauce (page 233): 284 cals

Baked Marinated Salmon with Mustard-Dill Sauce (page 308): 324 cals

Spaghetti with Bolognese Sauce (page 328): 339 cals

CALORIE CUTS

Skipping the pine nuts will save 39 calories and 4 grams of fat per serving.

CHEESY SOUTHERN-STYLE SPOON BREAD

Serve this spoon bread alongside roasted or grilled vegetables, poultry, meats, or fish. It is ideal for a holiday table, or any table, for that matter. Some members of my family have been known to rewarm leftovers in a microwave oven for breakfast (yes, that's me). For more formal dinners, you can also bake the spoon bread in lightly greased 4- to 6-ounce (60 to 80 ml) ramekins. Bake for only 15 minutes, or until puffed and light golden. For a creamier spoon bread, add another ½ cup (125 ml) milk.

SERVES 6

Canola oil cooking spray

½ cup (180 g) fine stone-ground yellow cornmeal (see page 347)

2 teaspoons baking powder

½ teaspoon salt

½ teaspoon sugar

2 cups (500 ml) 2% milk

2 tablespoons unsalted butter

2 large eggs

Freshly ground pepper, to taste

⅓ cup (30 g) grated low-fat cheddar cheese or Parmesan cheese

2 tablespoons finely sliced fresh chives

Ground nutmeg, to taste, optional

1. Center an oven rack and preheat the oven to 350°F (180°C). Lightly grease a square 9-inch (23 cm) Pyrex or other baking dish with cooking spray; set aside.
2. In a small bowl, combine the cornmeal, baking powder, salt, and sugar; set aside.
3. In a medium saucepan, combine the milk and butter and heat over medium heat until the butter has melted. In the meantime, in a medium bowl, whisk the eggs until frothy. Add 1 cup of the warm milk-butter mixture to the eggs, whisking vigorously, then add the remaining milk mixture, whisking. Add the reserved cornmeal mixture and whisk until blended. Return the mixture to the saucepan and cook, stirring constantly, for 4 to 5 minutes, until the batter thickens to the consistency of oatmeal.
4. Stir in the pepper, cheddar cheese, chives, and nutmeg, if using, then transfer the batter to the prepared baking dish. (The spoon bread can be made up to this point 1 day in advance; cover and refrigerate. Bring to room temperature before baking, or add a few minutes to the baking time if baking cold.) Bake for 40 minutes, or until light brown and puffed. Serve promptly.

SWEET-AND-SOUR RED CABBAGE

Cooked red cabbage is always a winner with roasted chicken, pork loin, or other roasted meats. I like to serve it at Thanksgiving. I've omitted the traditional bacon to keep down the calories and fat count. This dish is even better the second day, after the vinegar has mellowed. If you don't have fennel seeds, it will still taste great.

SERVES 6

2 tablespoons vegetable oil

1 large onion, chopped

2 teaspoons fennel seeds

1½ pounds (720 g) red cabbage, cored and thinly sliced (about 8 cups, 2 liters)

1 large Granny Smith apple, peeled and coarsely grated

½ cup (125 ml) cider vinegar

½ cup (80 g) packed brown sugar

⅓ cup (80 ml) water

Salt and freshly ground pepper, to taste

1. In a large skillet, heat the vegetable oil over medium heat. Add the onions and sauté for 3 minutes, or just until they begin to turn golden. Add the fennel seeds and sauté for 30 seconds, then add the cabbage and apple and cook, stirring occasionally, for 5 minutes.

2. While the cabbage is cooking, in a small saucepan, combine the cider vinegar, brown sugar, and water and bring to a boil.

3. Pour the vinegar mixture over the cabbage, stir well, reduce the heat, and simmer, uncovered, for 20 to 30 minutes, until the liquid is almost gone and the cabbage is tender. Adjust the seasoning and serve promptly.

143 CALORIES IN

Protein: 2 g; Carbohydrates: 26 g; Fat: 5 g; Fiber: 3 g; Sodium: 224 mg; Carb Choices: 2; Diabetic Exchange: 1 Fruit, 2 Vegetable, 1 Fat

143 CALORIES OUT

Women: Walk: 35 minutes; Jog: 16 minutes

Men: Walk: 29 minutes; Jog: 14 minutes

CALORIE COMBOS

Grilled Lemony Lamb Chops (page 130): 177 cals

Beans and Rice Indian-Style (page 118): 189 cals

Roasted Pork Tenderloin with Mustard-Tarragon Marinade (page 127): 198 cals

Rosemary-and-Smoked-Paprika Chicken Kebabs (page 128): 199 cals

Everyone's Favorite Veggie Burgers (page 212): 223 cals

Minty Middle Eastern–Style Turkey Burgers (page 242): 231 cals

Memorable Meat Loaf (page 253): 233 cals

Roasted Chicken with Rosemary-Lemon-Garlic Rub (page 244): 244 cals

Aussie-Style BBQ Chicken (page 252): 279 cals

Baked Marinated Salmon with Mustard-Dill Sauce (page 308): 324 cals

SMASHED POTATOES WITH FRESH HERBS

These potatoes are a welcome break from traditional mashed potatoes, which more often than not are loaded with cream and butter. I like to use baby or new potatoes, smashed with their skins on, but any potatoes will do. If you have some Parsley Drizzle (page 144) on hand or in the freezer, it is wonderful with these potatoes. Just mix in a little to taste and skip the chives and parsley.

SERVES 6

144 CALORIES IN

Protein: 3 g; Carbohydrates: 24 g; Fat: 4 g; Fiber: 2 g; Sodium: 410 mg; Carb Choices: 1½; Diabetic Exchange: 1 Starch, 2 Vegetables

144 CALORIES OUT

Women: Walk:
35 minutes; Jog: 17 minutes

Men: Walk:
29 minutes; Jog: 14 minutes

CALORIE COMBOS

The Best Roasted Ratatouille (page 112): 130 cals

Grilled Lemony Lamb Chops (page 130): 177 cals

Roasted Pork Tenderloin with Mustard-Tarragon Marinade (page 127): 198 cals

Rosemary-and-Smoked-Paprika Chicken Kebabs (page 128): 199 cals

Memorable Meat Loaf (page 253): 233 cals

Roasted Chicken with Rosemary-Lemon-Garlic Rub (page 244): 244 cals

Cod Mediterranean-Style (page 225): 247 cals

Aussie-Style BBQ Chicken (page 252): 279 cals

French-Style Beef Stew (page 261): 286 cals

Baked Marinated Salmon with Mustard-Dill Sauce (page 308): 324 cals

1½ pounds (720 g) baby or new potatoes, scrubbed and halved

Sprinkle of salt

1 cup (250 ml) 2% milk, or to desired consistency

1½ tablespoons extra virgin olive oil

Freshly ground pepper, to taste

2 tablespoons thinly sliced fresh chives

⅓ cup (15 g) chopped fresh flat-leaf parsley

1. Place the potatoes in a large saucepan and add enough water to cover them by about 1 inch (3 cm). Add a sprinkle of salt and bring to a boil, then reduce the heat and simmer for about 15 minutes, or until soft. Drain and return the potatoes to the saucepan.

2. Using a potato masher, while the potatoes are still hot, mash them to a chunky consistency. Stir in the milk, salt, and pepper. Adjust to the desired consistency (adding more milk if needed), then mix in the chives and parsley, and serve hot.

POLENTA WITH HERBS AND CHEESE (📷 page 126)

Italian comfort food at its best. The herbs and cheeses make this dish. Feel free to play around with other cheeses: cheddar and Asiago are fantastic, and Stilton gives the polenta a tang (but may not be kid-friendly). Polenta is a wonderful alternative to mashed potatoes, and it is sublime topped with **The Best Roasted Ratatouille (page 112)** or **Grilled Vegetables (page 108)**. I also give instructions below for making polenta cakes, which I like to serve for formal dinners. Serve the cakes with grilled meat, poultry, or seafood.

SERVES 6

4 cups (1 liter) low-sodium fat-free stock	1 cup (170 g) polenta (not instant)	¼ cup (20 g) grated Parmesan cheese
1 cup (250 ml) 2% milk, or to desired consistency	1 teaspoon dried thyme	¼ cup (30 g) grated Swiss cheese
½ teaspoon salt	1 teaspoon minced fresh rosemary	½ teaspoon freshly ground pepper

1. Combine the stock, milk, and salt in a medium saucepan and bring to a boil over high heat. Add the polenta in a thin stream, whisking constantly to prevent lumps. Stir in the thyme and rosemary, then reduce the heat to a simmer and cook, stirring often, for 15 minutes, or until the polenta pulls away from the sides of the pan and is no longer gritty. The polenta should have a creamy texture, much like farina. If it is too thick, thin it with a bit more milk.

2. Add all of the remaining ingredients, mix well, and adjust the seasoning. Serve hot.

TO MAKE ROUND OR TRIANGULAR POLENTA CAKES:

1. Instead of serving after step 2 above, divide the warm cooked polenta evenly among 6 lightly greased cupcake cups or 4- or 6-ounce (60 or 80 ml) ramekins. Cover and refrigerate until firm. Or spread the cooked polenta in a greased 9-inch (23 cm) square baking pan, cover, and refrigerate. The polenta can be covered and refrigerated for up to 12 hours.

2. To unmold and reheat, slip the polenta out of the muffin cups or ramekins. Or if you used a baking pan, unmold the polenta and cut it into 3-inch (8 cm) squares, then cut each square into 2 triangles. Heat 1 tablespoon of vegetable oil in medium nonstick skillet over medium-high heat. The skillet must be hot to form a crust on the polenta, or the cheese will start to melt before the crust forms and the cakes will fall apart. Add the polenta cakes and cook until golden, about 2 minutes, then flip and cook the other side until golden, about 2 minutes longer. Reduce the heat to medium and cook until heated through. Serve hot.

146 CALORIES IN

Protein: 7 g; Carbohydrates: 21 g; Fat: 4 g; Fiber: 1 g; Sodium: 602 mg; Carb Choices: 1½; Diabetic Exchange: 1 Starch, 1 Very Lean Meat, 1 Fat

146 CALORIES OUT

Women: Walk: 36 minutes; Jog: 17 minutes

Men: Walk: 30 minutes; Jog: 14 minutes

CALORIE COMBOS

The Best Roasted Ratatouille (page 112): 130 cals

Vegetarian Chili (page 115): 156 cals

Grilled Lemony Lamb Chops (page 130): 177 cals

Roasted Pork Tenderloin with Mustard-Tarragon Marinade (page 127): 198 cals

Rosemary-and-Smoked-Paprika Chicken Kebabs (page 128): 199 cals

Memorable Meat Loaf (page 253): 233 cals

Roasted Chicken with Rosemary-Lemon-Garlic Rub (page 244): 244 cals

Cod Mediterranean-Style (page 225): 247 cals

Tuna with Tomato-Basil-Balsamic Dressing (page 227): 263 cals

Aussie-Style BBQ Chicken (page 252): 279 cals

147 CALORIES IN

Protein: 2 g; Carbohydrates: 26 g; Fat: 4 g; Fiber: 3 g; Sodium: 528 mg; Carb Choices: 2; Diabetic Exchange: 1 Starch, 1 Vegetable, 1 Fat

147 CALORIES OUT

Women: Walk:
36 minutes; Jog: 17 minutes

Men: Walk:
30 minutes; Jog: 14 minutes

CALORIE COMBOS

Crab Cakes with Super-Easy Tartar Sauce (page 119): 145 cals

Roasted Pork Tenderloin with Mustard-Tarragon Marinade (page 127): 198 cals

Rosemary-and-Smoked-Paprika Chicken Kebabs (page 128): 199 cals

Everyone's Favorite Veggie Burgers (page 212): 223 cals

Memorable Meat Loaf (page 253): 233 cals

Quinoa, Paneer, and Cabbage Patties (page 220): 235 cals

Roasted Chicken with Rosemary-Lemon-Garlic Rub (page 244): 244 cals

Indian-Spiced Broiled Salmon (page 226): 262 cals

Aussie-Style BBQ Chicken (page 252): 279 cals

Filet Mignon with Zesty Black Pepper Sauce (page 327): 307 cals

SWEET POTATO OVEN FRIES

The spices make these fries. If you do not like garam masala, or it does not work with the other foods you are serving, switch to chili powder or red pepper flakes, cinnamon, nutmeg, cloves, ginger, cumin, cardamom, or whatever you prefer. The oven must be very hot to get the caramelization going. You can keep the skin on these wedges; just scrub the potatoes really well. Please note that these fries are not crisp like traditional deep-fried French fries, but if you like sweet potatoes, they are yummy.

SERVES 5

1¼ pounds (600 g) sweet potatoes, cut into wedges about ½ inch (1.25 cm) thick

1½ teaspoons garam masala or other spices (see headnote above)

Pinch of cayenne, optional

Salt, to taste

2 tablespoons brown sugar

1½ tablespoons vegetable oil

1. Center an oven rack and preheat the oven to 450°F (230°C). Line a baking sheet with sides with foil. Place the sweet potatoes on the pan; sprinkle with the garam masala, cayenne, if using, salt, and brown sugar; add the vegetable oil; and toss until the potatoes are well coated. Spread the potatoes out so they are not touching each other.

2. Roast for 20 minutes, then turn the potatoes with a spatula and roast for another 10 to 15 minutes, until tender. If they are browning too quickly, reduce the oven heat to 400°F (200°C). Serve promptly.

GREAT GREEN COUSCOUS (📷 page 241)

Couscous is great because it takes literally about 10 minutes to cook from start to finish, and it goes with everything. In this recipe fresh herbs make it green. For even more color and vitamins, add thinly sliced or diced vegetables, such as green beans, corn, asparagus, zucchini, or red bell peppers. Grilled vegetables are a fantastic addition. You can substitute just about any cooked grain for the couscous: think quinoa, tabbouleh, or barley.

SERVES 4

1 cup (180 g) uncooked couscous

2 cups (80 g) loosely packed fresh cilantro leaves

½ cup (20 g) loosely packed fresh mint leaves

1 garlic clove, halved

½ teaspoon salt, or to taste

¼ cup (60 g) fat-free sour cream

¼ teaspoon red pepper flakes, optional

1. Cook the couscous according to the package directions. Fluff with a fork and set aside.

2. Combine the remaining ingredients in the bowl of a food processor and process until smooth, scraping down the sides of the bowl as needed. Mix the dressing into the couscous, adjust the seasoning, and transfer to a serving bowl. Serve promptly. (The bright green color will fade after a couple of hours, but the taste will not be affected.)

152 CALORIES IN

Protein: 5 g; Carbohydrates: 31 g; Fat: 0 g; Fiber: 2 g; Sodium: 258 mg; Carb Choices: 2; Diabetic Exchange: 2 Starch

152 CALORIES OUT

Women: Walk:
37 minutes; Jog: 17 minutes

Men: Walk:
31 minutes; Jog: 15 minutes

CALORIE COMBOS

Grilled Vegetables (page 108):
89 cals

The Best Roasted Ratatouille (page 112): 130 cals

Crab Cakes with Super-Easy Tartar Sauce (page 119): 145 cals

Rosemary-and-Smoked-Paprika Chicken Kebabs (page 128):
199 cals

Grilled Chicken Tandoori (page 236): 212 cals

Chicken, Mushroom, Red Bell Pepper, and Pineapple Kebabs (page 239): 224 cals

Indian-Spiced Broiled Salmon (page 226): 262 cals

Aussie-Style BBQ Chicken (page 252): 279 cals

Snapper with Olive-Artichoke-Tomato Tapenade (page 228):
279 cals

Glazed Flank Steak with Honey-Dijon Onions (page 259): 282 cals

CREAMED LEEKS AND SPINACH

For me, creamed leeks and spinach are the epitome of cozy comfort. Here I've cut some of the calories by using milk instead of heavy cream. You can adjust the leek–spinach ratio as you wish. I usually use frozen spinach for ease of preparation: it's almost as good as the fresh and saves tons of time. Ideally, make this dish a couple hours ahead to allow the flavors to develop. For a quick lesson on cleaning leeks, see the box below.

SERVES 6

2 tablespoons unsalted butter

3 tablespoons unbleached all-purpose flour

2 cups (500 ml) 2% milk, or as needed

12 ounces (360 g) thinly sliced leeks from 2 medium leeks (4 cups/1 liter sliced)

12 ounces (360 g) frozen spinach, thawed, drained, and excess liquid gently pressed out

⅓ cup (60 g) shredded Monterey Jack or Parmesan cheese

Dash of ground nutmeg, or to taste

Salt and freshly ground pepper, to taste

1. In a small saucepan, melt 1½ tablespoons of the butter over medium heat. Add the flour and whisk about 30 seconds. Add the milk, whisking constantly, and continue to whisk until you have a smooth sauce slightly thicker than whipping cream; then set aside. To prevent clumping, be sure to reach the inner edges of the pan as you whisk.

2. In a large saucepan or skillet, melt the remaining ½ tablespoon butter over medium heat. Add the leeks and sauté for 3 to 5 minutes, until they are soft but not browned. Push the leeks to the side, add the spinach, and continue to sauté until heated through. Add the reserved white sauce and cook, stirring constantly, until heated through.

3. Add the cheese and nutmeg and stir until the cheese melts. If the mixture is too thick, thin it with a bit more milk. Season with salt and pepper, and serve hot.

HOW TO WASH LEEKS

Leeks are a wonderful substitution for onions in soups, stir-fries, stews, and other vegetable dishes. They do, however, require diligent cleaning to remove any sand and dirt. The best way I've found to do this is to slice the leeks before washing them. Slice off the root end of each leek, and trim the greens to the point near the top where they begin to wilt or look fibrous. Slice the leeks according to the recipe you are using. Place the slices in a large bowl filled with water and rub the pieces with your fingers to dislodge any sand. Lift them out of the water and place in a colander; do not pour the leeks and water into the colander, or you will dump the sand back onto the leeks. Wash a second time, and drain thoroughly before cooking.

AROMATIC BROWN BASMATI RICE

Spices are the key to transforming plain rice into something much tastier. Garnish this rice with dried currants, slivered toasted almonds, cashews, or your favorite nuts. Be sure to warn your diners that there are whole spices, which I refer to as buried treasures, among the rice grains (assuming you do not remove them beforehand). This dish can be prepared up to 2 days in advance, covered, and refrigerated. Reheat in a microwave oven. Rice does not freeze well.

SERVES 6

- 1½ cups (300 g) uncooked brown basmati rice
- 1 tablespoon vegetable oil
- 1½ teaspoons cumin seeds
- 1 or 2 cinnamon sticks
- 6 whole green cardamom pods
- 3 bay leaves
- 7 whole cloves
- 1½ cups (240 g) thinly sliced onions
- 3½ cups (875 ml) boiling water
- ½ teaspoon salt, or to taste

1. Place the rice in a bowl, cover with water, and gently swish the rice with your fingers to remove the excess starch. Drain the rice in a sieve and repeat this procedure one more time, then soak the rice in cold water for 10 minutes. Drain and set aside.

2. Heat the vegetable oil in a large saucepan over medium heat until hot. Add the cumin seeds, cinnamon sticks, cardamom pods, bay leaves, and cloves, stir, and cook for 30 seconds, or until they give off their aromas. Add the onions and sauté, stirring frequently, until light golden brown, 5 to 7 minutes. If the onions are browning too fast, lower the heat.

3. Add the rice and sauté for 1 minute. Add the boiling water and salt, stir, and bring to a boil, then reduce the heat to low, cover, and gently simmer until almost all of the liquid has been absorbed and the grains are soft, about 15 to 17 minutes. Turn off the heat and let the rice sit, covered and undisturbed, for 10 minutes.

4. Using a fork, gently lift and separate the grains of rice. Adjust the seasoning and transfer to a serving bowl. Remove the whole spices, if desired, and serve.

184 CALORIES IN

Protein: 3 g; Carbohydrates: 36 g; Fat: 3 g; Fiber: 1 g; Sodium: 389 mg; Carb Choices: 2½; Diabetic Exchange: 2 Starch, 1 Vegetable

184 CALORIES OUT

Women: Walk: 45 minutes; Jog: 21 minutes

Men: Walk: 38 minutes; Jog: 18 minutes

CALORIE COMBOS

Paneer with Spinach, Tomatoes, and Spices (page 113): 143 cals

Grilled Lemony Lamb Chops (page 130): 177 cals

Grilled Chicken Tandoori (page 236): 212 cals

Minty Middle Eastern–Style Turkey Burgers (page 242): 231 cals

Classic Dal (page 217): 232 cals

Quinoa, Paneer, and Cabbage Patties (page 220): 235 cals

Indian-Spiced Broiled Salmon (page 226): 262 cals

Classic Chicken Curry with Coconut Milk (page 248): 266 cals

Chicken Thighs with Capers and Parsley (page 250): 273 cals

Butter Chicken Made Easy (page 251): 276 cals

GRILLED VEGETABLES

I love all kinds of grilled vegetables, sprinkled with a touch of balsamic vinegar and topped with chopped fresh basil leaves, flat-leaf parsley, or chives. They are scrumptious over piping-hot pasta, dusted with grated Parmesan cheese and a touch of Reduced-Fat Basil Walnut Pesto (page 156). Leftovers are fabulous in or alongside the Black Bean, Spinach, and Mushroom Quesadillas (page 301), the Broccoli, Mushroom, Cheddar, and Curry Frittata (page 216), or the Vegetarian Lasagna (page 303). One of my recipe testers used them in omelets the next morning. The grilling times listed following the recipe are meant as a guide; use your best judgment.

SERVES 6

Vegetables

1 medium zucchini, trimmed and halved lengthwise

1 medium yellow summer squash, trimmed and halved lengthwise

1 medium red bell pepper, cored, seeded, and halved

1 tablespoon extra virgin olive oil

1 tablespoon fresh lemon juice

1 garlic clove, minced

2 teaspoons dried oregano or Italian seasoning

Mushrooms

6 large portobello mushrooms, stems removed and caps wiped

2 tablespoons extra virgin olive oil

2 tablespoons balsamic vinegar

1 garlic clove, minced

1 teaspoon dried oregano or Italian seasoning

1 to 2 tablespoons balsamic vinegar, to taste

3 tablespoons chopped fresh basil

1. In a medium bowl, combine the zucchini, yellow squash, and red bell peppers. Add the olive oil, lemon juice, garlic, and oregano and mix until the vegetables are well coated. Set aside at room temperature for at least 30 minutes, and up to 1 hour, before grilling.

2. Meanwhile, in a second medium bowl, combine the mushrooms with the remaining ingredients and mix until well coated. Set aside at room temperature for at least 30 minutes, and up to 1 hour.

3. For a charcoal grill: Light a chimney starter filled with charcoal briquettes. When the coals are hot, spread them evenly over the bottom of the grill and set the cooking grate in place. Cover and heat until hot, about 5 minutes. For a gas grill: Turn all the burners to medium, cover, and heat until hot, about 10 minutes.

---

89 CALORIES IN

Protein: 3 g; Carbohydrates: 9 g; Fat: 5 g; Fiber: 3 g; Sodium: 16 mg; Carb Choices: ½; Diabetic Exchange: 2 Vegetable, 1 Fat

89 CALORIES OUT

Women: Walk:
22 minutes | Jog: 10 minutes

Men: Walk:
18 minutes | Jog: 9 minutes

CALORIE COMBOS

½ cup (80 g) plain boiled diced potatoes: 67 cals

2 cups (40 g) salad greens with 1 tablespoon Balsamic Vinaigrette (page 150): 73 cals

½ cup (80 g) plain white rice: 103 cals

½ cup (90 g) plain brown rice: 108 cals

½ cup (65 g) plain quinoa: 111 cals

Cheesy Southern-Style Spoon Bread (page 100): 127 cals

Spiced-Up Hash Browns (page 50): 133 cals

Smashed Potatoes with Fresh Herbs (page 102): 144 cals

Polenta with Herbs and Cheese (page 103): 146 cals

Beans and Rice Indian-Style (page 118): 189 cals

1 cup (100 g) plain egg noodles: 221 cals

Everyone's Favorite Veggie Burgers (page 212): 223 cals

Broccoli, Mushroom, Cheddar, and Curry Frittata (page 216): 229 cals

Quinoa, Paneer, and Cabbage Patties (page 220): 235 cals

Couscous Salad with Harissa Dressing (page 198): 241 cals

Black Bean, Spinach, and Mushroom Quesadillas (page 301): 388 cals

4. Oil the grill grate. Have a platter ready for the cooked vegetables. Grill the vegetables, including the mushrooms, turning to cook them on all sides, until crisp-tender, 7 to 10 minutes (see list). Adjust the heat and the position of the vegetables on the grill as needed to avoid burning. Remember that they will continue to cook slightly once off the heat.

5. Transfer the cooked vegetables to the serving platter. Or if you wish, transfer to a chopping board and cut into smaller pieces as desired, then transfer to the platter. Adjust the seasoning and sprinkle with the balsamic vinegar and basil. Serve warm or at room temperature.

GRILLING TIMES FOR VEGETABLES

- ▶ Zucchini and summer squash (sliced lengthwise in half): 8 to 10 minutes
- ▶ Bell peppers (cored, seeded, and cut in half): 7 to 9 minutes
- ▶ Portobello mushroom caps: 7 to 9 minutes, depending on their size
- ▶ Corn on the cob (husked): 8 to 10 minutes
- ▶ Sweet or regular onions (sliced about ½-inch/1.25 cm thick and skewered through the middle): 10 to 12 minutes
- ▶ Endive and radicchio (sliced lengthwise in half): 5 to 7 minutes

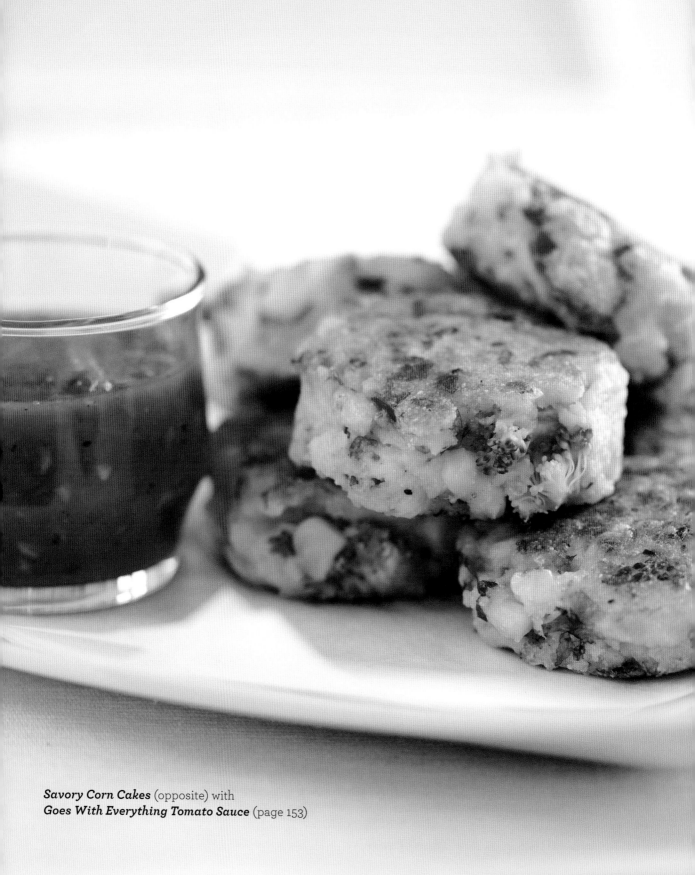

Savory Corn Cakes (opposite) with
Goes With Everything Tomato Sauce (page 153)

SAVORY CORN CAKES

Topped with a spoonful of Pico de Gallo (page 137), Fresh Mint, Cilantro, and Green Chile Chutney (page 143), or store-bought salsa, these corn cakes are fantastic served on their own, or as an accompaniment to just about anything. The red bell peppers and broccoli florets add color and vitamins, but they are not essential; for simpler cakes, omit them and increase the cornmeal by ¼ cup (30 g). Please note that stone-ground cornmeal and instant polenta are not the same thing (see page 347). If you substitute stone-ground cornmeal in this recipe, the cakes will be denser and drier.

MAKES ABOUT 15 CORN CAKES

½ cup (70 g) very small broccoli florets

¾ cup (90 g) instant polenta

½ cup (65 g) unbleached all-purpose flour

1 teaspoon baking soda

1 teaspoon salt, or to taste

Freshly ground pepper, to taste

1 large egg

1 cup (250 ml) low-fat buttermilk, or as needed

1 cup (100 g) fresh or frozen corn kernels

⅓ cup (50 g) finely diced red bell pepper

1 tablespoon minced fresh or jarred jalapeño, optional

3 tablespoons thinly sliced scallions

3 tablespoons chopped fresh cilantro

1 cup (100 g) coarsely grated reduced-fat Monterey Jack cheese or reduced-fat cheddar cheese

1 tablespoon canola oil

1. Boil or steam the broccoli florets in a small saucepan for 2 minutes, or until crisp-tender. Chop into very small pieces and set aside.

2. In a medium bowl, whisk together the polenta, flour, baking soda, salt, and pepper until well combined; set aside.

3. In another medium bowl, combine the egg and buttermilk and whisk until blended. Add the broccoli, corn, red bell peppers, jalapeños, if using, scallions, cilantro, and cheese. Mix gently, then add to the cornmeal mixture and stir until well combined. The batter should be thick, but if it seems too thick or dry, add up to 2 tablespoons more buttermilk.

4. Heat the canola oil in a large nonstick skillet over medium-low heat until hot. Add ¼-cup (60 ml) portions of the batter to the skillet and cook the cakes until the edges are set and the underside is golden brown, 2 to 3 minutes. Flip and cook for about 2 minutes more. Transfer the first batch to a plate and cook the remaining cakes. Serve warm. Refrigerate any leftovers, and reheat in a microwave oven or in an ungreased skillet over medium-low heat.

98 CALORIES IN

Protein: 5 g; Carbohydrates: 13 g; Fat: 3 g; Fiber: 1 g; Sodium: 305 mg; Carb Choices: 1; Diabetic Exchange: 1 Starch

98 CALORIES OUT

Women: Walk: 24 minutes | Jog: 11 minutes

Men: Walk: 20 minutes | Jog: 9 minutes

CALORIE COMBOS

Radish-Tomato-Cucumber Salsa (page 135): 12 cals

Pico de Gallo (page 137): 16 cals

Fresh Mint, Cilantro, and Green Chile Chutney (page 143): 30 cals

Broiled Zucchini with Parmesan (page 90): 49 cals

Tomato, Cucumber, and Radish Salad (page 76): 55 cals

Goes-with-Everything Fresh Tomato Sauce (page 153): 64 cals

2 cups (40 g) salad greens with 1 tablespoon Balsamic Vinaigrette (page 150): 73 cals

Yummy Guacamole (page 157): 86 cals

Grilled Vegetables (page 108): 89 cals

Caesar Salad with a Light Touch (page 83): 163 cals

Easy Black Bean Soup with Fixins (page 191): 295 cals

THE BEST ROASTED RATATOUILLE (📷 page 126)

(📷 page 126)

130 CALORIES IN

Protein: 3 g; Carbohydrates: 15 g; Fat: 7 g; Fiber: 5 g; Sodium: 402 mg; Carb Choices: 1; Diabetic Exchange: 3 Vegetable, 1 Fat

130 CALORIES OUT

Women: Walk: 32 minutes | Jog: 15 minutes

Men: Walk: 27 minutes | Jog: 12 minutes

CALORIE COMBOS

½ cup (80 g) plain boiled diced potatoes: 67 cals

2 cups (40 g) salad greens with 1 tablespoon Balsamic Vinaigrette (page 150): 73 cals

½ cup (80 g) plain white rice: 103 cals

½ cup (90 g) plain brown rice: 108 cals

½ cup (65 g) plain quinoa: 111 cals

Cheesy Southern-Style Spoon Bread (page 100): 127 cals

Spiced-Up Hash Browns (page 50): 133 cals

Smashed Potatoes with Fresh Herbs (page 102): 144 cals

Polenta with Herbs and Cheese (page 103): 146 cals

Beans and Rice Indian-Style (page 118): 189 cals

1 cup (100 g) plain egg noodles: 221 cals

Quinoa, Paneer, and Cabbage Patties (page 220): 235 cals

Couscous Salad with Harissa Dressing (page 198): 241 cals

This sublime ratatouille is as versatile as it is delicious: think topping for mashed potatoes, pasta, brown rice, whole grains, tofu, polenta, or spoon bread. You can fiddle around with the amounts and types of vegetables and seasonings. This dish freezes well. In fact, I always keep a batch in the freezer for I-don't-know-what-to-make-tonight meals. Put it on pasta with some Parmesan shavings, and you're good to go.

SERVES 6

1 large red bell pepper, cored, seeded, and cut into lengthwise into sixths

10 ounces (300 g) Japanese eggplants, cut into 1-inch (2.5 cm) slices

10 ounces (300 g) zucchini, cut into 1-inch (2.5 cm) slices on the diagonal

10 ounces (300 g) mushrooms, such as shiitakes, rinsed and stems removed

1 tablespoon dried oregano

1 tablespoon Italian seasoning

1 teaspoon salt, or to taste

Freshly ground pepper, to taste

1 tablespoon fresh lemon juice

3 tablespoons extra virgin olive oil

1 medium sweet onion, diced

2 garlic cloves, minced

12 ounces (360 g) ripe tomatoes, diced, or one 14.5-ounce (411 g) can diced tomatoes, drained

¼ cup (10 g) chopped fresh basil

Pinch of sugar

1 teaspoon balsamic vinegar, or to taste

1. Place the red bell pepper, eggplant, zucchini, and mushrooms on a large baking sheet with sides. Sprinkle the oregano, Italian seasoning, salt, pepper, lemon juice, and 2 tablespoons of the olive oil over them, then gently toss until all of the vegetables are well coated. Spread the vegetables out in an even layer and allow them to marinate at room temperature for 10 to 20 minutes.

2. Preheat the oven to 475°F (245°C). Place the baking sheet in the oven and roast the vegetables for 20 to 30 minutes, stirring them after 15 minutes of cooking. They are done when the eggplant and red bell peppers are just soft (don't overcook them, or they will be mushy).

3. While the vegetables are roasting, heat the remaining 1 tablespoon olive oil in a medium nonstick skillet over medium heat. Add the onions and sauté, stirring occasionally, for 5 to 7 minutes, until light golden. Add the garlic and sauté for 1 minute. Add the tomatoes and cook just until heated through; set aside.

4. Remove the vegetables from the oven and allow to cool slightly. Then, working in small batches, transfer them to a chopping board and cut into bite-size pieces. Place them in a serving bowl and pour any juices from the baking sheet into the bowl. Add the reserved tomato mixture, basil, sugar, and balsamic vinegar and gently mix. Adjust the seasoning and serve warm or at room temperature.

PANEER WITH SPINACH, TOMATOES, AND SPICES

No need to venture to an Indian restaurant for spinach paneer when you can make an amazing version at home. I like the spinach base more smooth than chunky, so I puree it, but you can skip that step if you prefer. As a substitute for the paneer, use an equal amount of firm tofu or tempeh. Any leftovers can be covered and refrigerated for up to 3 days; this dish does not freeze well.

SERVES 6

12 ounces (360 g) fresh spinach, trimmed, or 12 ounces (360 g) frozen whole spinach leaves

1½ tablespoons vegetable oil

1½ tablespoons minced peeled fresh ginger

1½ teaspoons cumin seeds or 1 teaspoon roasted ground cumin

1 onion, chopped

2 garlic cloves, minced

½ teaspoon turmeric

¼ teaspoon cayenne, or to taste

1 cup (160 g) diced ripe tomatoes

2 tablespoons minced seeded green chiles

2 teaspoons garam masala

1 teaspoon salt, or to taste

1 cup (250 ml) whole milk

8 ounces (240 g) paneer, drained and cut into ¼-inch (6 mm) cubes

1. If using fresh spinach, cook it in a large saucepan in 1 inch (2.5 cm) of water just until wilted, about 2 minutes. Drain, cool, and finely chop. If using frozen spinach, thaw or microwave it, place it in a colander to drain, then gently squeeze out the excess water. You should have at least 2 cups (500 ml) of spinach. Set aside.

2. In a large saucepan, heat the vegetable oil over medium heat. Add the ginger and cumin and sauté for 30 seconds, then add the onions and garlic and sauté, stirring, until the onions are light golden, 3 to 5 minutes.

3. Add the turmeric and cayenne, stir, and cook for 30 seconds, then add the tomatoes, green chiles, garam masala, and salt and cook, stirring occasionally, for 3 minutes. Add the spinach and milk, stir again, and cook over low heat until heated through, about 5 minutes. If you want a smooth spinach base, use an immersion blender, or transfer the mixture to a food processor or blender and process until fairly smooth, then return to the saucepan. Add the paneer, stir, and cook until heated through, 5 to 7 minutes. Adjust the seasoning and serve promptly.

143 CALORIES IN

Protein: 8 g; Carbohydrates: 11 g; Fat: 8 g; Fiber: 2 g; Sodium: 501 mg; Carb Choices: 1; Diabetic Exchange: 2 Vegetable, 1 High-Fat Meat

143 CALORIES OUT

Women: Walk: 35 minutes | Jog: 16 minutes

Men: Walk: 29 minutes | Jog: 14 minutes

CALORIE COMBOS

Radish-Tomato-Cucumber Salsa (page 135): 12 cals

Cucumber Yogurt Sauce (page 141): 19 cals

Indian-Style Cucumber Yogurt Salad (page 75): 45 cals

½ cup (80 g) plain boiled diced potatoes: 67 cals

½ cup (80 g) plain white rice: 103 cals

½ cup plain (90 g) brown rice: 108 cals

1 whole wheat chapati (Indian flatbread): 137 cals

Aromatic Brown Basmati Rice (page 107): 184 cals

Beans and Rice Indian-Style (page 118): 189 cals

Classic Dal (page 217): 232 cals

1 naan (Indian bread): 234 cals

HOW TO USE PANEER

Paneer (sometimes spelled *panir*) is a fresh, unripened Indian cheese akin to farmer cheese or pot cheese. The texture can vary from that of creamy ricotta to a firm, slightly dry, feta-like consistency. It is made from whole cow's or buffalo's milk that is curdled with lemon juice, vinegar, or whey from a previous batch of paneer, then left to drain or pressed to make a firm block. The best by far is homemade, and many Indian home cooks, particularly in northern India, make a batch of paneer at least once a week. Paneer can be sautéed like firm tofu and added to curries, vegetables dishes, or stews, or it can be crumbled and used in vegetable patties, as in the Quinoa, Paneer, and Cabbage Patties (page 221).

151 CALORIES IN

Protein: 10 g; Carbohydrates: 9 g; Fat: 10 g; Fiber: 2 g; Sodium: 243 mg; Carb Choices: ½; Diabetic Exchange: 2 Vegetable, 1 High-Fat Meat

151 CALORIES OUT

Women: Walk:
37 minutes | Jog: 17 minutes

Men: Walk:
31 minutes | Jog: 15 minutes

CALORIE COMBOS

Roasted Asparagus with Dill and Lemon Zest (page 88): 47 cals

Napa Cabbage with Ginger and Oyster Sauce (page 89): 48 cals

Tomato, Cucumber, and Radish Salad (page 76): 55 cals

Hot-and-Sweet Cucumber, Carrot, and Red Bell Pepper Salad (page 77): 61 cals

Japanese Eggplant in Sweet Chili Sauce (page 94): 86 cals

2 cups (40 g) salad greens with 1 tablespoon Benihana-Style Ginger-Sesame Dressing (page 155): 89 cals

Broccolini with Sesame and Spice (page 96): 99 cals

½ cup (80 g) plain white rice: 103 cals

½ cup (90 g) plain brown rice: 108 cals

½ cup (65 g) plain quinoa: 111 cals

Miso Soup with Tofu, Shiitakes, Noodles, and Baby Spinach (page 64): 139 cals

1 cup (200 g) plain udon noodles: 210 cals

SWEET-AND-SPICY FRIED TOFU

A Chinese-inspired dish that will make any tofu lover happy. I go back to this dish whenever I have a yen for tofu. You can make the sauce in advance and fry the tofu just before serving. This dish does not freeze well.

SERVES 3

Sweet-and-Spicy Sauce

2 tablespoons ketchup

1 tablespoon yellow miso

1 teaspoon brown sugar

¼ cup (60 ml) water

½ teaspoon cornstarch

1 teaspoon sriracha chili sauce, or to taste

½ tablespoon vegetable oil

1 tablespoon minced green or red chile, or to taste

1 tablespoon thinly sliced scallions, plus 2 tablespoons sliced scallions for garnish

2 teaspoons minced garlic

2 teaspoons minced peeled fresh ginger

Tofu

1 tablespoon vegetable oil

12 ounces (360 g) Silken Firm tofu, patted dry, cut into 1-inch (2.5 cm) squares or similar size rectangles, and patted dry again

3 tablespoons chopped fresh cilantro, for garnish

1. To make the sauce, in a small bowl, mix the ketchup, yellow miso, brown sugar, water, cornstarch, and sriracha sauce; set aside.

2. In a small skillet, heat the vegetable oil over medium heat until hot. Add the minced chile, 1 tablespoon of the scallions, garlic, and ginger and sauté for 1 minute, stirring constantly. Stir in the reserved ketchup mixture and cook for 1 minute; set aside.

3. When ready to fry the tofu, line a large plate with paper towels. In a large nonstick skillet, heat the vegetable oil over medium-high heat. Add the tofu and sauté, turning frequently, until lightly browned, about 5 minutes. Transfer to the prepared plate to drain briefly and then to a serving dish.

4. Spoon the sauce over the tofu and garnish with the remaining 2 tablespoons scallions and the cilantro. Serve promptly.

VEGETARIAN CHILI

Enjoy this flavor-packed chili over brown rice, quinoa, or polenta, or in a whole wheat wrap for lunch or dinner. If you are short on time, skip the bell peppers and jalapeños. I like to offer the following fixins: chopped cilantro and scallions, grated cheddar cheese, sour cream, and, of course, a bottle of hot sauce. I also like to freeze portions of chili to have on hand for an easy weeknight dinner. Note: Freeze it before adding the tofu.

SERVES 8

Chili

1½ tablespoons vegetable oil

1 large onion, chopped

3 garlic cloves, minced

6 ounces (180 g) shiitake mushrooms, rinsed, stems removed, and sliced

Salt and freshly ground pepper, to taste

1 medium red bell pepper, cored, seeded, and diced

1 to 3 tablespoons minced fresh or jarred jalapeños, optional

1 tablespoon chili powder, or to taste

1½ teaspoons roasted ground cumin

2 teaspoons dried oregano

1½ cups (375 ml) tomato sauce

One 14.5-ounce (411 g) can diced tomatoes, drained, or 1½ cups (375 ml) diced fresh tomatoes

One 15-ounce (425 g) can black beans, rinsed and drained (1½ cups, 375 ml)

2 teaspoons brown sugar

Optional Tofu

½ tablespoon vegetable oil

14 ounces (420 g) extra-firm tofu, cut into ½-inch (1.25 cm) cubes and blotted dry with paper towels

1. In a large nonstick skillet, heat 1 tablespoon of the vegetable oil over medium-high heat. Add the onions and sauté for about 3 minutes, stirring frequently, until light golden. Add the garlic, shiitake mushrooms, and a sprinkle of salt and pepper, and sauté for 3 minutes. Add the red bell peppers and jalapeños and sauté for 1 minute. Move the vegetables to one side of the skillet, add the chili powder, cumin, and oregano, and sauté for 30 seconds, then mix the spices with the vegetables.

2. Add the tomato sauce, diced tomatoes, black beans, and brown sugar, stir, and bring to a boil, then reduce the heat and gently simmer until the flavors come together, about 30 minutes.

3. While the chili is simmering, sauté the tofu, if using. Line a large plate with paper towels. In a large nonstick skillet, heat the vegetable oil over medium-high heat. Add the tofu and sauté, turning frequently, until lightly browned. Transfer to the lined plate and set aside.

4. When the chili is ready, adjust the seasoning and transfer it to a serving bowl. Add the tofu, if you have it, or serve it separately. Pass any fixins at the table.

TOFU AND BOK CHOY WITH CHILI SAUCE

I think you'll keep coming back to this fabulously simple method of preparing soft tofu by steaming it (if you don't have a steamer, see How to Design a Makeshift Steamer, below). If steamed tofu is not your thing, you can stir-fry firm tofu instead (see page 114 for instructions). Transform this tofu into a wonderful meal with brown rice or soba noodles. Asian cooks often steam tofu right on the serving platter, usually with the sauce or vegetables. This dish does not freeze well.

SERVES 3

174 CALORIES IN

Protein: 13 g; Carbohydrates: 13 g; Fat: 9 g; Fiber: 3 g; Sodium: 310 mg; Carb Choices: 1; Diabetic Exchange: 2 Lean Meat, 3 Vegetable

174 CALORIES OUT

Women: Walk:
42 minutes | Jog: 20 minutes

Men: Walk:
35 minutes | Jog: 17 minutes

CALORIE COMBOS

Napa Cabbage with Ginger and Oyster Sauce (page 89): 48 cals

Hot-and-Sweet Cucumber, Carrot, and Red Bell Pepper Salad (page 77): 61 cals

Japanese Eggplant in Sweet Chili Sauce (page 94): 86 cals

Broccolini with Sesame and Spice (page 96): 99 cals

½ cup (80 g) plain white rice: 103 cals

½ cup (90 g) plain brown rice: 108 cals

½ cup (65 g) plain quinoa: 111 cals

1 cup (200 g) plain udon noodles: 210 cals

Bok Choy

Pinch of salt

Pinch of sugar

10 ounces (300 g) baby bok choy, halved lengthwise, or quartered if large

Chili Sauce

½ cup (125 ml) water

½ teaspoon cornstarch

1 teaspoon toasted sesame oil

1 teaspoon vegetable oil

2 teaspoons minced garlic

2 teaspoons minced peeled fresh ginger

1½ tablespoons hoisin sauce

1 teaspoon lite soy sauce, or to taste

2 teaspoons Thai sweet chili sauce

1 teaspoon sugar

Tofu

12.3-ounce (349 g) package Morinaga Silken Tofu, or 14 ounces (420 g) soft tofu, drained

3 tablespoons chopped fresh cilantro

¼ cup (15 g) sliced scallions

1. To cook the bok choy, bring a pot of water to a boil and add the salt and sugar. Add the bok choy and boil for 2 minutes; drain well and set aside. (You can also steam the bok choy before you steam the tofu or, if your steamer is large, along with the tofu.)

2. To make the sauce, mix the water and cornstarch in a small cup until the cornstarch has dissolved; set aside. In a small skillet, heat the sesame and vegetable oils over medium heat. Add the garlic and ginger and cook, stirring, for 30 seconds. Add the remaining ingredients, stir, and simmer for 2 minutes. Set aside.

3. Steam the tofu in a steamer or large pot over medium-high heat until heated through. Depending on the thickness of the tofu and the temperature of your steamer, this can take from 7 to 15 minutes. To check, slide a thin knife or metal skewer into the middle of the block and then touch it to see if the tofu is hot throughout.

4. Transfer the tofu to a platter and arrange the bok choy around it. Spoon the sauce on top, garnish with the cilantro and scallions, and serve promptly.

HOW TO DESIGN A MAKESHIFT STEAMER

Steamers come in many different shapes and sizes, from simple collapsible stainless-steel versions (usually on three legs with a basket that opens up like a blooming rose) to stacked traditional bamboo baskets with lids, to electric steamers. I have all three. If I'm steaming something very big that does not fit into any of those steamers, like a whole fish, I make my own steamer. You can follow this same method to make a steamer of any size. You will need a saucepan with a lid, a cake rack (metal) with longish legs, and a heatproof serving platter or plate (the thick blue-and-white Chinese ones work well). When you're ready to steam, place the cake rack in the bottom of the saucepan and add water to below the level of the rack. Place your food on the heatproof platter or plate, cover, and bring the water to a boil, then reduce the heat and steam until cooked.

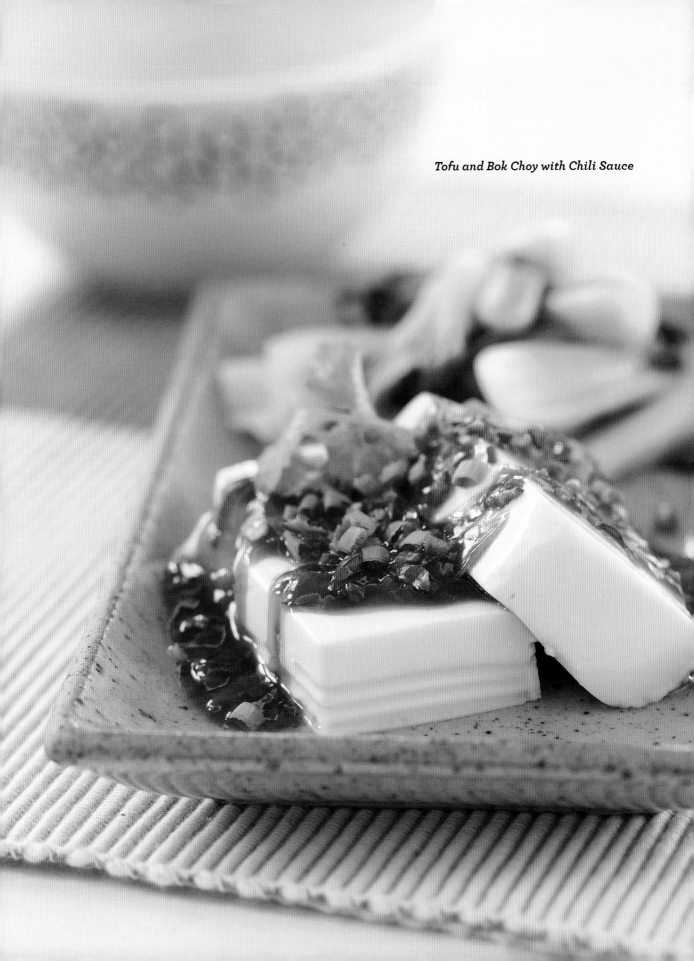

Tofu and Bok Choy with Chili Sauce

BEANS AND RICE INDIAN-STYLE

This rice and bean combo is packed with flavor. Use any Indian spices you have on hand. It's almost impossible to go wrong here, as every spice will be a bonus. I also like to add sliced shiitake or cremini mushrooms with the onions. Serve this with the Classic Dal, Paneer with Spinach, Tomatoes, and Spices, or a simple green salad. It is also fantastic with many of the nonvegetarian mains in this book. Reheat any leftovers in a microwave oven. This dish does not freeze well.

SERVES 8

1½ cups (300 g) white basmati rice

1 tablespoon vegetable oil

1 large onion, chopped

2 garlic cloves, minced

1 tablespoon minced peeled fresh ginger

½ teaspoon turmeric

2 teaspoons cumin seeds or 1½ teaspoons roasted ground cumin

1 teaspoon garam masala

3 whole green cardamom pods, optional

Pinch of cayenne, optional

1½ cups (375 ml) diced ripe tomatoes or one 14.5-ounce (411 g) can diced tomatoes, drained

One 14.5-ounce (411 g) can black-eyed peas, rinsed and drained

¼ teaspoon salt, or to taste

2¼ cups (560 ml) boiling water

3 tablespoons chopped fresh cilantro

1 tablespoon minced green chiles

1. Wash the rice in a sieve until the water is fairly clear, drain, and set aside. (There is no need to soak the rice before cooking.)

2. In a large nonstick saucepan or skillet (preferably with a lid), heat the vegetable oil over medium heat. Add the onions and sauté, stirring occasionally, for 5 minutes, or until light golden. Add the garlic and ginger and sauté for 1 minute. Add the turmeric, cumin, garam masala, cardamom pods and cayenne, if using, and cook for 30 seconds. Add the rice and sauté, stirring, for 1 minute.

3. Add the diced tomatoes, black-eyed peas, salt, and boiling water, stir, and bring to a boil. Reduce the heat, cover, and simmer for 20 minutes, or until the rice is cooked.

4. Fluff the rice with a fork. You can remove the cardamom pods, or warn diners that they are buried in the dish. Transfer the rice to a serving dish, sprinkle the cilantro and green chiles, and serve promptly.

CRAB CAKES WITH SUPER-EASY TARTAR SAUCE

Crabmeat can be expensive, especially the coveted jumbo lump meat. If your budget allows, by all means, use all jumbo lump, but if not, a mix of lump and backfin crabmeat is fine. Backfin has more shells and cartilage bits, so you will need to pick through it carefully. Once you taste my Super-Easy Tartar Sauce, you'll never buy bottled tartar sauce again. This lighter version has only 14 calories and zero fat. It is essential to use dill pickle relish; Vlasic is my preferred brand. Don't forget lemon wedges for serving.

SERVES 6

Super Easy Tartar Sauce
(makes about ½ cup/125 ml)

2 tablespoons nonfat mayonnaise

¼ cup (65 g) fat-free sour cream

1½ tablespoons dill pickle relish (not sweet pickle relish)

1 tablespoon drained medium capers, left whole or chopped

½ teaspoon grated lemon zest

1 teaspoon fresh lemon or lime juice, or to taste

Freshly ground pepper, to taste

Crab Cakes

1 pound (480 g) jumbo lump crabmeat (see headnote above), picked over to remove any shells and cartilage

½ cup (25 g) panko bread crumbs

3 tablespoons chopped fresh dill or cilantro, or a mixture

2 teaspoons grated lemon zest

2 teaspoons Dijon mustard

2 large eggs, lightly beaten

2 tablespoons light mayonnaise

2 tablespoons vegetable oil

1. To make the tartar sauce, combine all of the ingredients in a small bowl and mix well. Adjust the seasoning and transfer to a serving bowl. Cover and refrigerate until ready to use. The sauce can be made up to 3 days in advance.

2. To make the crab cakes, combine all of the ingredients except the vegetable oil in a bowl. Mix gently until well blended. Use a ⅓-cup (80 ml) measuring cup to portion out the cakes, shape them into patties, and place on a large plate. Cover and refrigerate until ready to cook; they can be formed up to 12 hours in advance.

3. When ready, heat the vegetable oil in a large nonstick skillet over medium heat. Add 3 or 4 cakes, to avoid overcrowding, and cook for about 3 minutes, or until golden brown on the bottom. Carefully flip and cook the other side for 3 minutes, or until thoroughly heated. (Note: You may need to adjust the heat if the crab cakes begin browning too quickly.) Transfer the crab cakes to a serving platter and cover loosely with foil to keep warm.

4. Cook the remaining crab cakes and serve with the tartar sauce.

196 CALORIES IN

Protein: 34 g; Carbohydrates: 1 g; Fat: 6 g; Fiber: 0 g; Sodium: 91 mg; Carb Choices: 0; Diabetic Exchange: 4 Lean Meat

196 CALORIES OUT

Women: Walk: 48 minutes | Jog: 22 minutes

Men: Walk: 40 minutes | Jog: 19 minutes

CALORIE COMBOS

Tomato, Cucumber, and Radish Salad (page 76): 55 cals

Lemony Dill Cabbage Slaw (page 78): 63 cals

2 cups (40 g) salad greens with 1 tablespoon Balsamic Vinaigrette (page 150): 73 cals

½ cup (80 g) plain white rice: 103 cals

½ cup (90 g) plain brown rice: 108 cals

½ cup (65 g) plain quinoa: 111 cals

Roasted New Potatoes (page 98): 118 cals

Creamed Leeks and Spinach (page 106): 156 cals

1 medium baked potato with 1 tablespoon fat-free sour cream: 173 cals

Aromatic Brown Basmati Rice (page 107): 184 cals

Lemony Basmati Rice (page 209): 210 cals

Couscous Salad with Harissa Dressing (page 198): 241 cals

Spinach Salad with Mushrooms, Fennel, and Avocado (page 201): 251 cals

Pasta Salad with Sun-Dried Tomato Pesto and Mozzarella Cheese (page 202): 264 cals

QUICK HERB-COATED TILAPIA

Simple and quick for weeknight dinners. You can use any white fish fillets, such as sole, flounder, or catfish. Monitor the heat when cooking to avoid burning the herbs; my advice is to err on the low-heat side. Serve with lemon or lime wedges on the side or, if you feel the need for a sauce, pair with any sauce in this book. One of my recipe testers scribbled this on her recipe: "I overnighted this in the fridge before cooking. So easy to prepare and cook. Great recipe!"

SERVES 4

1 cup (35 to 40 g) chopped fresh herbs, such as a combination of flat-leaf parsley, cilantro, and dill

1 tablespoon grated lemon zest

4 skinless tilapia fillets, about 6 ounces (180 g) each

Sprinkle of salt and freshly ground pepper

1 tablespoon vegetable or extra virgin olive oil

Fresh lemon or lime wedges, for garnish

1. In a small bowl, mix the herbs and lemon zest until well combined. Sprinkle the fillets with the salt and pepper, then gently press the herbs onto both sides of each fillet so they adhere. (Note: It's likely that not all the herbs will stick to the fish, but enough will adhere to impart a delicious flavor.) Place the fish on a large platter or tray.

2. In a large nonstick skillet, heat the oil over medium-low heat until hot. Cook the fish for 3 to 5 minutes on each side, depending on the thickness; if the heat is too high and the herbs are turning golden brown, reduce the heat. The finished fillets should have a dark green herb coating and should flake easily when the tip of a knife is inserted in the thickest part of the flesh.

3. Transfer the fish to a platter or individual plates and serve with the lemon or lime wedges.

SHRIMP WITH BROCCOLI AND RED BELL PEPPERS (page 122)

A quick and easy dish that goes well with plain brown basmati rice and a side of mixed greens topped with Benihana-Style Ginger-Sesame Dressing. All of the ingredients can be prepped in advance and then the stir-frying done at the last minute. Once the cooking starts, things move quickly, so make sure all of your ingredients are lined up. This dish does not freeze well.

SERVES 4

Shrimp

1½ pounds (720 g) peeled and deveined medium or large shrimp, rinsed (see How to Clean Shrimp, page 123)

Salt and freshly ground pepper, to taste

1 teaspoon cornstarch

Stir-Fry Sauce

¼ cup (60 ml) water

½ teaspoon cornstarch

2 teaspoons lite soy sauce, or to taste

Pinch of sugar

1 teaspoon fresh lime juice

Stir-Fry

1½ tablespoons vegetable oil

3 large garlic cloves, minced

1 small red bell pepper, cored, seeded, quartered, and thinly sliced

6 ounces (180 g) small broccoli florets

Salt and freshly ground pepper, to taste

2 tablespoons water

3 tablespoons chopped fresh cilantro

1. In a bowl, combine the shrimp with the salt, pepper, and cornstarch, stirring well to coat the shrimp. Set aside.

2. To make the sauce, in a small bowl, combine all of the ingredients and mix well; set aside.

3. In a large nonstick skillet, heat 1 tablespoon of the vegetable oil over medium heat. Add 1 teaspoon of the garlic and sauté for 30 seconds. Add the red bell peppers and broccoli and stir, then sprinkle with salt and pepper and sauté for 1 minute, stirring constantly. Add the water and continue to cook for about 3 minutes, just until the vegetables are crisp-tender. Transfer to a serving bowl and cover to keep warm. Do not rinse the skillet.

4. Add the remaining ½ tablespoon vegetable oil to the skillet and heat over medium-high heat. When the oil is hot, add the shrimp in a single layer and cook until pink and slightly golden on the first side, about 2 minutes, then flip the shrimp. Add the remaining garlic to the skillet and cook for 1 minute, then add the sauce and cook, stirring for 2 minutes, or until the sauce is slightly thickened and the shrimp are cooked through. Add the reserved cooked vegetables and any juices to the skillet and cook just until heated through.

5. Adjust the seasoning, garnish with the cilantro, and serve promptly.

198 CALORIES IN

Protein: 25 g; Carbohydrates: 8 g; Fat: 7 g; Fiber: 1 g; Sodium: 1,072 mg; Carb Choices: ½; Diabetic Exchange: 3 Lean Meat, 1 Vegetable

198 CALORIES OUT

Women: Walk: 48 minutes | Jog: 23 minutes

Men: Walk: 40 minutes | Jog: 19 minutes

CALORIE COMBOS

Napa Cabbage with Ginger and Oyster Sauce (page 89): 48 cals

Tomato, Cucumber, and Radish Salad (page 76): 55 cals

Lemony Dill Cabbage Slaw (page 78): 63 cals

Japanese Eggplant in Sweet Chili Sauce (page 94): 86 cals

2 cups (40 g) salad greens with 1 tablespoon Benihana-Style Ginger-Sesame Dressing (page 155): 89 cals

Broccolini with Sesame and Spice (page 96): 99 cals

½ cup (80 g) plain white rice: 103 cals

½ cup (90 g) plain brown rice: 108 cals

½ cup (65 g) plain quinoa: 111 cals

1 cup (200 g) plain udon noodles: 210 cals

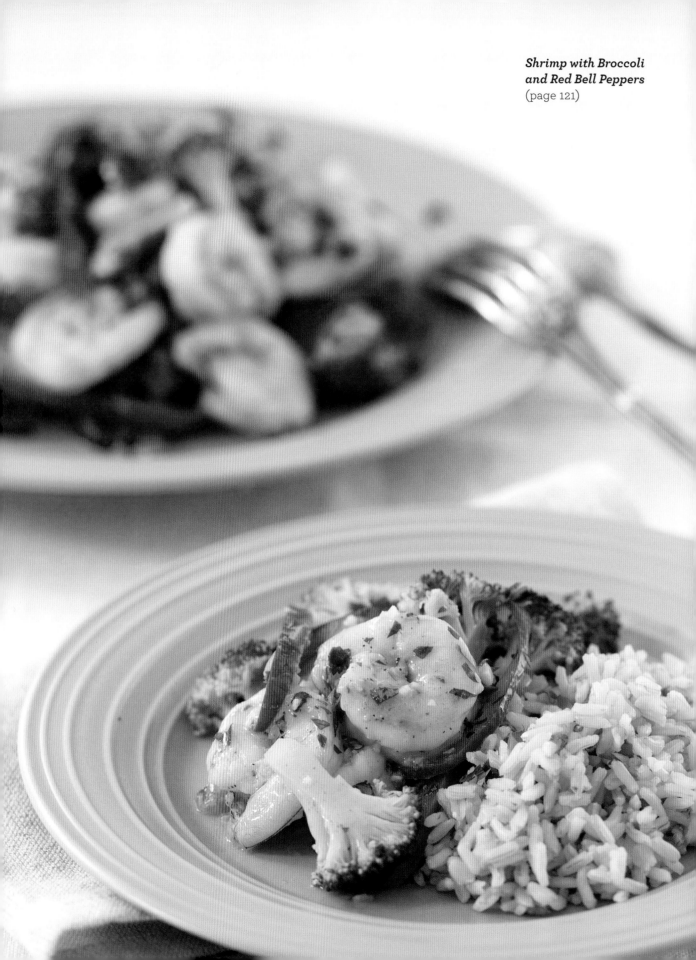

Shrimp with Broccoli and Red Bell Peppers
(page 121)

HOW TO CLEAN SHRIMP

If you want to save time, buy fresh shrimp that has already been cleaned, or frozen cleaned shrimp. If you have shrimp with the heads and/or shells intact, here is how to clean them: Twist off the heads. Then, working from the underside of the shrimp, where the legs are, peel apart the shell (a pulling action helps) in a outward motion. If the shells are tough, kitchen scissors can help. Gently pull off the shell at the tail end. (I say "gently," because sometimes you can pull off some meat with the tail.)

Rinse the shrimp under cold water and then devein them: using a sharp paring knife, lightly slit the arched back of the shrimp; do not cut too deep. Pull out the vein. Rinse the shrimp under cold water again, pat dry with paper towels, cover, and refrigerate until ready to use.

The shells and heads can be saved to make stock, or you can toss them. (Boiling them before throwing them out will prevent them from stinking up your garbage until trash pickup day.)

Here's another tip: If you want to avoid having your shrimp curl when you cook it, make three small slits on the underside of each one.

DIETER'S CHICKEN SKEWERS

Spices have practically zero calories, so not only are these skewers spiced-up delicious, they are just 154 calories per serving. You can grill or broil them, whichever is easier. If serving fewer people, the recipe can be cut on half, or you can make the whole recipe and freeze some of the uncooked marinated chicken. If you want a low-calorie sauce, try the Pico de Gallo or Cucumber Yogurt Sauce.

SERVES 6

Marinade

1½ teaspoons roasted ground cumin

1 teaspoon garlic powder

¼ teaspoon turmeric

Freshly ground pepper

2 teaspoons seasoned rice vinegar

1 tablespoon vegetable oil

¼ teaspoon salt, or to taste

Squeeze of fresh lime juice, or to taste

Dash of cayenne, optional

1½ pounds (750 g) chicken tenderloins

1. To make the marinade, in a medium bowl, combine all of the ingredients and mix well. Add the chicken and mix until well coated. Using a fork, prick the chicken to allow the seasoning to seep in. Cover and refrigerate for at least 3 hours, and up to 12 hours.

2. To prepare the skewers, thread 3 strips of chicken lengthwise onto each 8-inch (20 cm) metal or soaked bamboo skewer (see page 129). Leave enough room at the end of the skewers so you can hold them comfortably during grilling. Refrigerate until ready to cook.

3. If grilling the skewers, for a charcoal grill: Light a chimney starter filled with charcoal briquettes. When the coals are hot, spread them evenly over the bottom of the grill and set the cooking grate in place. Cover and heat until hot, about 5 minutes. For a gas grill: Turn all the burners to medium, cover, and heat until hot, about 10 minutes.

4. Have a platter ready for the cooked skewers. Oil the grill grate, then reduce the heat to medium-low, or allow the charcoal's heat to die down a bit, and grill the chicken skewers, uncovered, until nicely browned and cooked through, about 3 to 4 minutes, depending on your grill's temperature. They cook quickly, so watch carefully. Alternatively, broil the skewers on high, turning once or twice, for 3 to 4 minutes on each side, depending on the heat, until cooked through. Cut a piece of chicken in half to check for doneness. Transfer the skewers to the serving platter and serve promptly.

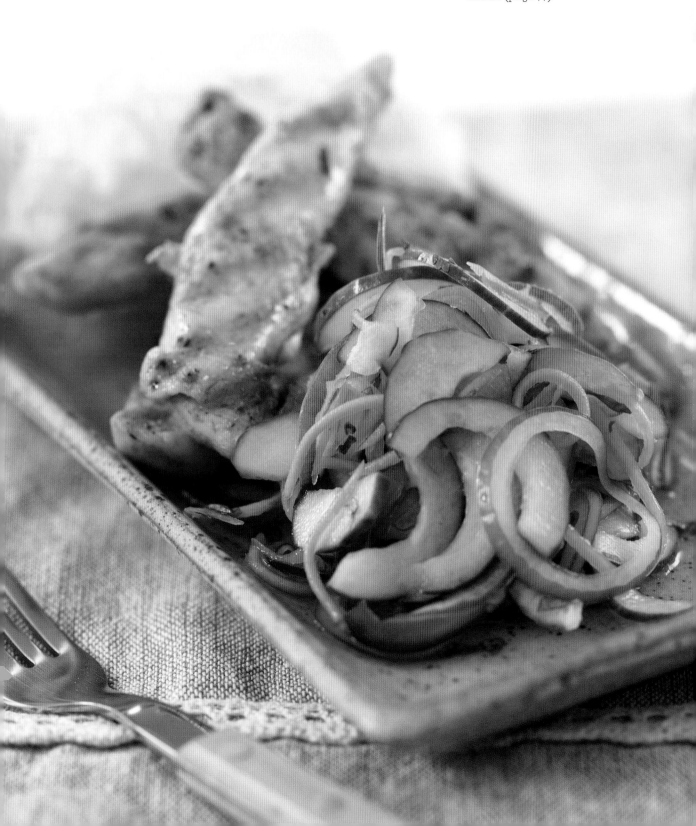

Dieter's Chicken Skewers with skewers removed (opposite), and *Hot-and-Sweet Cucumber, Carrot, and Red Bell Pepper Salad* (page 77)

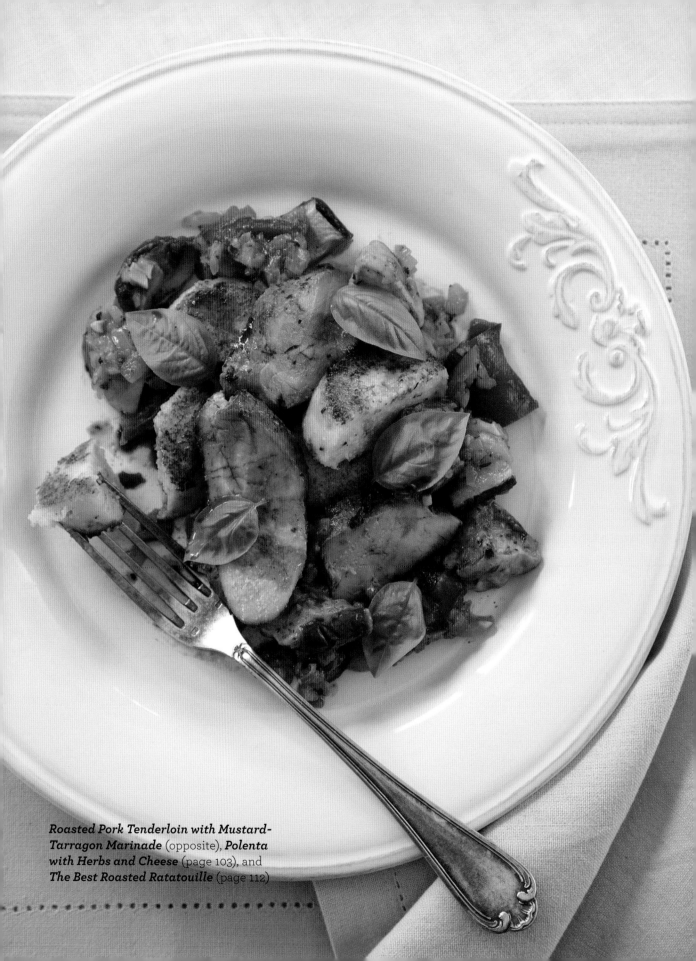

Roasted Pork Tenderloin with Mustard-Tarragon Marinade (opposite), **Polenta with Herbs and Cheese** (page 103), and **The Best Roasted Ratatouille** (page 112)

ROASTED PORK TENDERLOIN WITH MUSTARD-TARRAGON MARINADE

This tasty marinade also works well for chicken. Be careful not to overcook the pork tenderloin. Because there is almost no fat, it can dry out quickly. The serving possibilities are endless, but my favorite way to serve this is with Polenta with Herbs and Cheese and The Best Roasted Ratatouille. One of my recipe testers said that her teenage son ate half the tenderloin. Other mothers of teenage boys probably know this scenario well.

SERVES 5

Mustard-Tarragon Marinade

1 tablespoon vegetable oil

2 tablespoons lite soy sauce

2 tablespoons water

2½ tablespoons honey

3 tablespoons Dijon mustard

2 tablespoons chopped fresh tarragon

1 tablespoon dried tarragon

1 teaspoon garlic powder

Freshly ground pepper

2 pounds (1 kg) pork tenderloin (1 or 2 tenderloins, depending on the size)

1. To make the marinade, in a medium bowl, combine all of the ingredients and mix well. Add the pork tenderloin, turning to coat until it is well covered with the marinade, and poke the meat all over with a fork. Cover and refrigerate for at least 6 hours, and up to 24 hours. Flip once to make sure all sides are covered with the marinade.

2. When ready to cook, center an oven rack and preheat the oven to 400°F (200°C). Transfer the pork to a baking dish (reserve the marinade in the bowl) and roast for 25 to 30 minutes, depending on the thickness. As the pork cooks, baste it once or twice with the reserved marinade.

3. Once the pork is cooked, remove it from the oven and preheat the broiler to high. Broil for 5 minutes to give the outside a nice color, turning once during the cooking process, then cover with foil and let sit for 5 minutes before slicing and serving.

198 CALORIES IN

Protein: 38 g; Carbohydrates: 0 g; Fat: 4 g; Fiber: 0 g; Sodium: 96 mg; Carb Choices: 0; Diabetic Exchange: 5 Very Lean Meat

198 CALORIES OUT

Women: Walk:
48 minutes | Jog: 23 minutes

Men: Walk:
40 minutes | Jog: 19 minutes

CALORIE COMBOS

Broiled Zucchini with Parmesan (page 90): 49 cals

2 cups (40 g) salad greens with 1 tablespoon Balsamic Vinaigrette (page 150): 73 cals

Maple-Glazed Carrots (page 95): 98 cals

½ cup (80 g) plain white rice: 103 cals

½ cup (90 g) plain brown rice: 108 cals

½ cup (65 g) plain quinoa: 111 cals

Roasted New Potatoes (page 98): 118 cals

Cheesy Southern-Style Spoon Bread (page 100): 127 cals

Smashed Potatoes with Fresh Herbs (page 102): 144 cals

Polenta with Herbs and Cheese (page 103): 146 cals

Sweet Potato Oven Fries (page 104): 147 cals

Creamed Leeks and Spinach (page 106): 156 cals

Minty Basmati Rice and Potatoes (page 208): 206 cals

Endive, Radicchio, White Bean, and Blue Cheese Salad (page 207): 281 cals

ROSEMARY-AND-SMOKED-PAPRIKA CHICKEN KEBABS

The tasty combination of fresh rosemary (dried rosemary does not work here) and smoked paprika makes for fantastic kebabs. Ideally, the chicken should be marinated overnight to get the most flavor. This marinade can also be used with red meat, lamb, or even a meaty fish, such as swordfish or tuna. If you like, garnish the kebabs with lemon wedges and chopped fresh flat-leaf parsley.

MAKES 12 SKEWERS; SERVES 6

Rosemary-and-Smoked-Paprika Marinade

½ cup (135 g) nonfat plain Greek-style yogurt

1 tablespoon extra virgin olive oil

1 teaspoon garlic powder

3 to 4 tablespoons chopped fresh rosemary

2 teaspoons Italian seasoning

2 teaspoons smoked or plain paprika

1 teaspoon salt

Pinch of sugar

1 tablespoon balsamic vinegar

1½ pounds (720 g) boneless, skinless chicken breasts or chicken tenderloins, cut into 1-inch (2.5 cm) cubes

2 red bell peppers, cored, seeded, and cut into 1-inch (2.5 cm) pieces

1 sweet onion, cut into 1-inch (2.5 cm) pieces

1. To make the marinade, in a medium bowl, whisk together all of the ingredients. Add the chicken and stir until well coated, then, using a fork, prick the chicken to allow the marinade to seep in. Cover with plastic wrap and refrigerate for at least 3 hours, and up to 24 hours.

2. When ready to cook, thread the chicken, bell peppers, and onions, alternating them, onto twelve 12-inch (30 cm) metal or soaked bamboo skewers (see page 129). Leave enough room on the skewers so you can hold them comfortably during grilling. Reserve the extra marinade for basting the skewers.

3. For a charcoal grill: Light a chimney starter filled with charcoal briquettes. When the coals are hot, spread them evenly over the bottom of the grill and set the cooking grate in place. Cover and heat until hot, about 5 minutes. For a gas grill: Turn all the burners to high, cover, and heat until hot, about 10 minutes.

4. Have a serving platter ready for the cooked kebabs. Oil the grate, then reduce the heat to medium, or allow the charcoal's heat to die down a bit, and grill the kebabs, uncovered, basting occasionally with the reserved marinade toward the beginning of the cooking process, until the vegetables and chicken are nicely browned and the chicken is cooked through, about 5 minutes, turning and moving the pieces and adjusting the heat as needed. Cut a piece of chicken in half to check for doneness. Transfer the kebabs to the platter and serve promptly.

HOW TO GRILL SKEWERED FOOD EVENLY

One advantage of skewered chicken (and other meats) is that the proportion of meat to marinade is much higher than with whole chicken parts, where only the outer portion of the bigger pieces of meat comes in contact with the marinade. But one downside is that because the meat is cut into cubes, it can quickly get overcooked, so you need to keep a close eye on it. Here are three tips to remember when grilling skewered foods:

1. Don't jam the items on the skewers. Leave a tiny bit of space between the pieces of food so they can cook evenly and you don't end up with uncooked spots. Some people put the meat and vegetables on different skewers, but I like one to flavor the other, even if the veggies risk getting a little overcooked.
2. Oil your grill's grate when grilling foods not already marinated in an oil-containing marinade.
3. Maintain the heat at medium, not high. Parts of the meat can easily overcook and burn over high heat.
4. Metal skewers cook foods faster than bamboo ones, so pay attention to the cooking time and, more important, periodically test the meat for doneness.

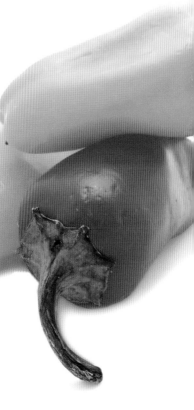

HOW TO SOAK BAMBOO SKEWERS FOR GRILLING

To avoid charred skewers, soak bamboo skewers in water for 1 to 2 hours before adding the food. If you don't have the time, even a few minutes of soaking is beneficial. After assembling the skewers, wrap a small piece of foil around each end of each skewer, or at least the end that you will use to hold the skewer—this will prevent the ends from charring and the skewer from breaking when you lift it off the grill.

GRILLED LEMONY LAMB CHOPS

Lemon, fresh herbs, and lamb are the perfect combo. Feel free to switch the herbs to your favorites; fresh oregano also works nicely. If you want a sauce, I would suggest the Fresh Mint, Cilantro, and Green Chile Chutney or the Salsa Verde. I like to serve these chops with the Glorious Greek Salad or the Couscous Salad with Harissa Dressing. A green salad is also terrific. Grilling the chops is ideal, but broiling works, too.

SERVES 6

Lemony Marinade

1 garlic clove, minced

2 teaspoons dried mint

3 tablespoons chopped fresh mint

2 tablespoons chopped fresh rosemary

1 teaspoon sugar

½ teaspoon freshly ground pepper

Pinch of salt

1 tablespoon extra virgin olive oil

1 tablespoon grated lemon zest, or to taste

1 to 2 tablespoons fresh lemon juice

6 bone-in lamb chops (1½ pounds, 720 g), about 1½ inches (4 cm) thick

1. To make the marinade, in a Pyrex baking dish large enough to hold the lamb chops, mix all of the ingredients. Poke the meat with a fork to allow the marinade to seep in. Press some of the marinade onto one side of each chop, then turn and do the same on the other side. Arrange the chops in a single layer in the dish, cover, and refrigerate for at least 6 hours, and up to 12 hours.

2. For a charcoal grill: Light a chimney starter filled with charcoal briquettes. When the coals are hot, spread them evenly over the bottom of the grill and set the cooking grate in place. Cover and heat until hot, about 5 minutes. For a gas grill: Turn all the burners to medium, cover, and heat until hot, about 10 minutes.

3. Have a serving platter ready for the cooked chops. Oil the grill grate. Grill the chops (reserving the marinade in the baking dish) to the desired doneness, 3 to 4 minutes per side for medium-rare, about 5 to 6 minutes per side for well done, depending on the thickness of the chops and the heat of your grill. Baste the chops with the reserved marinade occasionally toward the beginning of the cooking process, and move them around as necessary to ensure even cooking.

4. Transfer the chops to the platter, cover with foil, and let rest for 3 minutes before serving.

177 CALORIES IN

Protein: 23 g; Carbohydrates: 2 g; Fat: 8 g; Fiber: 0 g; Sodium: 74 mg; Carb Choices: 0; Diabetic Exchange: 3 Lean Meat

177 CALORIES OUT

Women: Walk: 43 minutes; Jog: 20 minutes

Men: Walk: 36 minutes; Jog: 17 minutes

CALORIE COMBOS

Fresh Mint, Cilantro, and Green Chile Chutney (page 143): 30 cals

Salsa Verde (page 145): 37 cals

2 cups (40 g) salad greens with 1 tablespoon Balsamic Vinaigrette (page 150): 73 cals

½ cup (75 g) plain couscous: 88 cals

Grilled Vegetables (page 108): 89 cals

½ cup (100 g) store-bought tabbouleh: 99 cals

Roasted New Potatoes (page 98): 118 cals

Great Green Couscous (page 105): 152 cals

Tomato, Artichoke Heart, Feta, and White Bean Salad (page 84): 168 cals

Minty Basmati Rice and Potatoes (page 208): 206 cals

Glorious Greek Salad (page 192): 210 cals

Couscous Salad with Harissa Dressing (page 198): 241 cals

Spinach Salad with Mushrooms, Fennel, and Avocado (page 201): 251 cals

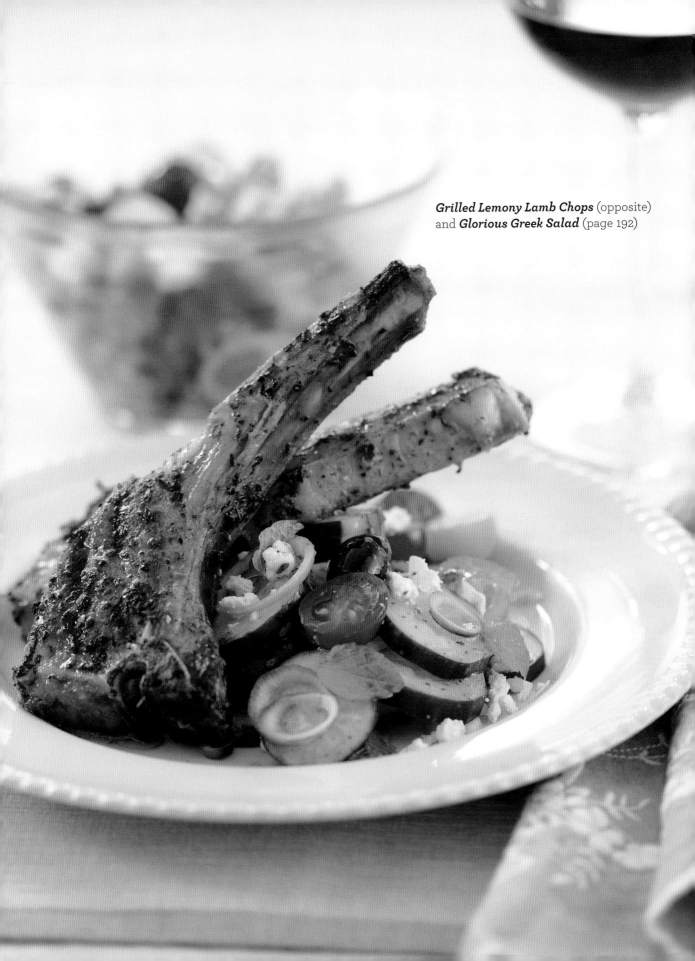

Grilled Lemony Lamb Chops (opposite)
and *Glorious Greek Salad* (page 192)

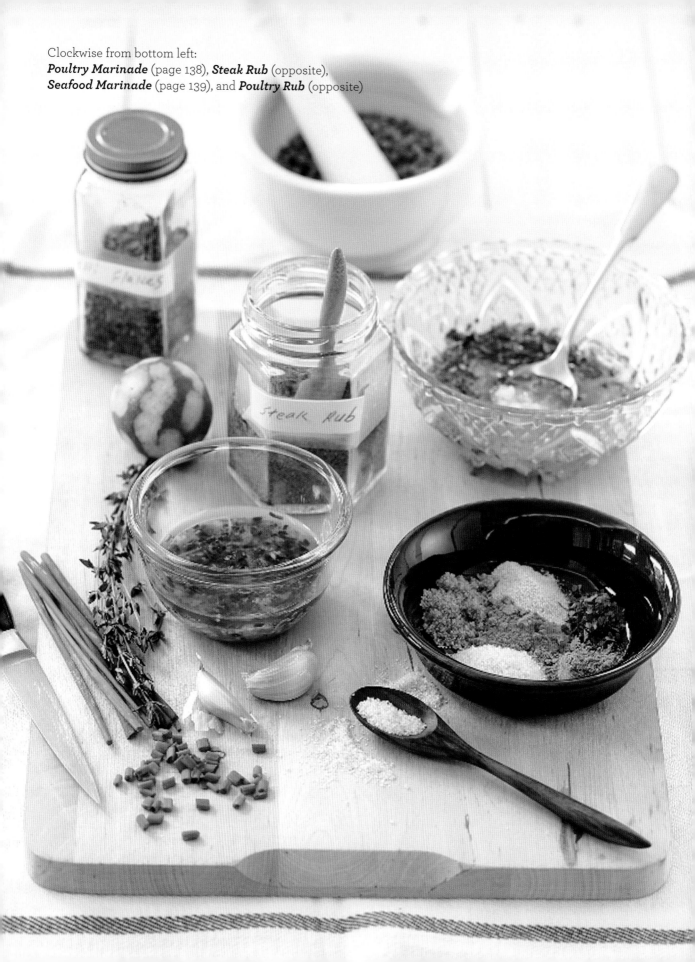

Clockwise from bottom left:
Poultry Marinade (page 138), **Steak Rub** (opposite),
Seafood Marinade (page 139), and **Poultry Rub** (opposite)

TWO ESSENTIAL RUBS

Here are two blueprints for rubs to which you can add cinnamon, allspice, black pepper, curry powder, chili powder, or anything else you want. See page 237 for instructions on How to Roast and Grind Spices. Both of these recipes can be doubled. Ideally, marinate the meat or chicken for at least 3 hours, and up to 24 hours.

POULTRY RUB

MAKES ENOUGH FOR UP TO 2 POUNDS (1 KG) CHICKEN

1 teaspoon brown sugar

2 teaspoons roasted ground coriander

1½ teaspoons garlic powder

¾ teaspoon ground ginger

½ teaspoon turmeric

Pinch of red pepper flakes

1 teaspoon salt

Combine all of the ingredients in a small bowl and mix until well blended. The rub will keep in a sealed container at room temperature for up to a month.

5 CALORIES IN

Protein: 0 g; Carbohydrates: 1 g; Fat: 0 g; Fiber: 0 g; Sodium: 292 mg; Carb Choices: 0; Diabetic Exchange: Free

5 CALORIES OUT

Women: Walk:
1 minute; Jog: 1 minute

Men: Walk:
1 minute; Jog: 1 minute

CALORIE COMBOS

4 ounces (120 g) boneless, skinless raw chicken breast: 129 cals

4 ounces (120 g) boneless, skinless raw chicken thigh: 135 cals

4 ounces (120 g) boneless, skinless raw chicken drumstick: 136 cals

STEAK RUB

MAKES ENOUGH FOR UP TO 2 POUNDS (1 KG) STEAK

1 tablespoon chili powder

1 teaspoon roasted ground cumin

1 teaspoon freshly ground pepper

½ teaspoon sugar

1 teaspoon garlic powder

2 teaspoons Worcestershire sauce

Combine all of the ingredients in a small bowl and mix until well blended. The rub will keep in a sealed container in the refrigerator for up to 2 weeks.

8 CALORIES IN

Protein: 0 g; Carbohydrates: 2 g; Fat: 0 g; Fiber: 0 g; Sodium: 22 mg; Carb Choices: 0; Diabetic Exchange: Free

8 CALORIES OUT

Women: Walk:
2 minute; Jog: 1 minute

Men: Walk:
2 minute; Jog: 1 minute

CALORIE COMBOS

4 ounces (120 g) raw flank steak: 186 cals

4 ounces (120 g) raw skirt steak: 186 cals

4 ounces (120 g) boneless raw beef chuck eye steak: 210 cals

4 ounces (120 g) raw filet mignon: 282 cals

WHITE BBQ SAUCE FOR CHICKEN

If you want a break from the traditional red BBQ sauce, this lemon-rosemary sauce will fit the bill. I use it on bone-in chicken thighs, breasts, or drumsticks, but you can also use it on boneless, skinless cuts. (FYI: The bone-in cuts are almost always sold with the skin on, so you will need to remove it.) I start cooking the chicken in the oven, then finish it off on the grill. This recipe can be easily halved. (Note: Dried rosemary does not work for this sauce.)

MAKES ENOUGH FOR UP TO 4 POUNDS (2 KG) BONE-IN CHICKEN

¼ cup (60 g) nonfat mayonnaise

Grated zest of 1 lemon

⅓ cup (80 ml) fresh lemon juice

2 tablespoons finely chopped fresh rosemary

2 teaspoons Dijon mustard

2 teaspoons honey or sugar

1½ teaspoons garlic powder

1 teaspoon salt

Freshly ground pepper, to taste

Combine all of the ingredients in a bowl and mix until well blended. Marinate the chicken for at least 12 hours, and up to 24 hours.

9 CALORIES IN

Protein: 0 g; Carbohydrates: 2 g; Fat: 0 g; Fiber: 0 g; Sodium: 191 mg; Carb Choices: 0; Diabetic Exchange: Free

9 CALORIES OUT

Women: Walk: 2 minutes; Jog: 1 minutes

Men: Walk: 2 minutes; Jog: 1 minutes

CALORIE COMBOS

12 ounces (360 g) bone-in, skinless raw chicken breast: 129 cals

7 ounces (210 g) bone-in, skinless raw chicken thigh: 135 cals

5 ounces (150 g) bone-in, skinless raw chicken drumstick: 136 cals

RADISH-TOMATO-CUCUMBER SALSA

Serve this salsa with grilled dishes, curries, quesadillas, or anything else that could benefit from a burst of freshness. To avoid soggy vegetables, prepare it no more than 2 hours in advance. Try to cut all of the vegetables approximately the same size, the smaller the better. For a sweet kick, skip the radish and instead add ½ cup (125 ml) diced pineapple.

MAKES ABOUT 2 CUPS (500 ML)

½ cup (60 g) sliced or diced red radishes

1 cup (160 g) diced ripe tomatoes

½ cup (75 g) diced seedless cucumber

1 tablespoon minced green chiles, optional

3 tablespoons chopped fresh cilantro

Squeeze of fresh lemon or lime juice, or to taste

1 teaspoon extra virgin olive oil

Pinch of sugar, or to taste

Salt and freshly ground pepper, to taste

Gently mix all of the ingredients in a serving bowl, then adjust the seasoning to taste. Let sit at room temperate for 15 minutes before serving, or cover and refrigerate if not serving promptly.

12 CALORIES IN | ¼ CUP (60 ML)

Protein: 0 g; Carbohydrates: 2 g; Fat: 0 g; Fiber: 0 g; Sodium: 77 mg; Carb Choices: 0; Diabetic Exchange: Free

12 CALORIES OUT

Women: Walk: 3 minutes; Jog: 1 minutes

Men: Walk: 2 minutes; Jog: 1 minutes

CALORIE COMBOS

Cucumber Yogurt Sauce (page 141): 19 cals

Dieter's Chicken Skewers (page 124): 154 cals

Grilled Lemony Lamb Chops (page 130): 177 cals

Beans and Rice Indian-Style (page 118): 189 cals

Grilled Chicken Tandoori (page 236): 212 cals

Everyone's Favorite Veggie Burgers (page 212): 223 cals

Classic Dal (page 217): 232 cals

Quinoa, Paneer, and Cabbage Patties (page 220): 235 cals

Indian-Spiced Broiled Salmon (page 226): 262 cals

Classic Chicken Curry with Coconut Milk (page 248): 266 cals

Chicken Curry Stir-Fry (page 317): 352 cals

Black Bean, Spinach, and Mushroom Quesadillas (page 301): 388 cals

CREAMY COCKTAIL SAUCE

Perfect for grilled seafood or anything else that goes well with the flavors of horseradish, lemon, and ketchup. You can adjust the amounts of all of the ingredients to suit your taste. This sauce can be made up to 3 days in advance.

MAKES ABOUT ¾ CUP (185 ML)

14 CALORIES IN | 1 TABLESPOON

Protein: 0 g; Carbohydrates: 3 g; Fat: 0 g; Fiber: 0 g; Sodium: 125 mg; Carb Choices: 0: Diabetic Exchange: Free

14 CALORIES OUT

Women: Walk: 3 minutes; Jog: 2 minutes

Men: Walk: 3 minutes; Jog: 1 minutes

CALORIE COMBOS

Crab Cakes with Super-Easy Tartar Sauce (page 119): 145 cals

Fish Sticks for Hale (page 230): 280 cals

Old Bay and Dill Salmon Patties (page 231): 283 cals

⅓ cup (80 ml) ketchup

1 tablespoon prepared horseradish

½ teaspoon grated lemon zest

1 tablespoon fresh lemon juice

1 teaspoon Worcestershire sauce

1 teaspoon nonfat mayonnaise

1 tablespoon fat-free sour cream

Combine all of the ingredients in a bowl and mix until well blended. Adjust the seasoning, cover, and refrigerate until ready to serve.

PICO DE GALLO

Fresh, tasty, low-cal perfection. From northern Mexico, *pico de gallo* is literally translated as "rooster's beak," which alludes to the sharpness or spiciness of the flavor. It is a zero-fat sauce that marries well with just about everything from grilled meats to seafood. Chips are tempting, of course, but high in fat and low in nutrients, so go easy, and choose whole grain chips if possible. (Note: The sauce can also be made by hand. Try to chop everything as finely as possible, and yes, it's a lot of work.) This sauce is best the day it is made; it can become watery if it sits for too long.

MAKES 2 CUPS (500 ML)

2 ripe tomatoes, cored, seeded, and chopped (2 cups, 500 ml)

1 to 2 tablespoons minced fresh serrano chiles or jalapeños (fresh or jarred)

3 tablespoons chopped white onion

¼ cup (10 g) packed fresh cilantro leaves

Greens from 1 scallion, sliced

1 small garlic clove, halved

Pinch of sugar

1 tablespoon fresh lime or lemon juice, or to taste

Salt, to taste

Combine all of the ingredients in the bowl of a food processor or in a blender and process to the desired consistency, from fairly chunky to semi-smooth; scrape down the sides of the bowl as needed. Adjust the seasoning, transfer to a bowl, and serve within 6 hours. Cover and refrigerate any leftovers.

16 CALORIES IN | 2 TABLESPOONS

Protein: 1 g; Carbohydrates: 4 g; Fat: 0 g; Fiber: 1 g; Sodium: 101 mg; Carb Choices: 0; Diabetic Exchange: Free

16 CALORIES OUT

Women: Walk: 4 minutes; Jog: 2 minutes

Men: Walk: 3 minutes; Jog: 2 minutes

CALORIE COMBOS

Savory Corn Cakes (page 111): 98 cals

7 whole wheat crackers: 120 cals

1 ounce (30 g) tortilla chips: 139 cals

Vegetarian Chili (page 115): 156 cals

Quick Herb-Coated Tilapia (page 120): 196 cals

Everyone's Favorite Veggie Burgers (page 212): 223 cals

Black Bean, Spinach, and Mushroom Quesadillas (page 301): 388 cals

THREE ESSENTIAL MARINADES

These three marinades are perfect for your everyday arsenal, when you want to add quick flavor to your food before grilling or broiling it. Each can be cut in half for a smaller yield.

STEAK MARINADE

MAKES ENOUGH FOR 4 POUNDS (2 KG) STEAK

17 CALORIES IN

Protein: 0 g; Carbohydrates: 2 g; Fat: 1 g; Fiber: 0 g; Sodium: 80 mg; Carb Choices: 0; Diabetic Exchange: Free

17 CALORIES OUT

Women: Walk: 4 minutes; Jog: 2 minutes

Men: Walk: 3 minutes; Jog: 2 minutes

CALORIE COMBOS

4 ounces (120 g) raw flank steak: 186 cals

4 ounces (120 g) raw skirt steak: 186 cals

4 ounces (120 g) boneless raw beef chuck eye steak: 210 cals

4 ounces (120 g) raw filet mignon: 282 cals

1 tablespoon vegetable oil

2 tablespoons lite soy sauce

2 tablespoons brown sugar

2 tablespoons Worcestershire sauce

1 teaspoon garlic powder

2 tablespoons minced shallots

Freshly ground pepper, to taste

Combine all of the ingredients in a bowl and mix until well blended. Marinate the steak for at least 3 hours, and up to 6 hours.

POULTRY MARINADE (page 132)

MAKES ENOUGH FOR 4 POUNDS (2 KG) POULTRY

17 CALORIES IN

Protein: 0 g; Carbohydrates: 0 g; Fat: 2 g; Fiber: 0 g; Sodium: 146 mg; Carb Choices: 0; Diabetic Exchange: Free

17 CALORIES OUT

Women: Walk: 4 minutes; Jog: 2 minutes

Men: Walk: 3 minutes; Jog: 2 minutes

CALORIE COMBOS

4 ounces (120 g) boneless, skinless raw chicken breast: 129 cals

4 ounces (120 g) boneless, skinless raw chicken thigh: 135 cals

4 ounces (120 g) boneless, skinless raw chicken drumstick: 136 cals

2 tablespoons extra virgin olive oil

2 tablespoons minced fresh herbs, such as thyme, tarragon, basil, and/or parsley

2 tablespoons thinly sliced fresh chives or scallions

1 teaspoon grated lemon zest

1 tablespoon fresh lemon juice

1 garlic clove, minced

1 teaspoon sugar

1 teaspoons salt

¼ teaspoon red pepper flakes

2 tablespoons water

Combine all of the ingredients in a bowl and mix until well blended. Marinate the chicken or other poultry for at least 3 hours, and up to 24 hours.

SEAFOOD MARINADE (📷 page 132)

MAKES ENOUGH FOR 4 POUNDS (2 KG) SEAFOOD

1 tablespoon seasoned rice vinegar

2 tablespoons canola oil

1 tablespoon fresh lime juice

1 tablespoon grated peeled fresh ginger

1 garlic clove, minced

½ teaspoon sugar

2 tablespoons finely sliced fresh chives

½ teaspoon salt

Pinch of red pepper flakes

Combine all of the ingredients in a bowl and mix until well blended. Marinate the seafood for at least 1 hour, and up to 3 hours.

18 CALORIES IN

Protein: 0 g; Carbohydrates: 1 g; Fat: 2 g; Fiber: 0 g; Sodium: 88 mg; Carb Choices: 0; Diabetic Exchange: Free

18 CALORIES OUT

Women: Walk:
4 minutes; Jog: 2 minutes

Men: Walk:
4 minutes; Jog: 2 minutes

CALORIE COMBOS

6 ounces (180 g) raw Atlantic cod fillet: 139 cals

4 ounces (120 g) raw swordfish steak: 163 cals

4 ounces (120 g) raw bluefin tuna steak: 163 cals

6 ounces (120 g) raw tilapia fillet: 163 cals

6 ounces (180 g) raw wild Atlantic salmon fillet: 242 cals

6 ounces (180 g) raw farmed Atlantic salmon fillet: 354 cals

18 CALORIES IN | 1 TABLESPOON

Protein: 0 g; Carbohydrates: 1 g; Fat: 2 g; Fiber: 0 g; Sodium: 30 mg; Carb Choices: 0; Diabetic Exchange: Free

18 CALORIES OUT

Women: Walk:
4 minutes; Jog: 2 minutes

Men: Walk:
4 minutes; Jog: 2 minutes

CALORIE COMBOS

3 red radishes: 2 cals

¼ cup (40 g) sliced celery: 2 cals

3 tablespoons sliced cucumber: 3 cals

2 tablespoons grated carrot: 3 cals

¼ cup (35 g) diced red bell pepper: 8 cals

2 cups (50 g) baby spinach: 13 cals

2 cups (40 g) sliced butterhead lettuce (Boston or Bibb): 14 cals

5 cherry tomatoes: 15 cals

2 cups (40 g) bagged mixed salad greens, Italian blend: 20 cals

2 cups (40 g) sliced iceberg lettuce: 20 cals

2 cups (40 g) sliced romaine: 20 cals

¼ cup (12 g) plain croutons: 31 cals

¼ cup (35 g) diced avocado: 47 cals

¼ cup (60 g) low-fat cottage cheese: 49 cals

ALMOST-FAT-FREE DIETER'S LEMONY DRESSING

What makes this dressing low-fat? Using water in place of most of the oil; the percentage is really up to you. This is particularly good on a salad of romaine lettuce with chickpeas, tomatoes, and fresh herbs.

MAKES ABOUT ½ CUP (125 ML)

¼ cup (60 ml) water

2 to 3 tablespoons fresh lemon juice, to taste

½ teaspoon sugar

1 tablespoon extra virgin olive oil

2 teaspoons Dijon mustard

Salt and freshly ground pepper, to taste

1 small garlic clove, smashed and peeled

Combine all of the ingredients in a bowl and mix until well blended. Adjust the seasoning, transfer to a jar if desired, cover, and refrigerate. Whisk or shake before serving. (You need not remove and discard the garlic, but it is used only to flavor the dressing; it should not be consumed.)

CUCUMBER YOGURT SAUCE

This sauce is perfect for any grilled dish or as an accompaniment to spicy Indian foods. Feel free to use ½ teaspoon (or more) roasted ground cumin instead of the mix of cumin and coriander. You can adjust all of the spices to taste. The cucumber can be omitted or replaced with finely chopped seeded ripe tomatoes. Add minced green chiles to ramp up the heat. Yogurt lovers might want to double this recipe.

MAKES ABOUT ½ CUP (125 ML)

½ cup (120 g) low-fat or nonfat plain Greek-style yogurt

3 tablespoons finely grated seedless cucumber

1 to 2 teaspoons fresh lemon juice, or to taste

¼ to ½ teaspoon minced garlic

¼ teaspoon roasted ground cumin

¼ teaspoon roasted ground coriander

¼ teaspoon dried mint

Pinch of cayenne

Pinch of sugar

Salt, to taste

Combine all of the ingredients in a bowl and mix until well blended. Adjust the seasoning, transfer to a serving bowl, cover, and refrigerate until ready to serve.

19 CALORIES IN | 2 TABLESPOONS

Protein: 3 g; Carbohydrates: 2 g; Fat: 0 g; Fiber: 0 g; Sodium: 11 mg; Carb Choices: 0; Diabetic Exchange: Free

19 CALORIES OUT

Women: Walk: 5 minutes; Jog: 2 minutes

Men: Walk: 4 minutes; Jog: 2 minutes

CALORIE COMBOS

Dieter's Chicken Skewers (page 124): 154 cals

Grilled Lemony Lamb Chops (page 130): 177 cals

Beans and Rice Indian-Style (page 118): 189 cals

Grilled Chicken Tandoori (page 236): 212 cals

Everyone's Favorite Veggie Burgers (page 212): 223 cals

Classic Dal (page 217): 232 cals

Quinoa, Paneer, and Cabbage Patties (page 220): 235 cals

Indian-Spiced Broiled Salmon (page 226): 262 cals

Classic Chicken Curry with Coconut Milk (page 248): 266 cals

Chicken Curry Stir-Fry (page 317): 352 cals

ALL-AMERICAN BBQ SAUCE

A brilliant combo of spices and flavors that is sure to be a hit at your next BBQ. Adjust the ingredients as you wish: some like more heat, others prefer a sweeter sauce. The recipe can be cut in half, but I recommend making a whole batch and freezing what you don't use, ready for whenever you need it. Don't forget to prick or score your chicken to maximize the flavor. (See How to Score Bone-In Chicken Parts, page 245.) This sauce is also delicious on ribs!

MAKES ABOUT 2 CUPS (500 ML), ENOUGH FOR 4 POUNDS (2 KG) CHICKEN

29 CALORIES IN | 2 TABLESPOONS

Protein: 0 g; Carbohydrates: 5 g; Fat: 1 g; Fiber: 1 g; Sodium: 162 mg; Carb Choices: 0; Diabetic Exchange: 1 Vegetable

29 CALORIES OUT

Women: Walk:
7 minutes; Jog: 3 minutes

Men: Walk:
6 minutes; Jog: 3 minutes

CALORIE COMBOS

4 ounces (120 g) boneless raw chicken breast: 129 cals

4 ounces (120 g) boneless raw chicken thigh: 135 cals

12 ounces (360 g) bone-in, skinless raw chicken breast: 129 cals

7 ounces (210 g) bone-in, skinless raw chicken thigh: 135 cals

5 ounces (150 g) bone-in, skinless raw chicken drumstick: 136 cals

1 tablespoon vegetable oil

1 small onion, minced

2 garlic cloves, minced

One 14.5-ounce (411 g) can diced tomatoes, with their juices

½ cup (125 ml) cider vinegar

¼ cup (60 ml) orange juice

¼ cup (40 g) packed brown sugar

2 teaspoons chipotle chile powder or regular chili powder

1 teaspoon ground ginger

2 teaspoons smoked or regular paprika

1 teaspoon salt

1 teaspoon freshly ground pepper

1. In a medium saucepan, heat the oil over medium-high heat. Add the onions and sauté for 7 minutes, or until golden brown. Add the garlic and cook for 30 seconds, then add all the remaining ingredients and bring to a boil. Reduce the heat and simmer for 10 minutes. Let cool slightly before pureeing.

2. Puree the sauce in a blender or food processor. Store, covered and refrigerated, for up to 1 week, or freeze for up to 1 month. Marinate the chicken for at least 6 hours, and up to 24 hours.

FRESH MINT, CILANTRO, AND GREEN CHILE CHUTNEY

I love this Indian-style green sauce, commonly called *pudina* chutney, and I eat it with just about anything from flatbreads and steamed vegetables to curries, rice, and dals. If you don't want the heat, omit the green chile. The chutney sauce is best served on the day it is made, but it can be prepared up to a day in advance; the green color will fade a bit, but the taste will not be affected. A mini food processor or blender with a small pitcher is perfect for making this. One recipe tester commented that she served this with corn fritters and her friends loved it. Another said that it was "fancy and tasty, and super easy."

MAKES ABOUT ½ CUP (125 ML)

1 tablespoon chopped peeled fresh ginger

1 garlic clove, halved

1 tablespoon minced seeded green chile, or to taste

⅓ cup (80 g) fat-free sour cream or nonfat plain Greek-style yogurt, or as needed

1½ cups (60 g) tightly packed fresh cilantro leaves

½ cup (20 g) tightly packed fresh mint leaves

½ teaspoon sugar, or to taste

Pinch of cayenne, optional

1 tablespoon fresh lemon juice, or to taste

Salt, to taste

Place the ginger, garlic, and green chile in a blender or mini food processor and pulse a few times to chop. Add the sour cream, cilantro, mint, sugar, cayenne, if using, and lemon juice and process, scraping down the sides of the bowl as necessary, until smooth. If you find the sauce too thick to process, add a tablespoon more sour cream. Adjust the seasoning and transfer to a serving bowl. Cover with plastic wrap pressed flush against the surface of the sauce to prevent discoloration and refrigerate until ready to serve.

30 CALORIES IN | 2 TABLESPOONS

Protein: 2 g; Carbohydrates: 6 g; Fat: 0 g; Fiber: 1 g; Sodium: 21 mg; Carb Choices: 0; Diabetic Exchange: 1 Vegetable

30 CALORIES OUT

Women: Walk: 7 minutes; Jog: 3 minutes

Men: Walk: 6 minutes; Jog: 3 minutes

CALORIE COMBOS

Dieter's Chicken Skewers (page 124): 154 cals

Grilled Lemony Lamb Chops (page 130): 177 cals

Aromatic Brown Basmati Rice (page 107): 184 cals

Beans and Rice Indian-Style (page 118): 189 cals

Lemony Basmati Rice (page 209): 210 cals

Grilled Chicken Tandoori (page 236): 212 cals

Everyone's Favorite Veggie Burgers (page 212): 223 cals

Classic Dal (page 217): 232 cals

Quinoa, Paneer, and Cabbage Patties (page 220): 235 cals

Indian-Spiced Broiled Salmon (page 226): 262 cals

Classic Chicken Curry with Coconut Milk (page 248): 266 cals

PARSLEY DRIZZLE

CALORIE COMBOS

½ cup (90 g) plain brown rice: 108 cals

1 cup (100 g) plain whole wheat spaghetti: 174 cals

4 ounces (120 g) boneless chicken breast, roasted: 187 cals

1 cup (130 g) cheese ravioli: 191 cals

6 ounces (180 g) Australian lamb chop, broiled: 213

4 ounces (120 g) flank steak, broiled: 260 cals

Chicken-Zucchini Burgers with Ricotta and Sun-Dried Tomatoes (page 247): 261 cals

6 ounces (180 g) wild Atlantic Salmon fillet, roasted or grilled: 310 cals

6 ounces (180 g) formed Atlantic Salmon fillet, roasted or grilled: 350 cals

CALORIE CUTS

Add more water in place of some of the oil.

You'll find yourself drizzling this green oil on everything from salads and mashed potatoes to grilled meat and vegetables. The parsley can be substituted with an equal amount of cilantro leaves, or you can use a mix of fresh herbs, as I sometimes do. A mini food processor is ideal for this small job. Covered and refrigerated, leftovers keep for up to 5 days. They can also be frozen for up to 1 month.

MAKES ABOUT ½ CUP (125 ML)

1 cup (70 g) tightly packed fresh flat-leaf parsley leaves

¼ cup (60 ml) canola oil or very light extra virgin olive oil

2 tablespoons water

1 garlic clove, halved, or to taste

Salt and freshly ground pepper, to taste

In the bowl of a mini food processor, combine all the ingredients and process until smooth. Adjust the seasoning, transfer to a serving bowl, cover, and refrigerate until ready to serve. Whisk before serving.

SALSA VERDE

Salsa verde, literally translated as green sauce, will brighten up any grilled steak, poultry, or meaty fish, such as tuna or swordfish. I like to mix cilantro and flat-leaf parsley in this Italian sauce, as it results in a more dynamic taste than just using one herb. For easy thawing and serving, freeze in small portions for up to 3 months.

MAKES ABOUT I CUP (250 ML)

1½ cups (60 g) packed fresh cilantro leaves and some of the stems

½ cup (25 g) packed fresh flat-leaf parsley leaves

2 or 3 anchovy fillets or 1 to 2 teaspoons anchovy paste, to taste

1½ tablespoons medium capers, drained, or to taste

1 garlic clove, halved

1½ tablespoons fresh lemon juice, or to taste

Pinch of sugar

2 tablespoons extra virgin olive oil

1 tablespoon water

Freshly ground pepper, to taste

Combine all of the ingredients in the bowl of a food processor and process until fairly smooth, scraping down the sides of the bowl as needed. Transfer to a serving bowl. Cover with plastic wrap, pressed flush against the surface of the sauce to prevent discoloration, and refrigerate if not serving immediately.

37 CALORIES IN | I TABLESPOON

Protein: 1 g; Carbohydrates: 1 g; Fat: 4 g; Fiber: 0 g; Sodium: 106 mg; Carb Choices: 0; Diabetic Exchange: 1 Fat

37 CALORIES OUT

Women: Walk:
9 minutes; Jog 4 minutes

Men: Walk:
8 minutes; Jog: 4 minutes

CALORIE COMBOS

4 ounces (120 g) boneless chicken breast, roasted: 187 cals

6 ounces (180 g) Australian lamb chop, broiled: 213 cals

4 ounces (120 g) flank steak, broiled: 260 cals

6 ounces (180 g) wild Atlantic salmon, roasted or grilled: 310 cals

6 ounces (180 g) farmed Atlantic salmon, roasted or grilled: 350 cals

CLASSIC RED WINE VINAIGRETTE

If you are looking for an everyday salad dressing for all kinds of greens or other salad mediums such as pasta, rice, couscous, or whole grains, this recipe fits the bill. The vinaigrette has a long shelf life, so feel free to double it. You can mix it by hand, or if you are making a big batch, use a handheld blender for a perfect emulsion. If you like fresh herbs in your dressing, it's best to add them after the blending. One of my recipe testers shared my sentiments in this comment: "I hate store-bought dressings, so it's always nice to have a good recipe."

MAKES ABOUT ⅓ CUP (80 ML)

1 teaspoon Dijon mustard, or to taste

Salt and freshly ground pepper, to taste

Pinch of sugar

2 tablespoons red wine vinegar

3 tablespoons water

2 tablespoons canola oil, or a mix of canola and extra virgin olive oil

1 garlic clove, smashed and peeled

Combine the mustard, salt, pepper, sugar, vinegar, and water in a small bowl and mix until well combined. In a slow stream, whisk in the canola oil until emulsified. Adjust the seasoning, transfer to a jar if desired, and add the smashed garlic. Cover and refrigerate for up to 2 weeks. Whisk or shake before serving. (Do not remove and discard the garlic; it is used only to flavor the dressing; it should not be consumed.)

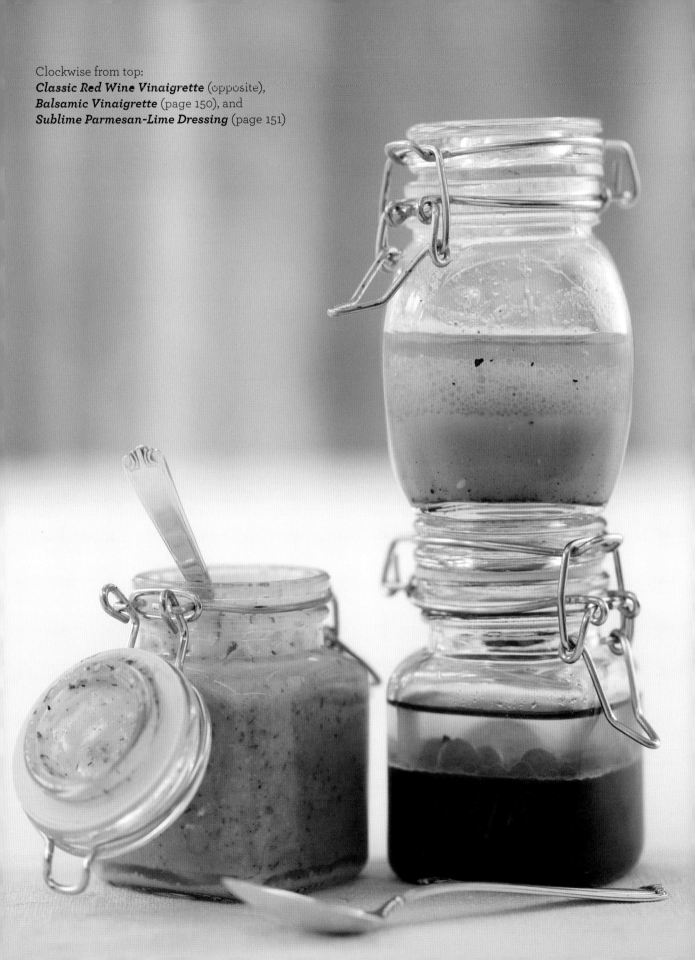

Clockwise from top:
Classic Red Wine Vinaigrette (opposite),
Balsamic Vinaigrette (page 150), and
Sublime Parmesan-Lime Dressing (page 151)

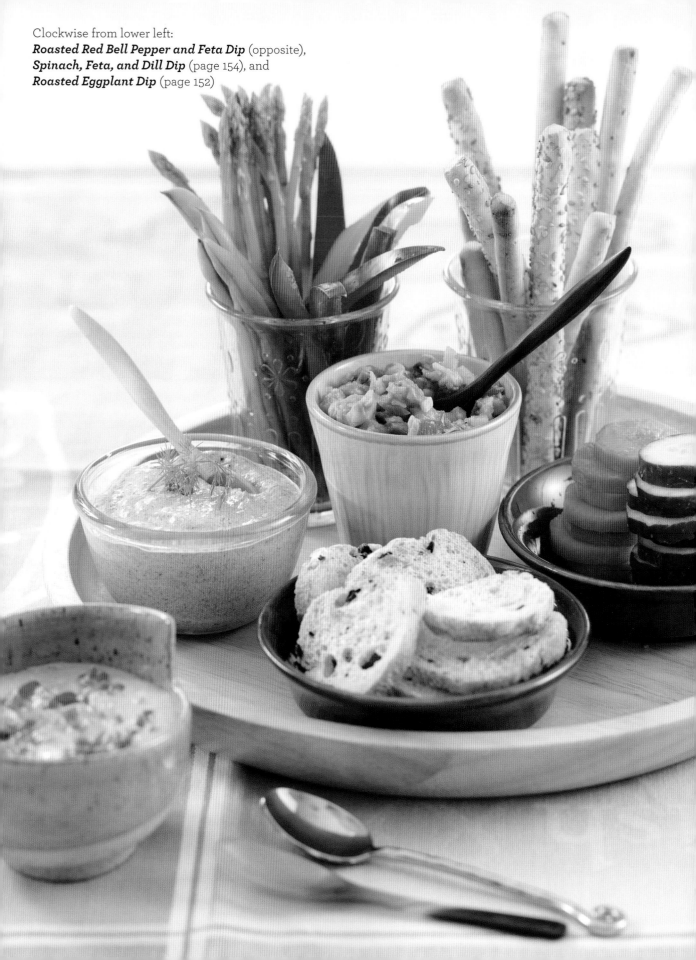

Clockwise from lower left:
Roasted Red Bell Pepper and Feta Dip (opposite),
Spinach, Feta, and Dill Dip (page 154), and
Roasted Eggplant Dip (page 152)

ROASTED RED BELL PEPPER AND FETA DIP

This is probably one of the easiest and tastiest dips you will ever make. I use three cheeses to achieve a tangy yet creamy outcome. See Calorie Combos for suggestions for dipping choices and their calorie counts.

MAKES ABOUT ¾ CUP (180 ML)

¼ cup (40g) reduced-fat feta cheese

¼ cup (50 g) part-skim ricotta cheese

3 tablespoons reduced-fat cream cheese

½ cup (90 g) jarred roasted red bell peppers, coarsely chopped

Salt and freshly ground pepper, to taste

Place all of the ingredients in the bowl of a food processor and process until fairly smooth, scraping down the sides of the bowl as necessary. Adjust the seasoning, transfer to a serving bowl, cover, and refrigerate until ready to use.

46 CALORIES IN | 2 TABLESPOONS

Protein: 3 g; Carbohydrates: 2 g; Fat: 3 g; Fiber: 0 g; Sodium: 275 mg; Carb Choices: 0; Diabetic Exchange: 1 Fat

46 CALORIES OUT

Women: Walk:
11 minutes; Jog: 5 minutes

Men: Walk:
9 minutes; Jog: 4 minutes

CALORIE COMBOS

4 celery sticks: 2 cals

4 broccoli florets: 5 cals

4 asparagus spears: 6 cals

4 carrot sticks: 6 cals

4 cucumber sticks: 8 cals

4 green beans: 9 cals

4 red bell pepper sticks: 12 cals

2 plain thin, crisp breadsticks: 25 cals

6 pita chips: 60 cals

7 whole wheat crackers: 120 cals

1 whole wheat chapati (Indian flatbread): 137 cals

1 ounce (30 g) tortilla chips: 139 cals

1 naan (Indian bread): 234 cals

Protein: 0 g; Carbohydrates: 1 g;
Fat: 6 g; Fiber: 0 g; Sodium: 21
mg; Carb Choices: 0; Diabetic
Exchange: 1 Fat

53 CALORIES OUT

Women: Walk:
13 minutes; Jog: 6 minutes

Men: Walk:
11 minutes; Jog: 5 minutes

CALORIE COMBOS

3 red radishes: 2 cals

¼ cup (40 g) sliced celery: 2 cals

3 tablespoons sliced cucumber:
3 cals

2 tablespoons grated carrot: 3 cals

¼ cup (35 g) diced red bell pepper:
8 cals

2 cups (40 g) baby spinach: 13 cals

2 cups (40 g) sliced butterhead
lettuce (Boston or Bibb): 14 cals

5 cherry tomatoes: 15 cals

2 cups (40 g) bagged mixed salad
greens, Italian blend: 20 cals

2 cups (100 g) sliced iceberg
lettuce: 20 cals

2 cups (100 g) sliced romaine:
20 cals

¼ cup (12 g) plain croutons: 31 cals

¼ cup (35 g) diced avocado:
47 cals

¼ cup (60 g) low-fat cottage
cheese: 49 cals

BALSAMIC VINAIGRETTE (📷 page 147)

If you want a slightly sweet, rich vinaigrette to dress greens with traces of bitter
undertones, such as endive, arugula, mizuna, and watercress, look no further. This
dressing is also good drizzled over the classic combination of juicy ripe tomatoes
and mozzarella cheese with fresh basil leaves. Either white or dark balsamic can
be used. A trick for any balsamic dressing is to add a bit of fresh lemon or lime
juice to offset the sweetness. This dressing has a long shelf life, so feel free to
double it.

MAKES ABOUT ⅓ CUP (80 ML)

1 teaspoon Dijon mustard

**Salt and freshly ground
pepper, to taste**

**2 tablespoons balsamic
vinegar**

**2 teaspoons fresh lemon
juice, or to taste**

2 tablespoons water

2½ tablespoons canola oil

**1 small garlic clove,
smashed and peeled**

Combine the mustard, salt, pepper, vinegar,
lemon juice, and water in a small bowl and mix
until well combined. In a slow stream, whisk
in the canola oil until emulsified. Adjust the
seasoning, and add the smashed garlic. Keep
in the bowl or transfer to a jar if desired, cover
and refrigerate for up to 2 weeks. Whisk or
shake before serving. (You need not remove
and discard the garlic; it is used only to flavor
the dressing; it should not be consumed.)

SUBLIME PARMESAN-LIME
DRESSING (📷 page 147)

You're sure to fall in love with this bright green dressing, bursting with fresh herbs and sunny citrus flavor. It's perfect for a plate of simple greens or a fancy salad. Or drizzle it over sliced smoked salmon—that's one of my favorite ways to serve it. This dressing is best used within 3 or 4 days. The bright green color will eventually fade, but that will not affect the taste.

MAKES ABOUT ½ CUP (125 ML)

3 to 4 tablespoons grated Parmesan cheese

2 heaping tablespoons chopped fresh flat-leaf parsley, dill, or a mix of both

1 small garlic clove, halved

1 tablespoon sliced fresh chives or scallion greens

1 tablespoon cider vinegar or distilled vinegar

1 tablespoon fresh lime juice

2 tablespoons water

1 tablespoon canola oil

2 tablespoons extra virgin olive oil

1 teaspoon Dijon mustard

Pinch of sugar

Salt and freshly ground pepper, to taste

Combine all of the ingredients in the bowl of a mini food processor and puree until smooth, scraping down the sides of the bowl as needed. Adjust the seasoning, transfer to a bowl or jar, cover, and refrigerate. Whisk or shake before serving.

56 CALORIES IN | 1 TABLESPOON

Protein: 1 g; Carbohydrates: 1 g; Fat: 6 g; Fiber: 0 g; Sodium: 45 mg; Carb Choices: 0; Diabetic Exchange: 1 Fat

56 CALORIES OUT

Women: Walk:
14 minutes; Jog: 6 minutes

Men: Walk:
11 minutes; Jog: 5 minutes

CALORIE COMBOS

3 red radishes: 2 cals

¼ cup (40 g) sliced celery: 2 cals

3 tablespoons sliced cucumber: 3 cals

2 tablespoons grated carrot: 3 cals

¼ cup (35 g) diced red bell pepper: 8 cals

2 cups (40 g) baby spinach: 13 cals

2 cups (40 g) sliced butterhead lettuce (Boston or Bibb): 14 cals

5 cherry tomatoes: 15 cals

2 cups (40 g) bagged mixed salad greens, Italian blend: 20 cals

2 cups (100 g) sliced iceberg lettuce: 20 cals

2 cups (100 g) sliced romaine: 20 cals

¼ cup (12 g) plain croutons: 31 cals

¼ cup (35 g) diced avocado: 47 cals

¼ cup (60 g) low-fat cottage cheese: 49 cals

62 CALORIES IN | ¼ CUP (60 ML)

Protein: 1 g; Carbohydrates: 4 g;
Fat: 5 g; Fiber: 1 g; Sodium: 76
mg; Carb Choices: 0; Diabetic
Exchange: 1 Vegetable, 1 Fat

62 CALORIES OUT

Women: Walk:
15 minutes; Jog: 7 minutes

Men: Walk:
13 minutes; Jog: 6 minutes

CALORIE COMBOS

4 celery sticks: 2 cals

4 broccoli florets: 5 cals

4 carrot sticks: 6 cals

4 asparagus spears: 6 cals

4 cucumber sticks: 8 cals

4 green beans: 9 cals

4 red bell pepper sticks: 12 cals

2 plain thin, crisp breadsticks: 25
cals

6 pita chips: 60 cals

7 whole wheat crackers: 120 cals

1 whole wheat chapati (Indian
flatbread): 137 cals

1 ounce (30 g) tortilla chips: 139
cals

1 naan (Indian bread): 234 cals

CALORIE CUTS

Use cooking oil spray for broiling
the eggplant, reducing the amount
of olive oil by 2 tablespoons. This
will save 30 calories and 3.5 grams
of fat per serving.

ROASTED EGGPLANT DIP (📷 page 148)

This fabulous dip was inspired by my Indian friend Manju Saigal, who serves it
with her incredible homemade naan, chapati, and crackers. Cut-up veggies, whole
wheat or rosemary-flavored flatbreads, or rye crackers are perfect for dipping. The
eggplant can be cooked in advance, the skin removed, and the pulp frozen for
up to 1 month. When you are ready to make the dip, thaw it and proceed with the
recipe. See Calorie Combos for more suggestions for dipping choices and their
calorie counts.

MAKES ABOUT 2 CUPS (500 ML)

3 tablespoons extra virgin
olive oil

8 ounces (270 g) Japanese
eggplants, stems trimmed
and halved lengthwise

1 medium onion, finely
chopped

1 garlic clove, minced

1 teaspoon roasted ground
cumin

½ teaspoon roasted ground
coriander

Pinch of cayenne, or to taste

1 cup (100 g) diced ripe
tomatoes

1 to 2 tablespoons minced
green chiles, optional

Salt, to taste

3 tablespoons chopped fresh
cilantro

1. Preheat the broiler to medium or high,
depending on its strength. Smear 2
tablespoons of the olive oil on a baking
sheet with sides. Add the eggplant halves
and turn them in the oil to coat all sides.
Arrange the eggplants cut side down on
the baking sheet. Place under the broiler
and cook for about 5 minutes on each side,
or until the eggplant pulp is soft. Remove
from the broiler.

2. When the eggplant is cool enough to
handle, using a dull knife or spoon, scrape
the pulp from the skin and place it in a
bowl. Mash it to a chunky consistency and
set aside.

3. Heat the remaining 1 tablespoon olive oil
in a medium nonstick skillet over medium-
high heat. Add the onions and sauté for
3 minutes, or until light golden. Add the
garlic and sauté for 30 seconds, then add
the cumin, coriander, and cayenne and
sauté for another 30 seconds. Add the
tomatoes and green chiles, if using, and
cook for 2 minutes. Add the reserved
eggplant pulp, season with salt, and cook
over low heat, stirring occasionally, for 3
minutes, or until the oil begins to separate.

4. Remove from the heat, mix in the chopped
cilantro, and adjust the seasoning. Transfer
to a serving bowl and serve warm or at
room temperature.

GOES-WITH-EVERYTHING FRESH TOMATO SAUCE (📷 page 110)

The Spanish call this simple tomato sauce a *sofrito* and use it as a base for a wide range of dishes, from paella to a simple and light red sauce for fish. Use it in place of ketchup, salsa, or anytime you need a tomato sauce. I usually double the recipe and keep what I don't use in the freezer to serve later with pasta. Add whatever you like, from chopped olives or capers to sliced jarred artichoke hearts or diced jarred red bell peppers. It can be made up to 2 days in advance. One of my recipe testers used this sauce on pizza and said her friends loved it.

MAKES ABOUT 1¼ CUPS (310 ML)

- 1½ tablespoons extra virgin olive oil
- ⅓ cup (70 g) finely chopped onion
- 2 bay leaves
- 1 garlic clove, minced
- 2 teaspoons Italian seasoning or dried oregano
- 3 cups (480 g) diced ripe tomatoes
- 2 teaspoons tomato paste, or to taste
- ¼ cup (60 ml) water
- Pinch of sugar
- Salt and freshly ground pepper, to taste
- 3 tablespoons sliced fresh basil leaves

1. Heat the olive oil in a small skillet over medium heat. Add the onions and bay leaves and sauté for 3 minutes, or until the onions begin to turn golden brown. Add the garlic and Italian seasoning and sauté for 1 minute. Add the tomatoes, tomato paste, water, sugar, salt, and pepper, stir, and bring to a boil, then reduce the heat and gently simmer for 5 to 7 minutes, until the sauce thickens to a thick salsa consistency.

2. Add the basil and adjust the seasoning. Transfer to a bowl and serve warm or at room temperature. Cover and refrigerate any leftovers.

64 CALORIES IN | ¼ CUP (60 ML)

Protein: 1 g; Carbohydrates: 6 g; Fat: 4 g; Fiber: 2 g; Sodium: 23 mg; Carb Choices: ½; Diabetic Exchange: 1 Vegetable, 1 Fat

64 CALORIES OUT

Women: Walk: 16 minutes; Jog: 7 minutes

Men: Walk: 13 minutes; Jog: 6 minutes

CALORIE COMBOS

Savory Corn Cakes (page 111): 98 cals

½ cup (80 g) plain white rice: 103 cals

½ cup (90 g) plain brown rice: 108 cals

½ cup (65 g) plain quinoa: 111 cals

Cheesy Southern-Style Spoon Bread (page 100): 127 cals

Polenta with Herbs and Cheese (page 103): 146 cals

1 cup (100 g) plain spinach pasta: 166 cals

1 cup (100 g) plain whole wheat spaghetti: 174 cals

1 cup (130 g) cheese ravioli: 191 cals

Broccoli, Mushroom, Cheddar, and Curry Frittata (page 216): 229 cals

Fish Sticks for Hale (page 230): 280 cals

SPINACH, FETA, AND DILL DIP (📷 page 148)

A wonderfully healthy dip that marries well with whole wheat crackers, baked whole wheat flatbread, or cut-up veggies. The spinach and dill give it a bright green color, while the cheeses add flavor and creaminess. The full-fat version of this dip clocks in at 105 calories and 10 grams of fat per serving, compared to the 65 calories and 3 grams of fat in this one. See Calorie Combos for more suggestions for dipping choices and their calorie counts.

MAKES ABOUT I CUP (250 ML)

⅓ cup (65 g) tightly packed chopped cooked spinach, well drained

2 tablespoons sliced scallions

3 tablespoons chopped fresh dill

1 tablespoon nonfat mayonnaise

2 tablespoons fat-free sour cream

3 tablespoons reduced-fat cream cheese

⅓ cup (60 g) reduced-fat feta cheese

1 teaspoon Dijon mustard

Salt and freshly ground pepper, to taste

Combine all of the ingredients in the bowl of a food processor and process until smooth, or to the desired consistency, scraping down the sides of the bowl as needed. Adjust the seasoning and transfer to a serving bowl. Cover and refrigerate if not serving promptly.

BENIHANA-STYLE GINGER-SESAME DRESSING

If you like the standard come-with-your-meal salad at the Benihana chain of Japanese restaurants, you'll love this creamy golden dressing. It is especially good drizzled over salads made with grilled shrimp, seafood, chicken, beef, or tofu. I use it in my Quinoa, Corn, Edamame, and Snow Pea Salad (page 196). My kids love it; I hope yours will, too. This dressing is a bit high in calories, so feel free to lighten it by substituting some of the canola oil with water. One of my recipe testers wrote that she uses her handheld immersion blender for salad dressings, so this was super easy. Another tester suggested adding toasted sesame seeds, which is a great idea. You can double the recipe; it keeps for 2 weeks, refrigerated.

MAKES ABOUT ½ CUP (125 ML)

2 teaspoons chopped peeled fresh ginger

1 garlic clove, halved

2 tablespoons cider vinegar

1½ tablespoons lite soy sauce

½ teaspoon brown sugar

1 teaspoon toasted sesame oil

¼ cup (60 ml) canola oil

2 tablespoons water

Combine all of the ingredients in the bowl of a mini food processor, or use an immersion blender, and puree until smooth, scraping down the sides of the bowl as needed. Adjust the seasoning, transfer to a bowl or jar, cover, and refrigerate. Whisk or shake before serving.

---

69 CALORIES IN | I TABLESPOON

Protein: 0 g; Carbohydrates: 0 g; Fat: 7 g; Fiber: 0 g; Sodium: 108 mg; Carb Choices: 0; Diabetic Exchange: 1½ Fat

69 CALORIES OUT

Women: Walk: 17 minutes; Jog: 8 minutes

Men: Walk: 14 minutes; Jog: 7 minutes

CALORIE COMBOS

3 red radishes: 2 cals

¼ cup (40 g) sliced celery: 2 cals

2 tablespoons grated carrot: 3 cals

¼ cup (30 g) sliced cucumber: 5 cals

¼ cup (35 g) diced red bell pepper: 8 cals

2 cups (40 g) baby spinach: 13 cals

2 cups (40 g) sliced butterhead lettuce (Boston or Bibb): 14 cals

5 cherry tomatoes: 15 cals

2 cups (40 g) bagged mixed salad greens, Italian blend: 20 cals

2 cups (100 g) sliced iceberg lettuce: 20 cals

2 cups (100 g) sliced romaine: 20 cals

¼ cup (12 g) plain croutons: 31 cals

¼ cup (35 g) diced avocado: 47 cals

¼ cup (60 g) low-fat cottage cheese: 49 cals

REDUCED-FAT BASIL WALNUT PESTO

76 CALORIES IN | I TABLESPOON

Protein: 2 g; Carbohydrates: 1 g; Fat: 8 g; Fiber: 0 g; Sodium: 112 mg; Carb Choices: 0; Diabetic Exchange: 2 Fat

76 CALORIES OUT

Women: Walk: 19 minutes; Jog: 9 minutes

Men: Walk: 16 minutes; Jog: 7 minutes

CALORIE COMBOS

½ cup (80 g) plain white rice: 103 cals

½ cup (90 g) plain brown rice: 108 cals

½ cup (65 g) plain quinoa: 111 cals

1 cup (100 g) plain spinach pasta: 166 cals

1 cup (100 g) plain whole wheat spaghetti: 174 cals

4 ounces (120 g) boneless chicken breast, roasted: 187 cals

1 cup (130 g) cheese ravioli: 191 cals

6 ounces (180 g) Australian lamb chop, broiled: 213 cals

4 ounces (120 g) flank steak, broiled: 260 cals

Chicken-Zucchini Burgers with Ricotta and Sun-Dried Tomatoes (page 247): 261 cals

6 ounces (180 g) wild Atlantic salmon fillet, roasted or grilled: 310 cals

6 ounces (180 g) farmed Atlantic salmon fillet, roasted or grilled: 350 cals

CALORIE CUTS

Substitute 2 tablespoons water for 2 tablespoons of the olive oil and save 30 calories per serving and 3.5 grams of fat.

A lovely pesto to toss with pasta or put some on top of grilled fish or chicken. Add a tiny spoonful to soups or use it in sandwiches instead of mayonnaise. To lighten the fat, I substituted water for some of the oil; feel free to reduce the oil even further. This sauce keeps refrigerated for up to 3 days and can be frozen for up to 1 month. Freeze it in small batches so you can thaw it quickly as needed.

MAKES ABOUT I CUP (250 ML)

2 cups (80 g) tightly packed fresh basil leaves

3 tablespoons extra virgin olive oil or canola oil, or a mix of both

3 tablespoons water

¼ cup (20 g) grated Parmesan cheese

3 tablespoons chopped toasted walnuts

1 garlic clove, cut into 3 pieces

Salt and freshly ground pepper, to taste

In the bowl of a food processor, combine all of the ingredients and puree until fairly smooth, scraping down the sides of the bowl as needed. Adjust the seasoning and consistency, if necessary, and transfer to a bowl. If not serving promptly, cover with plastic wrap pressed flush against the surface of the sauce to prevent discoloration and refrigerate.

YUMMY GUACAMOLE (📷 page 213)

This is a super dip for sliced vegetables or baked tortilla chips (try not to eat too many!). It can also be a great substitute for mayonnaise in sandwiches or burgers. Keep it plain or jazz it up. I find the easiest way to mash avocados is to place the pulp in a pie plate and mash it with a fork. Forgo the food processor or blender, as these give the avocado a pasty consistency. Because the only caloric item in this dip is the avocados (670 calories total), the only way to cut back is to eat less, as hard as that may be. Guacamole is best served soon after it is made.

MAKES ABOUT 2 CUPS (500 ML)

3 ripe (1 pound, 500 g) avocados, preferably Hass (1½ cups, 375 ml pulp)

1 to 2 tablespoons minced white or red onion

¼ cup (40 g) finely diced ripe tomato

2 teaspoons fresh lime juice, or to taste

2 tablespoons chopped fresh cilantro, or to taste

1 small garlic clove, minced, or ¼ teaspoon garlic powder, or to taste

Dash of hot sauce, optional

Salt, to taste

1. Cut the avocados in half and remove the pits. Scoop out the pulp with a spoon into a pie plate or on a deep plate. Using the back of a fork, mash the avocados to a chunky consistency.
2. Transfer to a serving bowl, add the remaining ingredients, and mix until well combined. Season to taste, and serve as soon as possible. If not serving promptly, cover with plastic wrap pressed flush against the surface of the sauce to prevent discoloration and refrigerate.

86 CALORIES IN | 2 TABLESPOONS

Protein: 1 g; Carbohydrates: 5 g; Fat: 8 g; Fiber: 4 g; Sodium: 77 mg; Carb Choices: 0; Diabetic Exchange: 2 Fat

86 CALORIES OUT

Women: Walk: 21 minutes; Jog: 10 minutes

Men: Walk: 18 minutes; Jog: 8 minutes

CALORIE COMBOS

4 celery sticks: 2 cals

4 broccoli florets: 5 cals

4 asparagus spears: 6 cals

4 carrot sticks: 6 cals

4 cucumber sticks: 8 cals

4 green beans: 9 cals

4 red bell pepper sticks: 12 cals

Savory Corn Cakes (page 111): 98 cals

7 whole wheat crackers: 120 cals

1 ounce (30 g) tortilla chips: 139 cals

Vegetarian Chili (page 115): 156 cals

Everyone's Favorite Veggie Burgers (page 212): 223 cals

Black Bean, Spinach, and Mushroom Quesadillas (page 301): 388 cals

HOW TO PREVENT AN AVOCADO HALF FROM BROWNING

You are not going to believe how easy and fat-free this tip is: simply run the avocado half under water and then wrap it in plastic wrap or put it in a plastic bag. No oil needed. Leave the pit in the half, if possible. This should prevent browning for at least 12 hours.

DESSERTS

CHOCOLATE WALNUT MERINGUES

These cookies are the perfect sweet splurge. The only problem is that they are addictive! Ideally, the sugar should be superfine, as it dissolves quickly. You can substitute the walnuts with pecans. The instant coffee is optional because kids might not like it. Silpats are ideal for lining the baking sheets, but baking paper works well, too. These cookies keep at room temperature in an airtight container for 1 week; they do not freeze well.

MAKES SIXTY 2-INCH (5 CM) COOKIES

2 cups walnuts (6.5 ounces/ 200 g), lightly toasted and completely cooled

3 tablespoons plus ¼ cup (90 g) sugar, preferably superfine

Pinch of salt

½ cup (3 ounces/90 g) semisweet chocolate chips

2 large egg whites

¼ teaspoon cream of tartar

2 to 3 teaspoons instant coffee crystals, optional

1. Center an oven rack and preheat the oven to 225°F (100°C). Line 2 large baking sheets with baking paper or Silpats and set aside.

2. Combine 1 cup (100 g) of the walnuts, 3 tablespoons of the sugar, and the salt in the bowl of a food processor and pulse about 7 times, until the nuts are ground to the consistency of coarse cornmeal with a few lumps; do not process to a paste. Transfer the nut mixture to a bowl. (Do not rinse the food processor bowl.) Add the chocolate to the bowl and process until chopped into small bits; again, avoid making a paste. Add the remaining walnuts and the reserved nut mixture and pulse about 3 times. Set aside.

3. In a large bowl, combine the egg whites and cream of tartar and beat with an electric mixer on low speed for 30 seconds. Increase the speed to medium and beat for 30 seconds more, until frothy bubbles begin to appear. Add the remaining sugar, increase the speed to high, and continue beating until soft, glossy peaks form, about 3 minutes. Gently fold in the reserved nut mixture and instant coffee, being careful not to deflate the whites. The mixture does not have to be thoroughly blended.

4. Drop the batter by the teaspoonful about 1½ inches (4 cm) apart onto the prepared baking sheets (about 30 cookies per sheet). Bake for 55 minutes, or until the cookies are hard. Remove the cookies and cool completely on a rack, then store in an airtight container.

MINI CHOCOLATE CUPCAKES (📷 page 161)

Homemade cupcakes are the best. I decided to include a less caloric, mini version of my favorite chocolate cupcakes in this book. The trick is beets. They result in supremely moist cupcakes and allow for a generous reduction of the butter. Here I used only 4 tablespoons of butter; my original recipe (which is totally amazing) calls for 10 tablespoons. For convenience, I call for canned beets, but you can use fresh. Cook and puree enough beets to yield ¾ cup pureed pulp (180 ml). Any extras can be tossed into a salad. (Note: If you puree the entire can of beets you will need to discard 2 tablespoons of the beet puree to equal ¾ cup.) Go easy on the frosting or skip it if you need to cut back on calories. The frosted cupcakes can be covered and refrigerated for up to 5 days; unfrosted cupcakes can be frozen for up to 1 month (frost before serving, if desired).

MAKES 48 MINI-CUPCAKES

2½ cups (325 g) unbleached all-purpose flour

3 tablespoons Dutch-processed unsweetened cocoa powder

¼ teaspoon salt

2 large eggs

½ cup (125 ml) low-fat buttermilk

1 teaspoon vanilla extract

1 teaspoon baking soda

2 teaspoons cider vinegar or distilled vinegar

4 tablespoons (60 g) unsalted butter, at room temperature

1 cup (230 g) sugar

One 15-ounce (425 g) can sliced red beets, finely pureed (about ¾ cup, 180 ml)

Creamy Chocolate Frosting (recipe follows; optional)

1. Center an oven rack and preheat the oven to 350°F (180°C). Line 4 mini-size 12-cup cupcake pans with mini cupcake liners; set aside.

2. Sift together the flour, cocoa powder, and salt into a bowl; set aside.

3. In a second bowl or a measuring cup, mix the eggs, buttermilk, vanilla extract, baking soda, and vinegar; set aside.

4. In a medium bowl, cream the butter and sugar with an electric mixer on medium speed until light, about 3 minutes. Add half of the egg mixture and half of the flour mixture and beat on low speed for about 30 seconds. Add the remaining egg and flour mixtures and beat again, then add the pureed beets and beat until well incorporated.

5. Divide the batter evenly among the cupcake cups, using a teaspoonful per cupcake to fill each one about three-quarters full; do not overfill. Bake 2 pans at a time for 13 minutes, or until a toothpick inserted in the center of a cupcake comes out clean. Remove from the oven and transfer the cupcakes to a cake rack to cool completely before frosting.

55 CALORIES IN | 1 CUPCAKE WITHOUT FROSTING

Protein: 1 g; Carbohydrates: 10 g; Fat: 1 g; Fiber: 0 g; Sodium: 38 mg; Carb Choices: ½; Diabetic Exchange: ½ Starch

55 CALORIES OUT

Women: Walk: 13 minutes; Jog: 6 minutes

Men: Walk: 11 minutes; Jog: 5 minutes

78 CALORIES IN | 1 CUPCAKE WITH FROSTING

Protein: 1 g; Carbohydrates: 13 g; Fat: 3 g; Fiber: 0 g; Sodium: 44 mg; Carb Choices: 1; Diabetic Exchange: 1 Starch

78 CALORIES OUT

Women: Walk: 19 minutes; Jog: 9 minutes

Men: Walk: 16 minutes; Jog: 7 minutes

23 CALORIES IN | FROSTING FOR 1 MINI CUPCAKE

Protein: 0 g; Carbohydrates: 3 g; Fat: 1g; Fiber: 0 g; Sodium: 6 mg; Carb Choices: 0; Diabetic Exchange: Free

23 CALORIES OUT

Women: Walk: 6 minutes; Jog: 3 minutes

Men: Walk: 5 minutes; Jog: 2 minutes

CALORIE CUTS

Skip the frosting and save 23 calories and 1 gram of fat per mini cupcake.

CREAMY CHOCOLATE FROSTING

Apply this lovely chocolate frosting sparingly and enjoy every bite. I do not use nonfat cream cheese, as it is too runny and does not hold its shape well.

MAKES ABOUT 1 CUP (250 ML)

½ cup (90 g) semisweet chocolate chips

1 tablespoon unsalted butter

2 ounces (60 g) reduced-fat cream cheese, at room temperature

1 cup (140 g) confectioners' sugar, or as needed

1. In a small bowl, microwave the chocolate and butter just until melted, stirring once or twice, then set aside. It should only take a few seconds; do not overheat, or the chocolate might turn grainy.

2. In a medium bowl, beat the cream cheese with an electric mixer on medium speed until smooth, about 1 minute. Add the melted chocolate mixture and the confectioners' sugar and beat until well blended. If the frosting is too runny, add more confectioners' sugar 1 tablespoon at a time. Use right away, or cover and refrigerate.

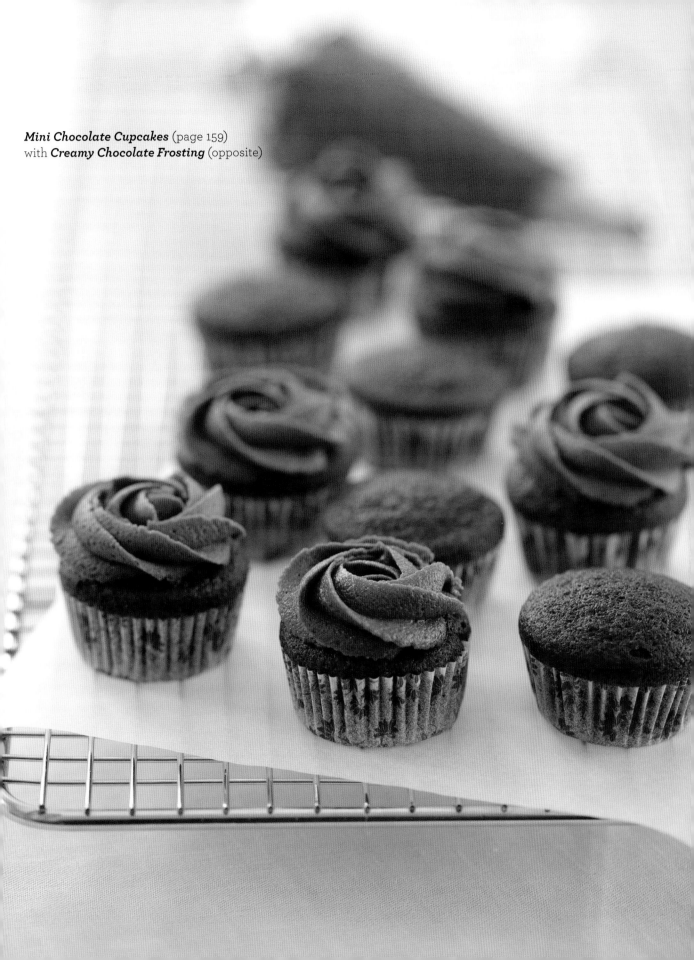

Mini Chocolate Cupcakes (page 159)
with *Creamy Chocolate Frosting* (opposite)

WALNUT CRANBERRY BISCOTTI (📷 page 164)

These orange-and-star-anise-laced biscotti will fill your kitchen with amazing aromas as they bake. They are perfect for dipping in a cup of coffee or in a glass of Italian vin santo. Make a double batch to give as gifts during the holidays. Don't be afraid of the seven-step instructions; making biscotti is actually easy. Once you make them, you will understand the bake-slice-bake process. The biscotti will keep for 4 weeks at room temperature in an airtight container and can be frozen for up to 3 months. Sometimes I bake one log and freeze the other log to bake when I run out of biscotti.

MAKES ABOUT FORTY 3½-INCH (9 CM) COOKIES

1 cup (100 g) walnut halves

2½ cups (325 g) unbleached all-purpose flour

1⅓ cups (300 g) sugar

½ teaspoon salt

1 teaspoon baking powder

2 teaspoons ground star anise, or to taste

1½ tablespoons grated orange zest

3 large eggs, lightly beaten

1 tablespoon vanilla extract

½ cup (70 g) dried cranberries

1. Center a rack in the oven and preheat the oven to 300°F (150°C). Spread the walnuts on a baking sheet and toast in the oven for 8 minutes, or until they emit a nutty aroma. (This is just a light toast, as they will be baked in the biscotti.) Remove from the oven and cool.

2. In a large bowl, combine the flour, sugar, salt, baking powder, star anise, and orange zest, and whisk until combined.

3. Add the eggs and vanilla extract and mix well with a wooden spoon; the batter will be stiff. Add the cranberries and reserved walnuts and mix again; make sure that all the ingredients are well blended and no flour is left in the bottom of the bowl. The dough will be sticky, but if it is so sticky that it is too difficult to work with, add 1 tablespoon of flour at a time. Just remember, though, the more flour you add, the harder your finished cookies will be.

DESSERTS

4. To shape the loaves, place two 15-inch (38 cm) pieces of plastic wrap on a work surface. Scoop half of the dough in a loaf shape down the center of one piece; it should be about 12 inches (30 cm) long and 3 inches (8 cm) wide. Lift the two long sides of the plastic wrap and bring them together, pressing the dough into a neat log shape. Fold the plastic over the log. Then lift the dough by the two ends of the plastic wrap, and twirl to tighten into a log shape. Repeat with the second portion of dough. Place the logs in the freezer for at least 2 hours or up to 1 month. (Note: Freezing the logs helps them hold their shape as they bake.)

5. To bake the biscotti, center an oven rack and preheat the oven to 350°F (180°C). Line a large baking sheet with baking paper. Unwrap one log of dough by unwinding both ends of the plastic wrap and then peeling it back. Flip the log onto baking sheet and peel off the rest of the wrap. Repeat with the remaining log, leaving 3 to 4 inches (8 to 10 cm) between them. (Note: If you can't fit both logs on 1 sheet, bake the logs one at time or use 2 sheets.)

6. Bake for 15 minutes, then reduce the oven temperature to 325°F (160°C) and bake for 15 minutes longer. Remove the baking sheet from the oven and reduce the oven temperature to 250°F (120°C).

7. Allow the logs to cool for 5 minutes, then transfer one log to a chopping board. Slice the log ½ inch (1.25 cm) thick, getting 17 to 20 cookies per log. Transfer the sliced cookies to the baking sheet, arranging them cut side down in rows. Repeat with the remaining log. Bake for 20 minutes, then flip the cookies and bake for another 20 minutes. Cool completely (they will harden as they cool). Store in an airtight container at room temperature for up to 2 weeks.

HOW TO KEEP NUTS FRESH

The best way to ensure you get fresh nuts is to buy them from a source with a high turnover, and always read the expiration dates. If you are planning to use the nuts within 2 weeks after purchase, store them at room temperature; if not, freeze them for up to 3 months. When I buy nuts such as pecans or walnuts in bulk, I like to toast them (see the box on page 93) before I freeze them. This saves me a step when I'm cooking or baking.

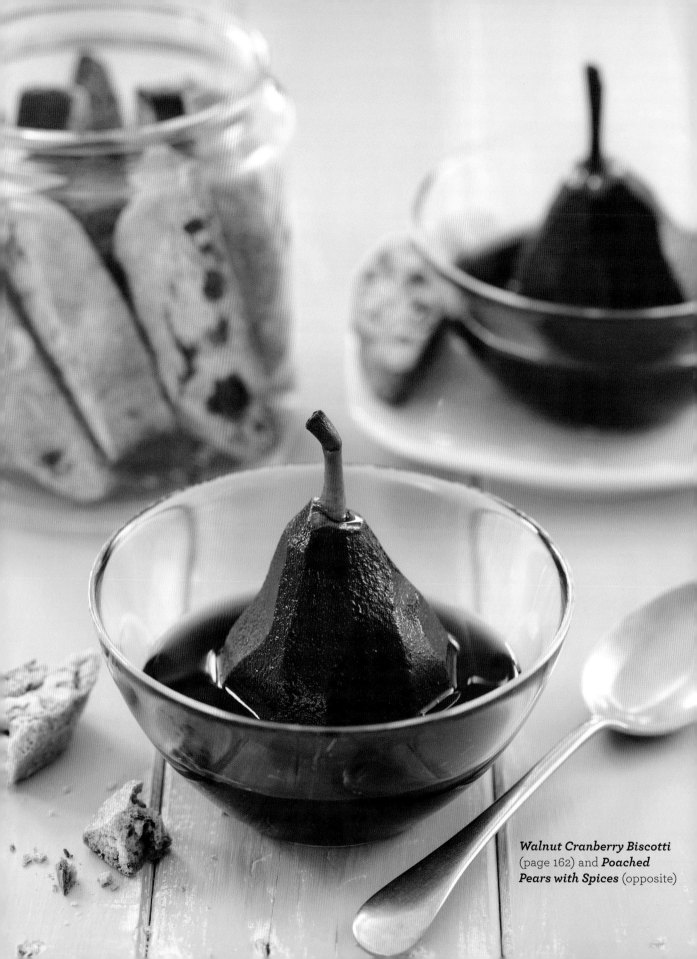

Walnut Cranberry Biscotti (page 162) and **Poached Pears with Spices** (opposite)

POACHED PEARS WITH SPICES

Poached pears are sublimely easy and tasty. The best pears for poaching are just-ripe Bosc pears. The type of wine is important, but it does not have to be expensive. Use a Merlot or Cabernet Sauvignon or, for a more fruity effect, a Syrah or Zinfandel. If you prefer a white wine, try a Sauternes. The spices are up to you. You can also add dried fruit to the poaching liquid, such as figs, apricots, or prunes. Ideally, the cooked pears should soak in the syrup overnight, and they can stay soaking, refrigerated, for up to 5 days. I serve these pears with the Walnut-Cranberry Biscotti (page 162).

SERVES 6

1 bottle (750 ml) red or white wine

½ cup (115 g) sugar

1 cinnamon stick

2 whole star anise

3 whole green cardamom pods, slightly crushed

Zest of 1 small orange, removed in strips with a vegetable peeler

2 teaspoons vanilla extract

2 pounds (1 kg) firm smallish Bosc pears (about 6), peeled and cored (stems intact for presentation, if desired)

1. In a medium nonreactive saucepan, combine all of the ingredients except the pears and bring to a simmer. Add the pears; they should be submerged. If not, add just enough water to submerge them completely. Bring to a simmer, then reduce the heat and gently simmer for 30 minutes, or until the pears are somewhat tender; they will continue to soften off the heat. Pierce with a toothpick or the tip of a knife to check.

2. Transfer the pears and poaching liquid to a bowl, cover, and refrigerate for at least 12 hours, and ideally 24 hours, for the pears to absorb the flavors.

3. Serve at room temperature or chilled with some of the poaching liquid. Refrigerate any leftovers.

96 CALORIES IN

Protein: 1 g; Carbohydrates: 26 g; Fat: 0 g; Fiber: 5 g; Sodium: 2 mg; Carb Choices: 2; Diabetic Exchange: 1½ Fruit

96 CALORIES OUT

Women: Walk: 23 minutes; Jog: 11 minutes

Men: Walk: 20 minutes; Jog: 9 minutes

CREAMY CHOCOLATE POTS

In France, these decadent creamy pots (*pots de crème* is their fancy name) are made with an equal mix of heavy cream and milk, and, boy, are they rich. In this version, I've reduced the fat and calories by using only whole milk (reduced-fat milk just doesn't cut it). You can use any small ovenproof molds; ¼- to ⅓-cup (60 to 80 ml) capacity is ideal. In this recipe I use ¼-cup molds. Espresso or demitasse cups or small ramekins are all great choices. If you use larger ⅓-cup molds, you will get 8 servings and each will have 222 calories and 12 grams of fat. The egg whites left over from this recipe can be frozen (see below), or they can be used in the Chocolate Walnut Meringues (page 158). Use the best-quality chocolate you can find: Ghirardelli, Scharffen Berger, Frey, and Lindt are excellent brands. This dessert is best served at room temperature on the day it is made. One of my recipe testers commented on how deliciously rich the taste was without any cream. She's right!

MAKES TWELVE ¼-CUP (60 ML) PORTIONS

2 cups (500 ml) whole milk	broken or chopped into small pieces	4 large egg yolks
7 ounces (210 g) high-quality dark chocolate,	1 teaspoon vanilla extract	Fresh raspberries, for garnish
	2 tablespoons sugar	Fresh mint, for garnish

1. Center an oven rack and preheat the oven to 300°F (150°C). Arrange twelve ¼-cup (60 ml) cups or ramekins in a large deep baking pan. Bring a kettle of water to a boil for a water bath.

2. In a medium saucepan, bring the milk to a boil, then turn off the heat and add the chocolate. Stir gently with a whisk until the chocolate has completely melted; the mixture will thicken as you stir. Set aside.

3. In a heatproof bowl, whisk the vanilla extract, sugar, and egg yolks. Slowly add the hot chocolate mixture, whisking gently until well combined. Strain the mixture through a fine-mesh sieve into a large measuring cup (this facilitates pouring into the small cups). Divide the chocolate mixture evenly among the cups. Add enough hot water to the baking pan to reach halfway up the sides of the cups; do not overfill, or you will risk spilling water into the cups.

4. Bake until the custard has set, about 30 minutes; the custard should still jiggle a bit when done. Carefully remove the baking dish from the oven and allow the cups to cool in the water bath for 15 minutes, then remove and cool to room temperature. The cups can sit, lightly covered, at room temperature for up to 6 hours. If longer, cover and refrigerate; ideally, bring to room temperature before serving. Garnish each cup with fresh raspberries and mint.

HOW TO FREEZE EGG WHITES

If you use a lot of egg yolks but not whites, you may want to freeze the whites. Be sure to label the container with the number of egg whites and/or the amount of measured egg whites. The white from an average large egg equals about ⅓ cup (80 ml). Fresh egg whites can be frozen for up to 1 month; they can also be refrigerated for up to 3 days.

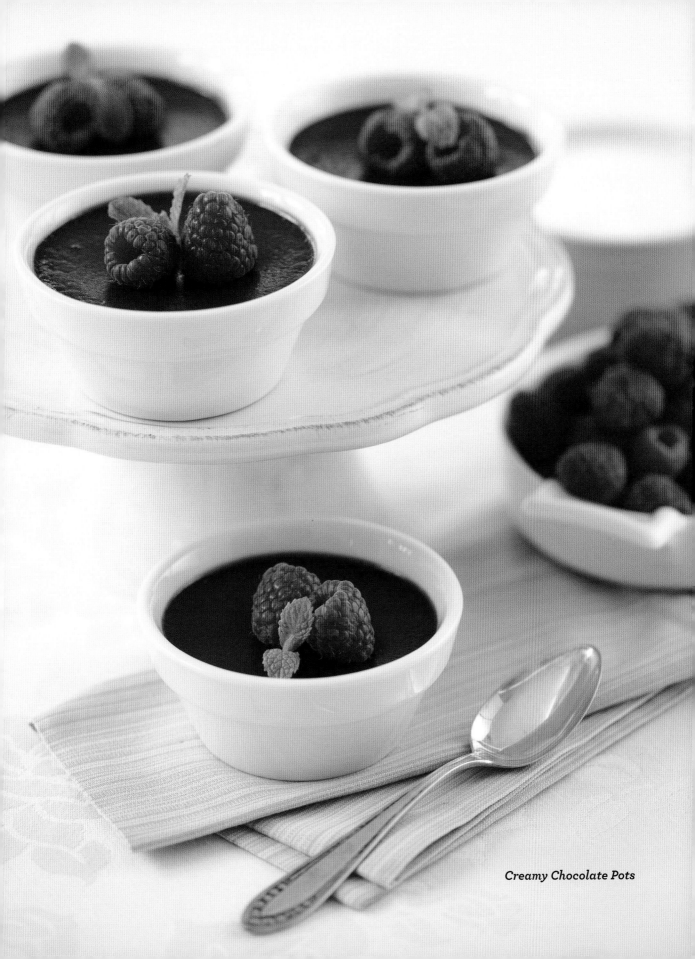

Creamy Chocolate Pots

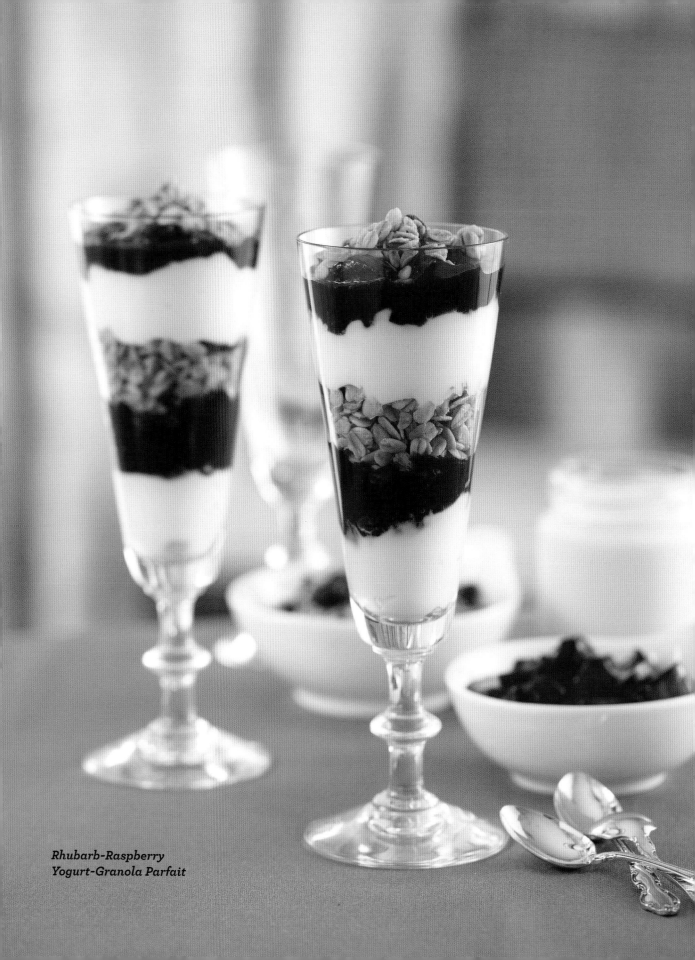

*Rhubarb-Raspberry
Yogurt-Granola Parfait*

RHUBARB-RASPBERRY YOGURT-GRANOLA PARFAIT

Parfaits may appear deliciously healthy, but they can be caloric, especially store-bought ones. The best way to control the calories is to make them yourself. If the Rhubarb-Raspberry Sauce is not your thing, try this with the Blueberry-Plum Sauce (page 47), or even just your favorite fresh fruits or berries. While this dish is in the dessert section, it is lovely for breakfast or as a snack at any time of day.

SERVES 2

1 cup (240 g) nonfat plain Greek-style yogurt

¼ cup (60 ml) Rhubarb-Raspberry Sauce (page 46) or about 1½ cups (375 ml) cut-up fresh fruit or berries

¼ cup (20 g) store-bought low-fat granola or Best-Ever Homemade Granola (page 184)

In 2 glasses or small bowls, make layers of the yogurt, sauce, and granola. Serve promptly.

156 CALORIES IN

Protein: 9 g; Carbohydrates: 25 g; Fat: 3 g; Fiber: 2 g; Sodium: 96 mg; Carb Choices: 1½; Diabetic Exchange: 1 Skim Milk, 1 Fruit

156 CALORIES OUT

Women: Walk: 38 minutes; Jog: 18 minutes

Men: Walk: 32 minutes; Jog: 15 minutes

CALORIE CUTS

Omit the sauce and save 26 calories per serving. Use a low-sugar jam or fresh fruit instead. Reduce or omit the granola. Best-Ever Homemade Granola clocks in at 127 calories and 6 grams of fat per ¼ cup.

MOIST AND DELICIOUS BANANA BREAD

One thin slice of this banana bread, infused with nuts, is all you need. If you do not have whole wheat flour, substitute an equal amount of unbleached all-purpose flour. Pecans can be substituted for the walnuts, or the nuts can be left out. Or, if you're not worried about calories, add chocolate chips instead. Store leftovers in an airtight container at room temperature for up to 3 days, refrigerate for up to 1 week, or freeze for up to 1 month. I've gone as low as I can go with sugar and fat; the small amount of butter gives it the nice crumb.

MAKES 2 LOAVES; SERVES 20

Canola oil cooking spray

1 cup (130 g) unbleached all-purpose flour, plus extra for flouring the pans

1 cup (130 g) whole wheat flour

1 teaspoon baking soda

Pinch of salt

1 cup (230 g) sugar

¼ cup (60 ml) canola oil

3 tablespoons unsalted butter, at room temperature

2 large eggs

4 overripe bananas, peeled and mashed (about 1½ cups, 375 ml)

3 tablespoons 2% milk

1 teaspoon vanilla extract

1 cup (100 g) chopped toasted walnuts or pecans, optional

1. Center an oven rack and preheat the oven to 375°F (190°C). Grease two 8½ x 4½ x 2½-inch (21 x 12 x 7 cm) loaf pans with cooking spray and lightly flour; set aside.

2. Sift together the flours, baking soda, and salt into a bowl; set aside.

3. In a large bowl, combine the sugar, canola oil, and butter and beat with an electric mixer on medium speed until light and fluffy, about 3 minutes. Add the eggs one at a time, mixing for about 30 seconds after each addition.

4. Add the bananas, milk, and vanilla extract and mix on low speed until well blended. Add half of the reserved flour mixture and mix on low speed for 30 seconds, then add the remaining flour and mix just until blended. Using a rubber spatula, fold in the walnuts, if using.

5. Divide the batter evenly between the prepared loaf pans. Bake for 30 minutes, then reduce the oven temperature to 300°F (150°C) and bake for 25 to 30 minutes more, until a cake tester inserted into the center comes out clean. Remove from the oven and allow to cool for 10 minutes before unmolding. Cool completely before slicing.

HOW TO RIPEN BANANAS QUICKLY

Need your bananas to ripen within a day or two? Place them in a paper bag with a tomato or apple for up to 2 days. The fruit will emit ethylene gas, which speeds up the ripening process. Check your bananas after the first day to see how they are doing. Another option is to place the unpeeled bananas in a very low oven, about 170°F (77°C), for about an hour, or just until they start to develop brown spots or a brownish color. If, on the other hand, you have more ripe bananas than you can use at the moment, see How to Freeze Bananas (page 53).

CUCUMBER, MINT, LIME, AND GINGER JUICE (📷 page 172)

One of my recipe testers invented this refreshing light green drink, which I served to guests when I lived in Malaysia. The cooling concoction was the perfect answer to the sweltering tropical heat. I love fresh ginger, so I tend to add even more than what is called for in the recipe.

MAKES 2 CUPS (500 ML); SERVES 2

1 pound (480 g) cucumbers (not seedless)

⅓ cup (8 g) fresh mint leaves

2 tablespoons coarsely chopped peeled fresh ginger, or to taste

1 to 2 teaspoons sugar, to taste

1 to 2 tablespoons fresh lime juice, to taste

Combine all of the ingredients except the sugar in a juicer, and juice. Add the sugar and lime juice to taste, pour over ice, if desired, and serve.

54 CALORIES IN

Protein: 2 g; Carbohydrates: 13 g; Fat: 0 g; Fiber: 2 g;* Sodium: 10 mg; Carb Choices: 1; Diabetic Exchange: 1 Fruit

*Prejuicing fiber content; juicing will reduce fiber content.

54 CALORIES OUT

Women: Walk: 13 minutes; Jog: 6 minutes

Men: Walk: 11 minutes; Jog: 5 minutes

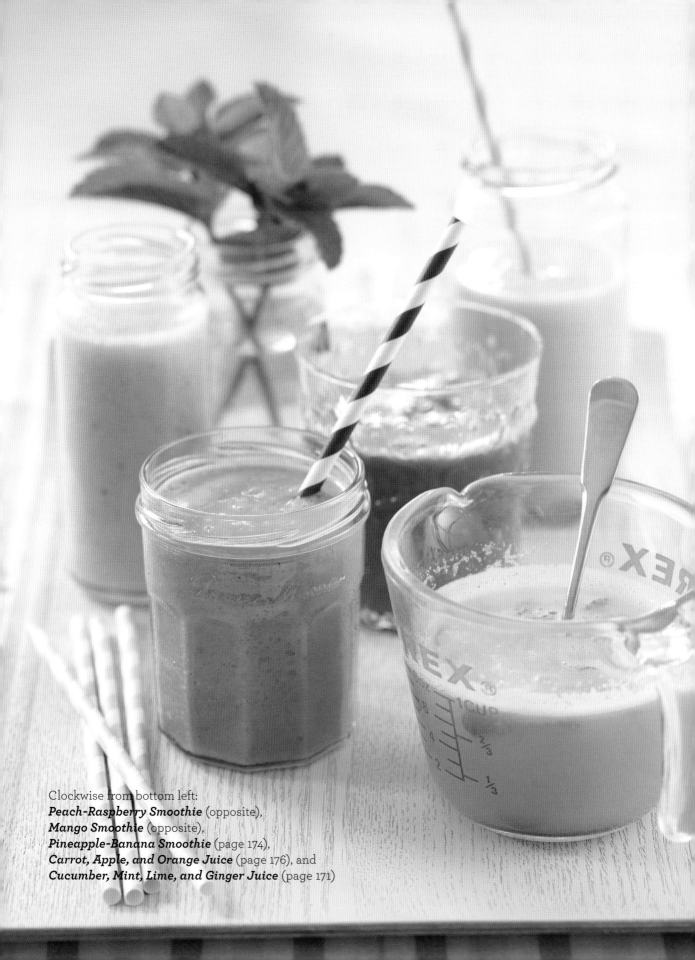

Clockwise from bottom left:
Peach-Raspberry Smoothie (opposite),
Mango Smoothie (opposite),
Pineapple-Banana Smoothie (page 174),
Carrot, Apple, and Orange Juice (page 176), and
Cucumber, Mint, Lime, and Ginger Juice (page 171)

THREE DELICIOUS FRUIT SMOOTHIES

Smoothies are a wonderful thing, but they can be extremely caloric. Some store-bought brands exceed 200 calories for an 8-ounce (250 ml) serving. They best way to control your calorie intake is to make them at home—and if your kids are old enough, teach them to make their own, too. As a baseline, keep in mind that ½ cup (125 ml, 120 g) of nonfat plain yogurt is about 72 calories. Refer to the Customized Fruit Salad on page 44 or the Appendix for calorie values of popular fruits. Optional Sweet Additions below will tell you how many calories various types of sweeteners contain. Lactose intolerant? Lactose-free or soy yogurt can be used. For a calcium boost, add nonfat powdered milk: 1 tablespoon will add 57 mg of calcium, plus 40 calories. Note: All nutritional breakdowns use nonfat plain yogurt.

EACH SMOOTHIE SERVES 2

Optional Sweet Additions

1 teaspoon sugar = 16 cals

1 teaspoon lite agave syrup = 20 cals

1 teaspoon honey = 21 cals

1 tablespoon frozen unsweetened apple juice concentrate = 29 cals

PEACH-RASPBERRY SMOOTHIE

½ cup (120 g) nonfat or low-fat plain yogurt

⅔ cup (150 g) sliced fresh peaches, canned peaches in lite syrup, drained, or frozen peaches

¼ cup (30 g) fresh or frozen raspberries

Place all of the ingredients in a blender and process until smooth. Serve over ice with a straw.

62 CALORIES IN | I SERVING

Protein: 3 g; Carbohydrates: 13 g; Fat: 0 g; Fiber: 1 g; Sodium: 40 mg; Carb Choices: 1; Diabetic Exchange: 1 Fruit

62 CALORIES OUT

Women: Walk: 15 minutes; Jog: 7 minutes

Men: Walk: 13 minutes; Jog: 6 minutes

MANGO SMOOTHIE

¾ cup (120 g) sliced fresh or frozen mango

½ cup (120 g) nonfat or low-fat plain yogurt

Place all of the ingredients in a blender and process until smooth. Serve over ice with a straw.

72 CALORIES IN | I SERVING

Protein: 3 g; Carbohydrates: 16 g; Fat: 0 g; Fiber: 1 g; Sodium: 41 mg; Carb Choices: 1; Diabetic Exchange: 1 Starch

72 CALORIES OUT

Women: Walk: 18 minutes; Jog: 8 minutes

Men: Walk: 15 minutes; Jog: 7 minutes

89 CALORIES IN | I SERVING

Protein: 3 g; Carbohydrates: 21 g; Fat: 0 g; Fiber: 1 g; Sodium: 41 mg; Carb Choices: 1½; Diabetic Exchange: 1 Starch

89 CALORIES OUT

Women: Walk:
22 minutes; Jog: 10 minutes

Men: Walk:
18 minutes; Jog: 9 minutes

PINEAPPLE-BANANA SMOOTHIE (📷 page 172)

½ cup (120 g) nonfat or low-fat plain yogurt

½ banana (120 g)

½ cup (70 g) fresh pineapple, chopped, or canned pineapple in natural juices, drained

Place all of the ingredients in a blender and process until smooth. Serve over ice with a straw.

HOW TO PEEL RIPE MANGOES

If you eat a lot of mangoes, you'll love this technique, which only works with ripe fruit. Place the mango either flat or on its side on a work surface and cut it horizontally more or less in half, cutting as close to the pit as possible. Once you have one side removed, remove the other side that same way, again slicing as close to the pit as possible. Then, to remove the skin, holding one mango half in one hand, insert the rim of a highball glass where the skin and pulp meet (you can start from either end). Wiggle the glass a bit, then slide it along the skin to the other end. The oval-shaped mango pulp should emerge intact inside the glass. Repeat with the second half.

MOJITO DE COLLEEN (📷 page 178)

This outstanding mojito was invented by Colleen Kemp, a friend of Elaine's. The orange vodka came about because she wanted a switch from the rum that is traditional in mojitos, and it was the only type of vodka she had. The best way to crush the mint is to place some crushed ice in the glass, about ⅓ cup (80 ml), then add the mint and crush it between the ice with the back of a tablespoon. This bruises the leaves just enough to release their oils.

SERVES 1

Crushed ice

½ cup (10 g) lightly packed fresh mint leaves

2 teaspoons lite agave syrup or simple syrup (see How to Make Simple Syrup, below)

2 tablespoons fresh lime juice

2 tablespoons Stoli orange vodka

Splash of club soda

Add some crushed ice to a sturdy glass. Then add the mint leaves and using a spoon, bruise and crush the leaves to release their flavors. Add the agave syrup, lime juice, and vodka and stir. Top off with a small splash of club soda to taste.

97 CALORIES IN

Protein: 1 g; Carbohydrates: 9 g; Fat: 0 g; Fiber: 1g;* Sodium: 17 mg; Carb Choices: ½; Diabetic Exchange: 2 Fat**

*The fiber comes from the mint, so it is not available.

**Note to diabetics: Alcohol can cause problems with blood sugar control; it should be consumed in moderation with meals or snacks.

97 CALORIES OUT

Women: Walk:
24 minutes; Jog: 11 minutes

Men: Walk:
20 minutes; Jog: 9 minutes

HOW TO MAKE SIMPLE SYRUP

Simple syrup is usually made by mixing equal amounts by volume of sugar and water: for example, ¼ cup (60 ml) water and ¼ cup (54 g) sugar makes ¼ cup simple syrup. For cocktails, sometimes less water is used to make the syrup so as not to dilute the drinks. Combine the sugar and water in a small saucepan and heat on the stove, or place in a Pyrex measuring cup and microwave. Stir to dissolve the sugar. Allow the syrup to cool before using. Store any unused syrup in a sealed container in the refrigerator for up to 1 month.

CARROT, APPLE, AND ORANGE JUICE (page 172)

If you need a break from green drinks, try this orange one. It is naturally sweet and a bit high in calories from the fruit, but the vitamins, especially vitamins A and C, may be worth it to you. Your kids might like this, too.

MAKES 2 CUPS (500 ML); SERVES 2

6 ounces (180 g) carrots

10 ounces (300 g) Granny Smith apples, cored

1 large orange, peeled and seeded

Combine all of the ingredients in a juicer, and juice. Pour over ice, if desired, and serve.

FIVE-A-DAY GREEN POWER DRINK

If you're looking for a blast of vitamins and antioxidants, look no further than this green elixir. "Five-a-day" refers to getting at least five daily servings of fruits and vegetables per day. Use any combination of fruits and vegetables you like—the possibilities are endless. If your children require a sweeter drink, add 1 to 2 teaspoons sugar or honey.

MAKES 2 CUPS (500 ML); SERVES 2

2 Granny Smith apples (30 g), cored

2 celery stalks (50 g), trimmed

4 cups (100 g) baby spinach

5 ounces (150 g) cucumber (not seedless)

⅓ cup (8 g) fresh mint or flat-leaf parsley leaves

Combine all of the ingredients in a juicer, and juice. Pour over ice, if desired, and serve.

FIVE-A-DAY PINK POWER DRINK

This is my favorite vitamin-powered drink, bar none. Ripe strawberries, papaya, pear, pineapple, and green apples are juiced into a gorgeous, light pink-peach, foamy, utterly delightful drink.

MAKES 4 CUPS (1 LITER); SERVES 4

8 ounces (240 g) fresh strawberries, hulled

10 ounces (300 g) papaya, peeled, seeded, and cubed

10 ounces (300 g) pears, cored

12 ounces (360 g) fresh or canned pineapple, cubed

8 ounces (240 g) Granny Smith apples, cored

Combine all of the ingredients in a juicer, and juice. Pour over ice, if desired, and serve.

157 CALORIES IN

Protein: 2 g; Carbohydrates: 41g; Fat: 1 g; Fiber: 6 g;* Sodium: 8 mg.; Carb Choices: 2½; Diabetic Exchange: 2 Starch

*Prejuicing fiber content; juicing will reduce the fiber content.

157 CALORIES OUT

Women: Walk: 38 minutes; Jog: 18 minutes

Men: Walk: 32 minutes; Jog: 15 minutes

PROSECCO WITH PEACHES (📷 page 178)

When I want a drink to celebrate, I always can count on this one. For a really peachy taste, puree a bit of fresh ripe peach and add it to the drink. Raspberries add a pretty touch.

SERVES 5

1 bottle (750 ml) Prosecco, chilled

5 to 10 tablespoons peach liqueur, to taste

1 ripe white or yellow peach, pitted and thinly sliced

Pour the Prosecco into champagne glasses. Add 1 to 2 tablespoons peach liqueur to each glass, along with a few peach slices. Adjust the taste with the liqueur and serve promptly.

170 CALORIES IN | 1 SERVING

Protein: 0 g; Carbohydrates: 11 g; Fat: 0 g; Fiber: 0 g; Sodium: 0 mg; Carb Choices: 1; Diabetic Exchange: ½ Starch, 3 Fat*

*Note to diabetics: Alcohol can cause problems with blood sugar control; it should be consumed in moderation with meals or snacks.

170 CALORIES OUT

Women: Walk: 41 minutes; Jog: 20 minutes

Men: Walk: 35 minutes; Jog: 16 minutes

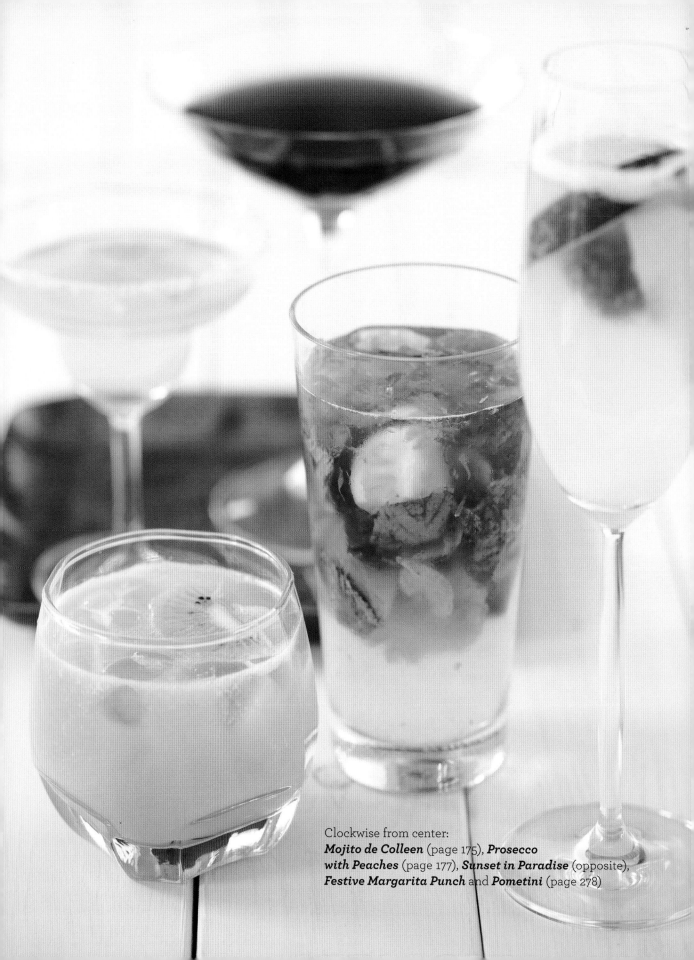

Clockwise from center:
Mojito de Colleen (page 175), *Prosecco with Peaches* (page 177), *Sunset in Paradise* (opposite), *Festive Margarita Punch* and *Pometini* (page 278)

SUNSET IN PARADISE

Picture yourself on a beach sipping this luscious tropical drink. Garnish with kiwi slices, if you like, and enjoy!

SERVES 2

1 heaping cup (240 g) fresh or frozen diced mango

½ cup (125 ml) passion fruit juice or pineapple juice

1 tablespoon fresh lime juice, or to taste

½ cup (125 ml) crushed ice

⅓ cup (80 ml) white or dark rum

Place all of the ingredients in a blender and process until smooth. Adjust the taste and serve chilled.

PART TWO

200 to 299

CALORIES PER SERVING

BAKED BLUEBERRY PANCAKE BLISS

Also called a Dutch or French pancake, this oven-baked bliss gets a boost of vitamins from fresh blueberries. Fresh raspberries are a fine substitute. For a family of four, like mine, you might want 2 pancakes, in which case, keep the oven on, and after the first pancake is served, wipe out the skillet with paper towels and whip up another batch. This pancake *must* be baked on the lowest oven rack to make it rise properly. This is not a sweet pancake, so add confectioners' sugar to taste. Kids usually pile it on as it is fun to watch the white powder go everywhere.

Cooking Note: The order in which you mix these ingredients is very important. The wet ingredients should be mixed before you add the dry ingredients, or the pancake may not rise sufficiently. A well-seasoned cast-iron skillet works best and allows you to cut the pancake in the pan without damaging the finish. If you do use an ovenproof skillet with a nonstick finish, transfer the pancake to a large plate or chopping board before slicing it. This pancake does not work well in a regular cake pan, so please don't attempt to use one (as one of my recipe testers found out the hard way).

SERVES 3

½ cup (125 ml) 2% milk, warmed

2 large eggs

½ cup (65 g) unbleached all-purpose flour

Pinch of ground cinnamon

½ teaspoon grated lemon zest, optional

1 tablespoon unsalted butter

½ cup (75 g) fresh blueberries

2 tablespoons confectioners' sugar, for dusting, or to taste

1. Position an oven rack on the lowest rung and preheat the oven to 425°F (220°C).
2. Whisk the milk and eggs in a bowl until foamy. Add the flour, cinnamon, and lemon zest, if using, and mix until smooth.
3. Melt the butter in a large (12-inch, 30 cm) ovenproof skillet over medium-high heat. Swirl it around the pan to make sure it coats the bottom and sides. Pour the batter into the pan, sprinkle it with the blueberries, and increase the heat to high. Cook for 1 minute, then transfer the skillet to the oven and bake for 15 minutes, or until puffed and golden brown.
4. Remove the pancake from the oven, sprinkle with the confectioners' sugar, and serve immediately.

WHOLE WHEAT PANCAKES

Light, airy, and delicious. I took my mother's original recipe and reduced the calories by cutting way back on the butter. My mother had written a note on the recipe saying, "Don't skip the butter and be sure to brown it to get that nutty flavor." So, I used a small portion of butter, but it's too little to be worth the trouble of browning. The pancake batter can be made up to 2 days in advance. Any leftover pancakes should be covered and refrigerated; reheat them in an ungreased nonstick skillet just until hot, 1 to 2 minutes per pancake. Don't use the microwave, which will make the pancakes unpleasantly rubbery. You can play around with different flours or flour blends. I sometimes mix all-purpose flour with an ancient grain flour blend by King Arthur Flour, which produces delicious pancakes. One of my recipe testers used buckwheat flour, which turned out really well, too.

MAKES ABOUT 12 PANCAKES; SERVES 4

1 large egg

1¼ cups (310 ml) 2% milk

½ teaspoon vanilla extract

½ cup (65 g) unbleached all-purpose flour

½ cup (65 g) whole wheat flour

2 teaspoons baking powder

Pinch of salt

2 tablespoons unsalted butter, melted

Canola oil or cooking spray

1. In a large bowl, whisk the egg, milk, and vanilla extract. Add the flours, baking powder, and salt and whisk until smooth. Add the melted butter and whisk until well incorporated.

2. Heat a medium nonstick skillet over medium to medium-high heat until hot. Using a heatproof brush, lightly grease the skillet with canola oil or cooking spray. Add a scant ⅓-cup (80 ml) of batter and immediately swirl the batter to form a pancake. Cook until the surface bubbles and sets and the underside is golden brown, usually a little longer than 1 minute. Flip the pancake with a wide spatula and cook for 1 minute more, or until cooked through. Transfer to a plate or platter.

3. Repeat this procedure with the remaining batter, lightly greasing the skillet as needed. You can keep the pancakes warm in a low oven.

216 CALORIES IN | 3 PANCAKES

Protein: 8 g; Carbohydrates: 27 g; Fat: 9 g; Fiber: 2 g; Sodium: 237 mg; Carb Choices: 2; Diabetic Exchange: 2 Starch 1 Fat

216 CALORIES OUT

Women: Walk: 53 minutes | Jog: 25 minutes

Men: Walk: 44 minutes | Jog: 21 minutes

CALORIE COMBOS

1 tablespoon diabetic-friendly, sugar-free strawberry jam (e.g., Polaner): 10 cals

Customized Fruit Salad (page 44): 23 to 57 cals

1 tablespoon low-sugar jam: 26 cals

Rhubarb-Raspberry Sauce (page 46): 26 cals

1 teaspoon unsalted butter: 34 cals

1 tablespoon maple syrup: 51 cals

½ cup (125 ml) orange juice: 56 cals

Blueberry-Plum Sauce (page 47): 57 cals

1 tablespoon honey: 64 cals

4 ounces (120 g) nonfat plain yogurt: 72 cals

4 ounces (120 g) low-fat plain yogurt: 77 cals

Five-a-Day Green Power Drink (page 176): 145 cals

Five-a-Day Pink Power Drink (page 177): 157 cals

CALORIE CUTS

Substitute 1 tablespoon canola oil for the butter and save 17 calories and 2 grams of fat per pancake. Skip sugary syrups and jams and instead top your pancakes with a low-calorie jam, fresh fruit, or a sprinkle of confectioners' sugar.

BEST-EVER HOMEMADE GRANOLA

Homemade granola doesn't get any better than this. This was the most requested recipe from my list among my recipe testers. One tester admitted to not sharing any of the finished granola with her family because it was so good. Her comment made me laugh. I make a batch of granola every week, tweaking the recipe according to what's in my cupboards. Feel free to use this recipe as a guide: add sunflower seeds, coconut flakes, pumpkin seeds, raisins, dried cherries, dried apples, and/or other freeze-dried or dried fruit. If you have a mix of grains on hand, add barley, rye or wheat flakes in place of or in addition to the oats. Now, you'll notice the addition of maple syrup, and yes, it's high in calories, but I prefer it to honey, which tends to produce a soft, sticky granola. Because the calorie counts of most granolas are high (some very high; please read the labels), one way to enjoy granola with fewer calories is to mix it with a healthy low-fat, whole-grain store-bought cereal (see suggestions in Calorie Combos).

MAKES ABOUT 5 CUPS (500 G)

OTHER POSSIBLE ADDITIONS

⅓ cup (65 g) dried apricots = 104 cals

⅓ cup (50 g) dried mango = 106 cals

⅓ cup (30 g) sweetened coconut flakes = 111 cals

⅓ cup (50 g) dried cherries = 132 cals

⅓ cup (50 g) raisins = 143 cals

⅓ cup (50 g) dried apples = 158 cals

286 CALORIES IN | ½ CUP

Protein: 6 g; Carbohydrates: 41 g; Fat: 12 g; Fiber: 4 g; Sodium: 34 mg; Carb Choices: 2½; Diabetic Exchange: 2½ Starch, 2 Fat

286 CALORIES OUT

Women: Walk: 70 minutes; Jog: 33 minutes

Men: Walk: 58 minutes; Jog: 27 minutes

CALORIE COMBOS

Customized Fruit Salad (page 44): 23 to 57 cals

½ cup (20 g) regular Cheerios: 55 cals

½ cup (25 g) Product 19: 50 cals

½ cup (125 ml) 2% milk: 61 cals

4 ounces (120 g) nonfat plain yogurt: 72 cals

½ cup (25 g) Kashi GoLean: 70 cals

4 ounces (120 g) low-fat plain yogurt: 77 cals

½ cup (35 g) All-Bran cereal: 80 cals

½ cup (35 g) Kashi GoLean Crisp: 120 cals

Five-a-Day Green Power Drink (page 176): 145 cals

Five-a-Day Pink Power Drink (page 177): 157 cals

CALORIE CUTS

Skip or reduce some of the optional dried fruit and nuts, which all tend to be high in calories.

Canola oil cooking spray

½ cup (125 ml) maple syrup

¼ cup (60 ml) canola oil

3½ cups (350 g) old-fashioned rolled oats

½ cup (50 g) chopped walnuts

⅓ cup (50 g) dried cranberries

⅓ cup (50 g) chopped dried mango, pineapple, apples, or other dried fruit (see Other Possible Additons for the calorie values of various additions)

1. Preheat the oven to 275°F (135°C). Lightly grease a large baking sheet with sides with cooking spray; set aside.

2. Combine the maple syrup and canola oil in a Pyrex measuring cup and place in a microwave oven to warm. Mound the rolled oats and walnuts on the greased baking sheet, then pour the maple syrup mixture over it and toss with 2 large spoons until well combined. Spread the granola evenly on the baking sheet.

3. Bake for about 20 minutes, then remove from the oven and carefully stir. Bake for another 20 minutes, or until light golden. The oats will still be a bit soft when they come out of the oven but will harden as they cool. Do not overbake or the granola may develop a bitter, burnt taste. Allow the granola to cool completely, then add the dried fruit and mix well. Store in an airtight container or Ziploc bag at room temperature.

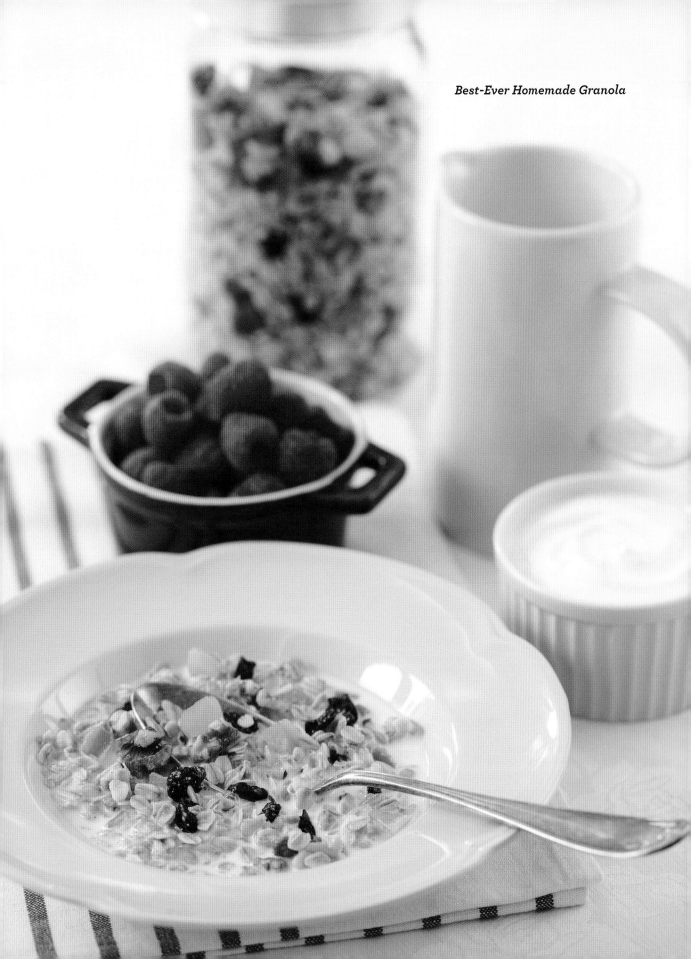

Best-Ever Homemade Granola

SOUPS

MEDITERRANEAN VEGETABLE SOUP

Think of this soup as a blank canvas: customize it to suit your own taste. Here are some pointers to bear in mind as you create your masterpiece: 1) Add vegetables that require a longer cooking time, such as potatoes, winter squash/gourds, or leeks, in Step 1. 2) Add quick-cooking vegetables, such as broccoli or cauliflower florets, sliced summer squash, corn, sliced green beans, or peas, in Step 2; add any greens, fresh or frozen, during the last 5 minutes of cooking. 3) Use any whole grain instead of pasta; cook the grains separately and then add them to the soup. Garnish with my Reduced-Fat Walnut-Basil Pesto (page 156), store-bought pesto, or sliced fresh basil leaves, along with freshly grated Parmesan cheese. This soup is even better on the second day, and it freezes well, though the vegetables tend to get a bit soggy.

SERVES 8

2 tablespoons vegetable oil

1 onion, chopped

2 garlic cloves, minced

2 carrots, cut lengthwise in half and thinly sliced

1 tablespoon dried oregano, basil, thyme, or Italian seasoning, or a mix, all to taste

1 teaspoon salt, or to taste

8 cups (2 liters) low-sodium fat-free stock, or as needed

1½ cups (375 ml) low-sodium V8 juice or tomato juice

One 14.5-ounce (411 g) can diced tomatoes, with their juices, or 2 cups (500 ml) diced ripe tomatoes

One 15.5-ounce (439 g) can great Northern, borlotti, or other beans, rinsed and drained

1 small zucchini, quartered and thinly sliced

¾ cup (120 g) ditalini, orzo, or other small pasta

8 ounces (240 g) baby spinach, Swiss chard, kale, or beet greens, stems removed, and thinly sliced

Freshly ground pepper, to taste

2 tablespoons plus 2 teaspoons Reduced-Fat Walnut-Basil Pesto (page 156) or store-bought pesto, optional

½ cup (45 g) grated Parmesan cheese, optional

1. Heat the vegetable oil in a large saucepan over medium-high heat until hot. Add the onions and sauté for 2 minutes. Add the garlic, carrots, and oregano and sauté for 3 minutes. Add the salt, stock, and V8 juice and bring to a boil, then reduce the heat and simmer, uncovered, for 15 minutes.

2. Add the tomatoes, beans, zucchini, and pasta and return to a boil, then reduce the heat and simmer for 15 to 20 minutes, until the pasta is completely cooked. Add the baby spinach during the last 5 minutes of cooking.

3. Season with the salt and pepper, and thin the soup with stock or water, if desired. Pass pesto and cheese at the table, if desired.

GREEN LENTIL SOUP WITH RICE AND VEGETABLES

This is my go-to soup when the weather turns chilly and I'm looking for a hearty but light meal to perk me up. Add your favorite vegetables and seasonings. A little balsamic vinegar splashed on the finished soup gives it a wonderful tang. This soup freezes well, but it will need to be thinned with water or stock before serving, as the lentils and rice absorb liquid like a sponge.

SERVES 8

2 tablespoons vegetable oil

1 medium onion, chopped, or 1 large leek, sliced

2 garlic cloves, minced

1 carrot, halved lengthwise, and thinly sliced

½ red bell pepper, cored, seeded, and diced

½ cup (100 g) uncooked brown or white rice

1 tablespoon dried thyme or Italian seasoning

7 cups (1.75 liters) low-sodium fat-free stock (6 cups/1.5 liters if using canned lentils), or as needed

1 cup (170 g) dried green lentils, picked over and rinsed, or 3 cups canned lentils (from two 14.5-ounce/411 g cans), rinsed and drained

6 ounces (180 g) baby spinach, baby kale, or your favorite greens, sliced

Salt and freshly ground pepper, to taste

Balsamic vinegar, for serving

1. Heat the vegetable oil in a large saucepan over medium heat. Add the onions and sauté for 2 minutes. Add the garlic, carrots, red bell peppers, rice, and thyme and sauté for 3 minutes.

2. Add the stock and lentils, stir, and bring to a boil. Skim off the foam with a spoon, then reduce the heat and simmer for 25 to 30 minutes, until the lentils are cooked. Stir the spinach into the soup and cook for 10 minutes more. If the soup is too thick, add a little more stock or water as necessary. (Note: If using canned lentils, complete Step 1, then add the lentils and simmer for 20 minutes, or until the rice is cooked; brown rice will take longer to cook than white, so add more water if necessary. Then stir in the spinach and cook for 10 minutes more.)

3. Adjust the seasoning and serve. Pass balsamic vinegar at the table.

214 CALORIES IN

Protein: 11 g; Carbohydrates: 34 g; Fat: 4 g; Fiber: 9 g; Sodium: 230 mg; Carb Choices: 2; Diabetic Exchange: 2 Starch, 1 Lean Meat

214 CALORIES OUT

Women: Walk: 52 minutes; Jog: 25 minutes

Men: Walk: 44 minutes; Jog: 21 minutes

CALORIE COMBOS

Roasted Red Bell Pepper and Feta Dip (page 149): 46 cals

Roasted Eggplant Dip (page 152): 62 cals

Spinach, Feta, and Dill Dip (page 154): 65 cals

1 whole wheat roll: 76 cals

7 whole wheat crackers: 120 cals

Everyone's Favorite Veggie Burgers (page 212): 223 cals

Quinoa, Paneer, and Cabbage Patties (page 220): 235 cals

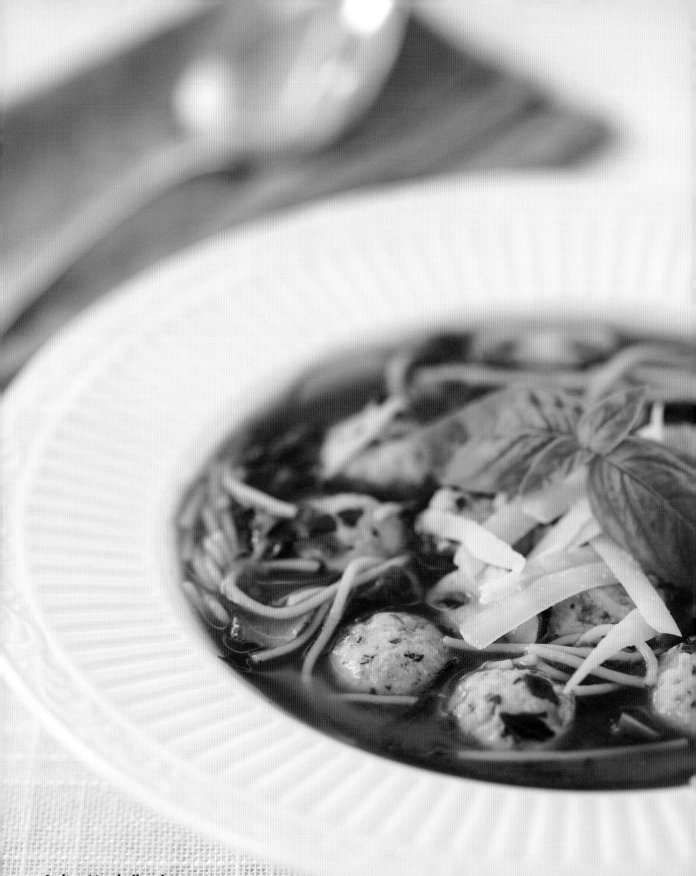

*Italian Meatball and
Noodle Soup with Greens*

ITALIAN MEATBALL AND NOODLE SOUP WITH GREENS

My husband loves this soup because it reminds him of a dish his mother used to make during his childhood. The mixture for the meatballs can be made up to 1 day in advance. Using only the egg white keeps them light. Any kind of small pasta, such as orzo, can be substituted for the angel hair. This soup does not freeze well.

SERVES 6

Chicken Meatballs (makes about 60 meatballs)

12 ounces (360 g) ground chicken

½ cup (35 g) panko bread crumbs

⅓ cup (30 g) grated Parmesan cheese

¼ cup (15 g) thinly sliced scallions

1 large egg white

½ teaspoon salt, or to taste

Freshly ground pepper, to taste

2 tablespoons minced jarred sun-dried tomatoes in oil, drained

1 teaspoon Italian seasoning

1 teaspoon dried thyme or oregano

2 tablespoons chopped fresh basil

2 tablespoons chopped fresh flat-leaf parsley

Soup

10 cups (2.5 liters) low-sodium fat-free stock

One 14.5-ounce (411 g) can diced tomatoes, with their juices

3 tablespoons tomato paste

1 cup (3 ounces/100 g) broken angel hair pasta (about 1-inch/2.5 cm long pieces)

4 cups (100 g) thinly sliced escarole, young kale, or your favorite greens, sliced

Optional Garnishes per Serving

Chopped fresh basil or 1 teaspoon Reduced-Fat Walnut-Basil Pesto (page 156)

1 tablespoon shredded or grated Parmesan cheese

1. To make the chicken meatballs, combine all of the ingredients in a large bowl and mix until well blended. Form the meatballs into teaspoon-size balls (or whatever size you like) and place them on a large plate or tray. Cover and refrigerate until ready to use.

2. To make the soup, bring the stock, diced tomatoes, and tomato paste to a boil in a large nonreactive pot, then reduce the heat to a simmer. Add the meatballs and cook for 10 minutes. Add the pasta and cook for 5 minutes, or until the meatballs and pasta are completely cooked. Add the greens and cook for 5 minutes.

3. Adjust the seasoning, and serve the soup garnished, if desired.

221 CALORIES IN | 1 SERVING SOUP WITHOUT GARNISHES

Protein: 20 g; Carbohydrates: 20 g; Fat: 7 g; Fiber: 4 g; Sodium: 530 mg; Carb Choices: 1; Diabetic Exchange: 1 Starch, 2 Medium-Fat Meat

221 CALORIES OUT

Women: Walk: 54 minutes; Jog: 2 minutes

Men: Walk: 45 minutes; Jog: 21 minutes

CALORIE COMBOS

1 tablespoon grated Parmesan cheese: 22 cals

1 teaspoon Reduced-Fat Basil Walnut Pesto (page 156): 25 cals

2 cups (40 g) salad greens with 1 tablespoon Balsamic Vinaigrette (page 150): 73 cals

Caesar Salad with a Light Touch (page 83): 163 cals

Spinach Salad with Mushrooms, Fennel, and Avocado (page 201): 251 cals

Endive, Radicchio, White Bean, and Blue Cheese Salad (page 207): 281 cals

CALORIE CUTS

Skip the Parmesan cheese in the meatballs and save about 25 calories per serving.

RED LENTIL SOUP WITH TOMATO-CUCUMBER SALSA

An earthy, minty, spicy soup lightened with a garnish of finely diced tomatoes, cucumbers, and green chile mixed with cilantro. The salsa adds only 7 calories per serving. To infuse the soup with even more flavor, I sometimes make a traditional Indian *tarka*, or spice-flavored oil; see How to Make a Basic Indian Tarka (page 210). Without the garnishes, the soup freezes well.

SERVES 6

2 tablespoons vegetable oil

1 medium onion, chopped

2 garlic cloves, minced

1 tablespoon minced peeled fresh ginger

2 medium carrots, halved lengthwise and thinly sliced

2 teaspoons dried mint

1½ teaspoons cumin seeds

Pinch of cayenne, optional

1½ cups (340 g) red lentils, rinsed and picked over

7½ cups (1 liter plus 775 ml) low-sodium fat-free stock, or as needed

Tomato-Cucumber Salsa

⅔ cup (130 g) diced cherry tomatoes

⅔ cup (100 g) diced seedless cucumber

1 tablespoon minced green chiles, optional

3 tablespoons chopped fresh cilantro, sliced fresh mint leaves, or a mix of both

Salt and freshly ground pepper, to taste

Squeeze of fresh lemon juice, or to taste

1. Heat the vegetable oil in a large saucepan over medium-high heat. Add the onions and sauté for 2 minutes. Add the garlic, ginger, carrots, dried mint, cumin seeds, and cayenne, if using, and sauté for 1 minute. Add the lentils and stock and bring to a boil. Reduce the heat and simmer, uncovered, for 30 minutes, or until the carrots are soft and the lentils are mushy.

2. While the soup is cooking, make the salsa: combine all of the ingredients in a small bowl and mix gently. Adjust the seasoning and set aside.

3. Remove the soup from the heat and cool slightly, then with an immersion blender, or using a regular blender, puree it to a slightly chunky consistency. If using a regular blender, you can puree half of the soup and then return it to the saucepan. Thin with a small amount of additional stock or water if necessary.

4. Before serving, reheat the soup and season with salt, pepper, and lemon juice to taste. Ladle into bowls, top each with a bit of the salsa, and serve promptly.

EASY BLACK BEAN SOUP WITH FIXINS (📷 page 70)

The key to a really good black bean soup is the fixins. Of course, the soup should be flavorful, maybe even on the spicy side, but the toppings are what make it great. Chipotle chile powder adds an intense depth of flavor. If you have chili oil, you can add a drop or two at the table. I call for canned black beans to keep this soup easy. One of my recipe testers added diced cooked chicken to the soup, which was a hit with her family. The soup, without the garnishes, freezes well.

SERVES 6

2 tablespoons vegetable oil

1 onion, chopped

1 carrot, chopped

½ red bell pepper, cored, seeded, and chopped

1 garlic clove, minced

2 teaspoons roasted ground cumin, or to taste

2 teaspoons dried oregano

1½ teaspoons chipotle or regular chili powder, or to taste

Two 15-ounce (425 g) cans black beans, rinsed and drained

5 cups (1¼ liters) low-sodium fat-free stock or water, or as needed

1 cup (250 ml) tomato juice or low-sodium V8 juice

½ teaspoon salt, or to taste

Freshly ground pepper, to taste

A couple of drops of balsamic vinegar, or to taste, optional

Fixins per Serving

1 tablespoon chopped fresh cilantro

½ ounce (15 g) reduced-fat cheddar cheese, grated

2 tablespoons diced avocado

1 teaspoon fat-free sour cream

2 tablespoons diced ripe tomatoes

1 tablespoon sliced scallions

1. Heat the vegetable oil in a large saucepan over medium-high heat until hot. Add the onions and sauté for 3 minutes. Add the carrots, red peppers, garlic, cumin, oregano, and chili powder and sauté for 3 minutes. Add the black beans, stock, and tomato juice and bring to a boil, then reduce the heat and simmer, uncovered, for 20 minutes, or until the carrots are tender.

2. Remove from the heat and allow the soup to cool slightly, then puree 3 cups (750 ml) of it. Return the pureed soup to the saucepan and stir. Add a little stock or water to thin the soup, if desired.

3. Season with salt and pepper, add the balsamic vinegar, if using, and serve promptly. Either garnish the soup, or pass the fixins at the table.

295 CALORIES IN | I SERVING SOUP WITH FIXINS

Protein: 14 g; Carbohydrates: 30 g; Fat: 13 g; Fiber: 10 g; Sodium: 453 mg; Carb Choices: 2; Diabetic Exchange: 2 Starch, 1 Medium-Fat Meat, 1 Fat

295 CALORIES OUT

Women: Walk: 72 minutes; Jog: 34 minutes

Men: Walk: 60 minutes; Jog: 28 minutes

CALORIE COMBOS

Roasted Red Bell Pepper and Feta Dip (page 149): 46 cals

¼ cup (35 g) diced avocado: 47 cals

Spinach, Feta, and Dill Dip (page 154): 65 cals

2 cups (40 g) salad greens with 1 tablespoon Balsamic Vinaigrette (page 150): 73 cals

1 whole wheat roll: 76 cals

Yummy Guacamole (page 157): 86 cals

Savory Corn Cakes (page 111): 98 cals

7 whole wheat crackers: 120 cals

1 ounce (30 g) tortilla chips: 139 cals

Caesar Salad with a Light Touch (page 83): 163 cals

Allie's Bruschetta (page 71): 172 cals

Cheese Toasts with Tomatoes, Cucumbers, and Greens (page 72): 175 cals

SALADS

GLORIOUS GREEK SALAD (📷 page 131)

(📷 page 131)

Who doesn't love a good Greek salad? The secret to making one lies in the quality of your ingredients, so buy the best you can afford. Feta cheese is imported from all around the globe these days, and the flavors and textures vary greatly. I call for reduced-fat feta here, but if you want to splurge with a full-fat one, go for it. The mint adds a wonderful freshness. If you have shallots on hand, add 1 to 2 tablespoons minced shallots for an oniony zing. Sliced or whole jarred peperoncini are great, too. The dressing can be made up to 3 days in advance, covered, and refrigerated. You will have a bit of leftover dressing, which is delicious on any greens.

SERVES 4

Greek Dressing

2 tablespoons red wine vinegar

1 tablespoon fresh lemon juice

1 tablespoon water

2 teaspoons Dijon mustard

½ teaspoon dried oregano

½ teaspoon dried mint

1 small garlic clove, smashed and peeled

¼ teaspoon salt, to taste

Freshly ground pepper, to taste

Pinch of sugar

3 tablespoons extra virgin olive oil

Salad

12 ounces (about 2 cups, 360 g) cherry tomatoes, halved, or ripe tomatoes, diced

1 cup (150 g) diced semi-peeled seedless cucumber

8 to 10 red radishes, thinly sliced

1 cup (160 g) crumbled reduced-fat feta

½ cup (80 g) pitted Kalamata or other brine-cured olives

2 tablespoons minced or thinly sliced red onion

3 tablespoons sliced fresh mint leaves

Squeeze of fresh lemon, or to taste

1. To make the dressing, in a small bowl, combine all of the ingredients except the olive oil and whisk. Slowly add the olive oil, whisking constantly until emulsified; set aside. Remove the garlic clove before serving.

2. In a large bowl, combine all of the salad ingredients except the lemon juice. Add about half of the dressing and gently toss. Adjust the seasoning, then add more dressing, if necessary, and a squeeze of lemon. Serve promptly.

HOW TO TAKE THE EDGE OFF RAW ONIONS

The best way to enjoy raw onions (usually in the form of slices) on a burger or in a salad without that stinging onion taste is to lightly salt them and soak in ice-cold water for 10 minutes. Drain, rinse well, and pat dry before serving. By doing this, you break down the cell walls and remove some of the harsh sulfur compounds. It's the sulfur molecules that make us cry while slicing or chopping onions.

---

210 CALORIES IN

Protein: 8 g; Carbohydrates: 8 g; Fat: 17 g; Fiber: 3 g; Sodium: 811 mg; Carb Choices: ½; Diabetic Exchange: 2 Vegetable, 1 High-Fat Meat, 1 Fat

210 CALORIES OUT

Women: Walk: 51 minutes | Jog: 24 minutes

Men: Walk: 43 minutes | Jog: 20 minutes

CALORIE COMBOS

1 whole wheat roll: 76 cals

1 whole wheat pita bread: 165 cals

Grilled Lemony Lamb Chops (page 130): 177 cals

2 ounces (60 g) focaccia: 180 cals

Roasted Pork Tenderloin with Mustard-Tarragon Marinade (page 127): 198 cals

Rosemary-and-Smoked-Paprika Chicken Kebabs (page 128): 199 cals

Easy Lime-Cilantro Grilled Chicken (page 238): 215 cals

Chicken-Zucchini Burgers with Ricotta and Sun-Dried Tomatoes (page 247): 261 cals

Aussie-Style BBQ Chicken (page 252): 279 cals

Glazed Flank Steak with Honey-Dijon Onions (page 259): 282 cals

Old Bay and Dill Salmon Patties (page 231): 283 cals

Beef and Vegetable Kebabs with Cilantro–Green Olive Drizzle (page 325): 304 cals

CALORIE CUTS

The feta and olives are the main sources of calories in the salad, so feel free to cut back on them. The feta has 70 calories and 5 grams of fat per serving; the olives are 19 calories and 2 grams of fat per serving.

BEET, FENNEL, AND GOAT CHEESE SALAD WITH ORANGE DRESSING

A dazzling salad bursting with vitamins. If you like beets, you're sure to make this one of your go-to recipes. See How to Cook Beets, (page 194) or to save time, pick up a package of cooked beets from the produce section of your grocery store or use canned or jarred beets. And pick up the orange segments, chickpeas, and crumbled feta from a salad bar. If you have them on hand, a light drizzle of walnut oil and some pomegranate seeds are superb additions. If you want more of any orangey taste, add some grated zest.

SERVES 4

Orange Dressing

¼ cup (60 ml) fresh orange juice

2 tablespoons canola oil

1 tablespoon water

1 teaspoon Dijon mustard

Salt and freshly ground pepper, to taste

Salad

6 cups (about 200 g) baby greens

2 cooked red beets (12 ounces/360 g), peeled and sliced into thin matchsticks

1 small fennel bulb, trimmed, halved, and thinly sliced

1 navel orange, cut into segments (see page 47)

¼ cup (40 g) crumbled goat cheese or reduced-fat feta cheese

2 tablespoons toasted sunflower or pumpkin seeds, or a mix of both

2 tablespoons chopped fresh dill

2 tablespoons thinly sliced scallions

1. To make the dressing, in a small bowl, combine all of the ingredients and whisk until emulsified; set aside.
2. On a serving platter or large plate, arrange the baby greens, beets, fennel, and orange segments, alternating them to contrast the colors. Sprinkle the cheese on top. Drizzle the dressing over the salad and garnish with the sunflower seeds, dill, and scallions. Serve promptly.

211 CALORIES IN

Protein: 6 g; Carbohydrates: 22 g; Fat: 12 g; Fiber: 6 g; Sodium: 205 mg; Carb Choices: 1½; Diabetic Exchange: 1 Starch, 1 Vegetable, 2 Fat

211 CALORIES OUT

Women: Walk:
51 minutes | Jog: 24 minutes

Men: Walk:
43 minutes | Jog: 20 minutes

CALORIE COMBOS

1 whole wheat roll: 76 cals

Savory Corn Cakes (page 111): 98 cals

1 whole wheat pita bread: 165 cals

Grilled Lemony Lamb Chops (page 130): 177 cals

2 ounces (60 g) focaccia: 180 cals

Quick Herb-Coated Tilapia (page 120): 196 cals

Rosemary-and-Smoked-Paprika Chicken Kebabs (page 128): 199 cals

Roasted Chicken with Rosemary-Lemon-Garlic Rub (page 244): 244 cals

Aussie-Style BBQ Chicken (page 252): 279 cals

Old Bay and Dill Salmon Patties (page 231): 283 cals

CALORIE CUTS

The goat cheese and sunflower seeds can be omitted. The cheese has 37 calories and 3 grams of fat per serving, and the sunflower seeds have 23 calories and 2 grams of fat per serving.

HOW TO COOK BEETS

I usually cook beets one of two ways: boiling or baking. To boil, fill a saucepan with enough water to cover the beets. Scrub the beets, but do not peel them. Slice off the tail and top ends. Boil gently until tender; the timing will depend on the size of your beets. A medium beet takes about 25 to 30 minutes. Check for doneness by sticking a sharp thin knife into a beet. It should be soft but still a bit firm.

To bake, preheat the oven to 400°F (200°C). Scrub the beets and trim them; leave the skin damp. Wrap each beet in a piece of aluminum foil. Place the beets on a baking sheet or directly on an oven rack and bake for about 45 minutes, or until tender.

Once cooled, peel the cooked beets and you're good to go. Be warned that the beet juice will stain your hands and anything else it comes in contact with (you may want to don an apron before handling cooked beets).

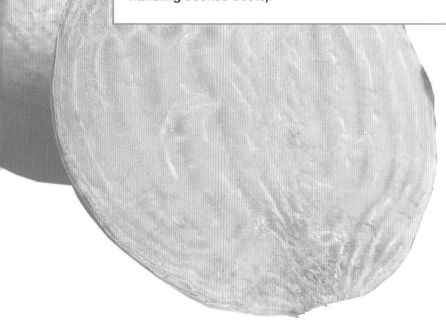

LEMONY TURKISH-STYLE CHICKEN SALAD

The crunch of the cucumbers and sweetness of the tomatoes perfectly round out the flavors and textures in this salad. A boiled whole chicken works well for this recipe, but a ready-roasted chicken from the grocery store is fine, too. Torn pieces of chicken will absorb more of the juices than knife-cut pieces. Marinate the salad in the olive oil and lemon juice for as long as possible, ideally up to 12 hours. One of my recipe testers mentioned that among her kids, some picked out the cucumbers while others picked out the tomatoes, but they all liked the chicken. Another tester mentioned using this for sandwiches the next day, and yet another enjoyed the leftovers with crackers. All good!

SERVES 6

4 cups (1½ pounds, 720 g) bite-size pieces (torn or cut) cooked chicken

2 tablespoons extra virgin olive oil

1 tablespoon grated lemon zest, or to taste

¼ cup (60 ml) fresh lemon juice, or to taste

1½ teaspoons dried mint

Salt and freshly ground pepper, to taste

Pinch of red pepper flakes, optional

1 cup (150 g) diced semi-peeled seedless cucumber

1 cup (160 g) diced ripe tomatoes or halved cherry tomatoes

½ cup (15 g) sliced scallions

⅓ cup (8 g) chopped fresh flat-leaf parsley

3 tablespoons light mayonnaise

1. In a large bowl, combine the chicken, olive oil, lemon zest, lemon juice, dried mint, salt, pepper, and red pepper flakes, if using. Toss gently and let sit at room temperature for at least 15 minutes, and ideally cover and refrigerate for up to 12 hours.

2. Just before serving, add the cucumbers, tomatoes, scallions, parsley, and mayonnaise and gently toss. Adjust the seasoning and serve.

234 CALORIES IN

Protein: 33 g; Carbohydrates: 4 g; Fat: 9 g; Fiber: 1 g; Sodium: 634 mg; Carb Choices: 0; Diabetic Exchange: 4 Lean Meat, 1 Vegetable

234 CALORIES OUT

Women: Walk: 57 minutes | Jog: 27 minutes

Men: Walk: 48 minutes | Jog: 22 minutes

CALORIE COMBOS

2 cups (40 g) salad greens (without dressing): 20 cals

Roasted Asparagus with Dill and Lemon Zest (page 88): 47 cals

Lemony Dill Cabbage Slaw (page 78): 63 cals

1 whole wheat roll: 76 cals

Grilled Vegetables (page 108): 89 cals

Gingery Squash Soup (page 63): 118 cals

7 whole wheat crackers: 120 cals

1 whole wheat pita bread: 165 cals

Great Green Couscous (page 105): 152 cals

Austrian-Style Potato Salad (page 82): 156 cals

Caesar Salad with a Light Touch (page 83): 163 cals

2 ounces (60 g) focaccia: 180 cals

Red Lentil Soup with Tomato-Cucumber Salsa (page 190): 253 cals

235 CALORIES IN

Protein: 10 g; Carbohydrates: 22 g;
Fat: 13 g; Fiber: 5 g; Sodium: 244
mg; Carb Choices: 1½; Diabetic
Exchange: 1 Starch, 1 Vegetable,
3 Fat

235 CALORIES OUT

Women: Walk:
57 minutes | Jog: 27 minutes

Men: Walk:
48 minutes | Jog: 23 minutes

CALORIE COMBOS

Thai-Style Hot-and-Sour Shrimp
Soup (page 59): 83 cals

Grilled Vegetables (page 108):
89 cals

Savory Corn Cakes (page 111):
98 cals

Quick Zucchini-Basil Soup
(page 62): 99 cals

Sweet-and-Spicy Fried Tofu
(page 114): 151 cals

Tofu and Bok Choy with Chili Sauce
(page 116): 174 cals

Grilled Lemony Lamb Chops
(page 130): 177 cals

Quick Herb-Coated Tilapia
(page 120): 196 cals

Roasted Pork Tenderloin with
Mustard-Tarragon Marinade
(page 127): 198 cals

Rosemary-and-Smoked-Paprika
Chicken Kebabs (page 128):
199 cals

Easy Lime-Cilantro Grilled Chicken
(page 238): 215 cals

Roasted Chicken with Rosemary-
Lemon-Garlic Rub (page 244):
244 cals

Chicken-Zucchini Burgers with
Ricotta and Sun-Dried Tomatoes
(page 247): 261 cals

CALORIE CUTS

Skip the optional peanuts and save
56 calories and 5 grams of fat per
serving.

QUINOA, CORN, EDAMAME, AND SNOW PEA SALAD

The sweet caramelized garlic oil is the perfect foil to the earthiness of the quinoa here. Using raw garlic simply would not have the same effect. The oil requires an extra step, but it really makes a difference. I like to use mixed quinoa (golden, red, and black), though you can use one type (see How to Cook and Freeze Quinoa, page 219). Fresh asparagus or green beans can be substituted for the snow peas. Simply quick-cook them and slice into ½-inch (1.25 cm) pieces. Adding grilled shrimp or diced cooked chicken will make this more of a main-course salad. (Note: The lime zest and vinegar will cause the bright green color of the snow peas and edamame to fade over time, but it will not affect the flavor.)

SERVES 5

½ cup (100 g) uncooked
quinoa, any kind

1 cup (160 g) cooked shelled
edamame

½ cup (70 g) frozen corn
kernels, thawed

1 teaspoon grated lime zest,
or to taste

1 tablespoon seasoned rice
vinegar or cider vinegar, or
to taste

5 ounces (150 g) snow peas,
ends trimmed

2 tablespoons vegetable oil

1 tablespoon minced garlic

Salt and freshly ground
pepper, to taste

⅓ cup (50 g) chopped salted
dry-roasted peanuts or
cashews, optional

3 tablespoons chopped fresh
cilantro

1. Cook the quinoa according to the package directions (for tips, see How to Cook and Freeze Quinoa, page 219), then place it in a serving bowl and fluff it. Add the edamame, corn, lime zest, and rice vinegar and toss gently. Set aside.

2. Boil the snow peas in salted water for 2 to 3 minutes, until crisp-tender. Drain in a sieve and rinse under cold water. Drain again and pat dry. Cut the snow peas into ½-inch (1.25 cm) slices on the diagonal, and add them to the quinoa mixture.

3. In a very small skillet, heat the vegetable oil over low heat. Add the garlic and cook for 30 seconds, or just until the garlic turns light golden; avoid burning the garlic, as it will turn bitter. Remove from the heat and allow the garlic to continue to cook to a deeper golden hue. Add the warm oil and garlic to the salad and toss gently. Adjust the seasoning, garnish with the peanuts, if using, and cilantro, and serve.

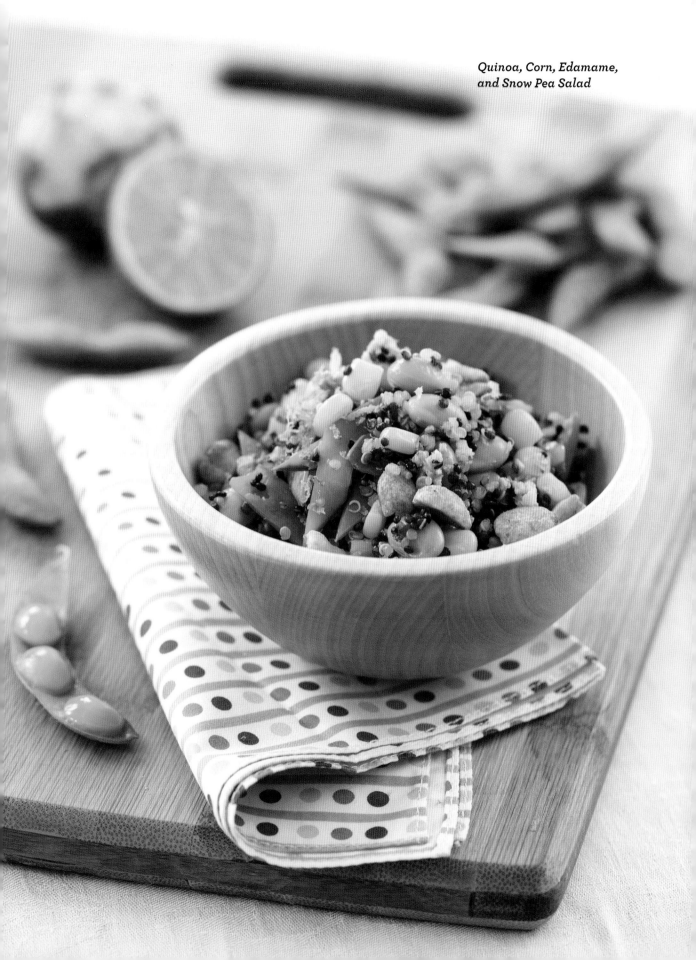

Quinoa, Corn, Edamame, and Snow Pea Salad

241 CALORIES IN

Protein: 7 g; Carbohydrates: 36 g;
Fat: 8 g; Fiber: 5 g; Sodium: 468
mg; Carb Choices: 2½; Diabetic
Exchange: 2 Starch, 1 Vegetable,
1 Fat

241 CALORIES OUT

Women: Walk:
59 minutes | Jog: 28 minutes

Men: Walk:
49 minutes | Jog: 23 minutes

CALORIE COMBOS

2 cups (40 g) salad greens (without
dressing): 20 cals

Grilled Vegetables (page 108):
89 cals

The Best Roasted Ratatouille
(page 112): 130 cals

Crab Cakes with Super-Easy Tartar
Sauce (page 119): 145 cals

Grilled Lemony Lamb Chops
(page 130): 177 cals

Quick Herb-Coated Tilapia
(page 120): 196 cals

Roasted Pork Tenderloin with
Mustard-Tarragon Marinade
(page 127): 198 cals

Rosemary-and-Smoked-Paprika
Chicken Kebabs (page 128):
199 cals

Easy Lime-Cilantro Grilled Chicken
(page 238): 215 cals

Roasted Chicken with Rosemary-
Lemon-Garlic Rub (page 244):
244 cals

COUSCOUS SALAD WITH HARISSA DRESSING

Harissa refers to a hot chili sauce from Northern Africa. This simple-to-make salad is one of my favorites. It goes well with almost anything. If you wish, swap the couscous with another grain, such as quinoa, farro, bulgur, or a mix. Other welcome additions include currants, pomegranate seeds, brined olives, brined fava beans, and sun-dried tomatoes. I sometimes add diced oranges or pineapple, along with toasted pine nuts. One of my recipe testers mentioned that this dish was a hit with her vegetarian friends.

SERVES 6

Couscous

1 cup (160 g) uncooked couscous

1 cup (200 g) canned chickpeas, rinsed and drained

1 teaspoon grated lemon zest, or to taste

Squeeze of fresh lemon juice, or to taste

Salt, to taste

1 cup (220 g) canned artichoke hearts, drained and sliced into thin wedges

Harissa Dressing

3 tablespoons canola oil

½ teaspoon chili powder, or to taste

¼ teaspoon garlic powder, or to taste

1 teaspoon dried oregano

2 teaspoons cumin seeds or 1½ teaspoons roasted ground cumin

Pinch of red pepper flakes, optional

1. Cook the couscous according to the package directions. Place it in a bowl and fluff with a fork. Add the remaining couscous ingredients and mix; set aside.

2. To make the harissa dressing, combine all of the ingredients in a very small skillet and heat over low heat (make sure it's low) just until the contents begin to sizzle, about 30 to 60 seconds. Do not cook too long, or the spices may burn and become bitter. Add the dressing to the couscous and mix gently until well blended. Adjust the seasoning and serve.

BROWN RICE AND LENTIL SALAD

The combo of lentils and brown rice is a classic. Cooked barley, farro, quinoa, bulgur, or just about any other whole grain, easily picked up at a salad bar, can be substituted for the brown rice. Add your favorite vegetables in place of the ones called for. To save time, use as many precut items from the salad bar as possible. Keep this tip in mind for other salads as well. The dressing can be made up to 3 days in advance, covered, and refrigerated.

SERVES 4

Dijon Dressing

2 tablespoons red wine vinegar

1 teaspoon Dijon mustard

1 garlic clove, minced

2 tablespoons extra virgin olive oil

Pinch of sugar

Salad

One 15.5-ounce (439 g) can green lentils, rinsed and well drained, or 1½ cups (375 ml) cooked lentils

1½ cups (270 g) cooked brown rice

⅓ cup (60 g) diced celery

⅓ cup (50 g) sliced or diced red radishes

15 cherry tomatoes, cut in half

2 tablespoons chopped fresh flat-leaf parley, dill, or a mix of both

¼ cup (15 g) thinly sliced scallions

½ teaspoon salt, or to taste

Freshly ground pepper, to taste

1. To make the dressing, combine all of the ingredients in a small bowl and whisk until emulsified.
2. In a serving bowl, combine all of the salad ingredients. Add the dressing and toss gently. Adjust the seasoning and serve promptly.

---

248 CALORIES IN

Protein: 10 g; Carbohydrates: 36 g; Fat: 8 g; Fiber: 9 g; Sodium: 344 mg; Carb Choices: 2½; Diabetic Exchange: 2 Starch, 1 Vegetable, 1 Fat

248 CALORIES OUT

Women: Walk:
60 minutes | Jog: 28 minutes

Men: Walk:
51 minutes | Jog: 24 minutes

CALORIE COMBOS

2 cups (40 g) salad greens (without dressing): 20 cals

Roasted Asparagus with Dill and Lemon Zest (page 88): 47 cals

Grilled Vegetables (page 108): 89 cals

Crab Cakes with Super-Easy Tartar Sauce (page 119): 145 cals

Grilled Lemony Lamb Chops (page 130): 177 cals

Quick Herb-Coated Tilapia (page 120): 196 cals

Roasted Pork Tenderloin with Mustard-Tarragon Marinade (page 127): 198 cals

Rosemary-and-Smoked-Paprika Chicken Kebabs (page 128): 199 cals

Easy Lime-Cilantro Grilled Chicken (page 238): 215 cals

Roasted Chicken with Rosemary-Lemon-Garlic Rub (page 244): 244 cals

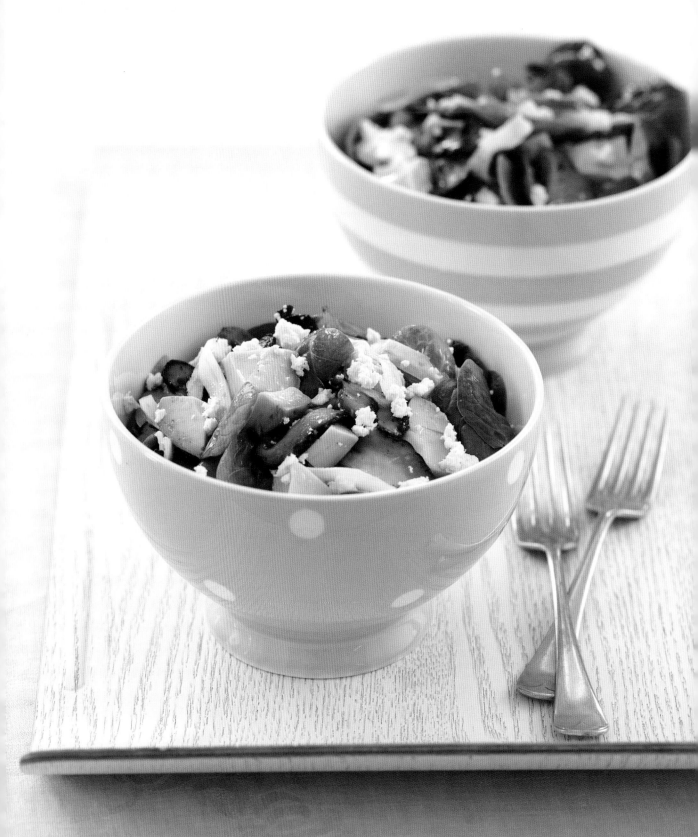

Spinach Salad with Mushrooms, Fennel, and Avocado

SPINACH SALAD WITH MUSHROOMS, FENNEL, AND AVOCADO

Some of my favorite ingredients come together in this salad. I cook the fennel just long enough to release its sweetness; if you prefer raw fennel, leave it uncooked. The avocado adds a welcome softness to the salad. Fresh mozzarella, Parmesan, or blue cheese can be used in place of the crumbled feta. To make this into a main course, add cooked chicken, shrimp, tofu, or tempeh. The mushrooms and fennel can be sautéed up to 2 days in advance and refrigerated. The dressing can be made up to 5 days ahead, covered, and refrigerated.

SERVES 4

Spinach Salad Dressing

2 tablespoons balsamic vinegar

1 teaspoon fresh lemon juice, or to taste

2 tablespoons extra virgin olive oil

1 tablespoon canola oil

1 tablespoon water

1 small garlic clove, smashed and peeled

Salt and freshly ground pepper, to taste

Salad

1 tablespoon extra virgin olive oil

1 teaspoon minced garlic

6 to 8 ounces (200 to 230 g) shiitake or cremini mushrooms, rinsed, stems removed, and sliced

Salt and freshly ground pepper, to taste

1½ cups (180 g) very thinly sliced fennel

⅓ cup (10 g) thinly sliced scallions

10 to 12 ounces (300 to 360 g) baby spinach

1 ripe avocado, halved, pitted, and cut into cubes or wedges

½ cup (80 g) crumbled reduced-fat feta cheese

1. To make the dressing, in a small bowl, whisk the ingredients until well blended. Let sit for 30 minutes at room temperature for the garlic flavor to develop. Remove the garlic before serving.

2. To make the salad, in a medium nonstick skillet, heat the olive oil over medium-high heat. Add the garlic and cook for 30 seconds. Add the mushrooms, season with salt and pepper, and cook, stirring occasionally, for 5 minutes, or until lightly browned. Add the fennel and scallions and cook for 1 minute. Transfer the contents of the skillet to a plate and cool to room temperature (or place the plate in the refrigerator if you are in a hurry).

3. Arrange the spinach on individual serving plates, or place it all in a large serving bowl. Top with the reserved mushroom mixture, followed by the avocado and feta cheese. Drizzle the dressing on top of the plated salads or, if serving in a salad bowl, gently mix with salad spoons. Serve promptly.

251 CALORIES IN

Protein: 8 g; Carbohydrates: 23 g; Fat: 16 g; Fiber: 10 g; Sodium: 558 mg; Carb Choices: 1½; Diabetic Exchange: 1 Low-Fat Milk, 2 Vegetable, 2 Fat

251 CALORIES OUT

Women: Walk:
61 minutes | Jog: 29 minutes

Men: Walk:
51 minutes | Jog: 24 minutes

CALORIE COMBOS

1 whole wheat roll: 76 cals

7 whole wheat crackers: 120 cals

Gingery Squash Soup (page 63): 118 cals

Crab Cakes with Super-Easy Tartar Sauce (page 119): 145 cals

Roasted Carrot and Fennel Soup (page 68): 159 cals

1 whole wheat pita bread: 165 cals

Grilled Lemony Lamb Chops (page 130): 177 cals

2 ounces (60 g) focaccia: 180 cals

Quick Herb-Coated Tilapia (page 120): 196 cals

Roasted Pork Tenderloin with Mustard-Tarragon Marinade (page 127): 198 cals

Rosemary-and-Smoked-Paprika Chicken Kebabs (page 128): 199 cals

Everyone's Favorite Veggie Burgers (page 212): 223 cals

Quinoa, Paneer, and Cabbage Patties (page 220): 235 cals

CALORIES CUTS

The avocado and feta cheese are the things to cut here. One quarter of a California avocado has 56 calories and 21 grams of fat; the feta cheese has 35 calories and 2 grams of fat per serving.

PASTA SALAD WITH SUN-DRIED TOMATO PESTO AND MOZZARELLA CHEESE

A colorful and delicious salad with an Italian flair. Try to find high-quality sun-dried tomatoes, as lower-quality ones tend to be leathery and tasteless. I'm partial to Pomodori Secchi D'Amico in oil. The Kalamata or brine-cured olives, peperoncini, and fresh basil all add a contrast of textures and flavors. The fresh mozzarella cheese and toasted pine nuts provide soft undertones (and, yes, some calories). Add Grilled Vegetables if you have leftovers; bell peppers and eggplant are particularly yummy. Cooked shrimp, chicken, or tofu can transform this salad into a main course; you may need to add a bit more dressing. My recipe testers loved this dish. One made it twice for houseguests and the second time added feta instead of mozzarella. The dressing can be made up to 3 days ahead, covered, and refrigerated.

SERVES 6

Sun-Dried Tomato Dressing

Heaping ½ cup (70 g) sun-dried tomatoes in oil, drained

1 small garlic clove

3 tablespoons hot water

2 tablespoons red wine vinegar, or to taste

Pasta

8 ounces (240 g) fusilli, bow-tie, orecchiette, or other bite-size pasta

⅓ cup (70 g) pitted Kalamata or a mix of brine-cured olives

⅓ cup (70 g) sliced jarred peperoncini or jarred red bell peppers

Pinch of red pepper flakes

About 1 cup (6 ounces/180 g) fresh mozzarella mini balls, cut in half

Salt and freshly ground pepper, to taste

3 to 4 tablespoons sliced fresh basil leaves, to taste

2 tablespoons toasted pine nuts

1. To make the dressing, in a mini food processor, pulse the sun-dried tomatoes, garlic, and hot water until they form a chunky puree; you may need to add a little more hot water. The yield should be a generous ⅓ cup (80 ml) dressing; if not, add a bit more water or oil. Set aside.

2. Cook the pasta according to the package directions. Drain (do not rinse it) and transfer to a serving bowl. While the pasta is still hot, toss with the dressing. Let cool slightly.

3. Add the olives, peperoncini, red pepper flakes, and mozzarella cheese to the pasta and toss again. (Note: Cover and refrigerate if not serving soon.) Adjust the seasoning, then garnish with the basil leaves and pine nuts and serve.

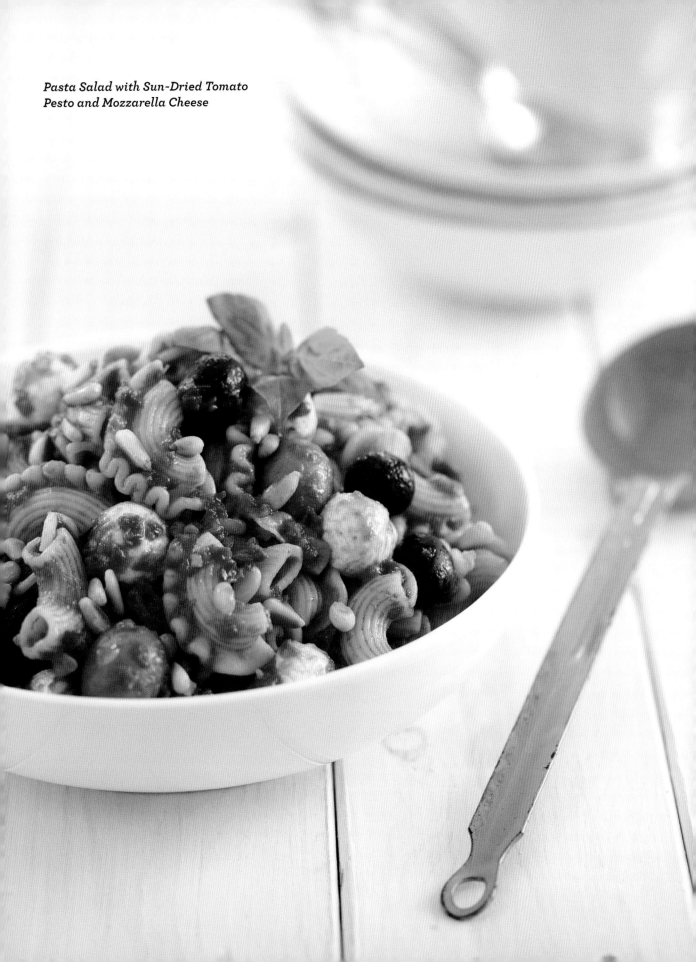

*Pasta Salad with Sun-Dried Tomato
Pesto and Mozzarella Cheese*

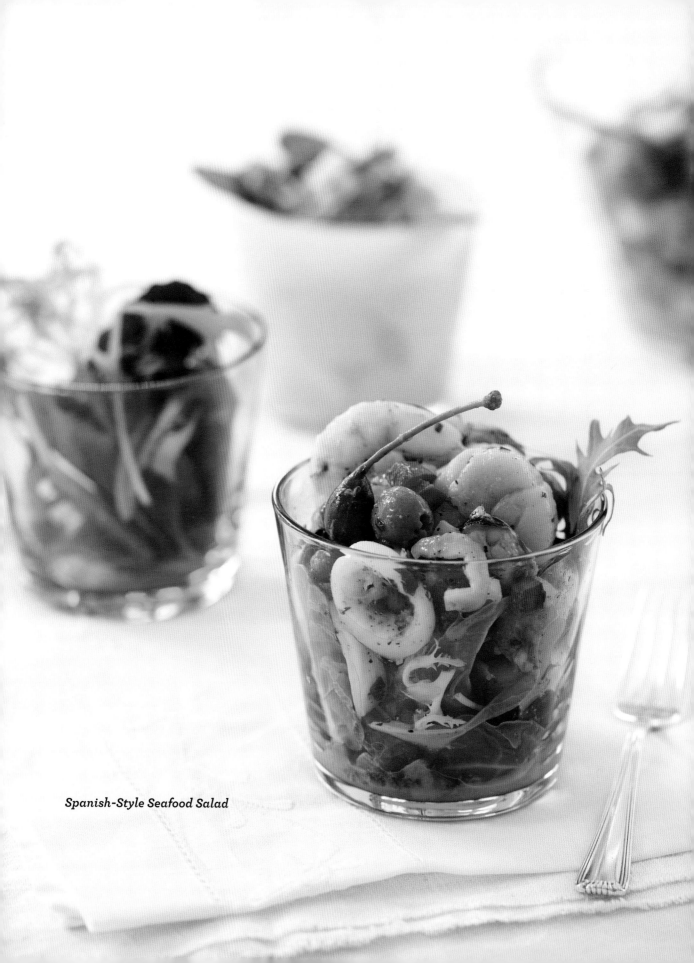

Spanish-Style Seafood Salad

SPANISH-STYLE SEAFOOD SALAD

A Mediterranean salad made with scallops, shrimp, mussels, and calamari, this is as healthy and tasty as it is beautiful. The only herb is flat-leaf parsley. There are no strong spices, but add some if you wish. I cook the different types of seafood separately (except for the mussels, which I called for cooked) because they have varying cooking times. If you're pressed for time, though, purchase ready-cooked seafood. Some markets, such as Whole Foods, feature seafood bars that offer cooked shrimp, mussels, and scallops. High-quality flash-frozen cooked or raw shellfish can also be used; frozen cooked seafood is a huge time saver.

SERVES 6

½ cup (120 g) diced or sliced celery

½ cup (60 g) thinly sliced fennel

½ cup (70 g) diced red bell pepper

½ cup (60 g) pitted black olives

½ cup (60 g) pitted green olives

2 tablespoons medium capers or about 15 caperberries, drained

¼ cup (60 g) thinly sliced sun-dried tomatoes in oil, drained

1 tablespoon grated lemon zest

3 tablespoons chopped fresh flat-leaf parsley

1 teaspoon Italian seasoning

3 tablespoons fresh lemon juice, or to taste

3 tablespoons extra virgin olive oil

8 ounces (240 g) medium shrimp, shelled, deveined, rinsed, cut lengthwise in half, and patted dry with paper towels (see How to Clean Shrimp, page 123)

Salt and freshly ground pepper, to taste

8 ounces (240 g) cleaned squid, rinsed, sliced into ¼-inch (6 mm) rings, and patted dry

8 ounces (240 g) sea scallops, tough side muscle removed, rinsed and patted dry

8 ounces (240 g) cooked mussels

Green Salad

6 cups (120 g) baby greens

2 to 3 tablespoons Classic Red Wine Vinaigrette, to taste (page 146)

1. In a large bowl, combine the celery, fennel, red bell peppers, black and green olives, capers, sun-dried tomatoes, lemon zest, parsley, Italian seasoning, and lemon juice and gently mix. Set aside.

2. In a large nonstick skillet, heat 1 tablespoon of the olive oil over medium-high heat. Season the shrimp with salt and pepper and sauté for 3 to 4 minutes, until cooked through. Transfer the shrimp and any juices to a heatproof bowl to cool. (Do not rinse the skillet.)

3. Add 1 tablespoon of the olive oil to the skillet and heat over medium-high heat. Season the squid and sauté for 3 to 5 minutes, until cooked through. Transfer the squid and any juices to the bowl with the shrimp.

(RECIPE CONTINUES)

268 CALORIES IN

Protein: 26 g; Carbohydrates: 14 g; Fat: 12 g; Fiber: 4 g; Sodium: 870 mg; Carb Choices: 1; Diabetic Exchange: 4 Lean Meat, 2 Vegetable

268 CALORIES OUT

Women: Walk: 65 minutes | Jog: 31 minutes

Men: Walk: 55 minutes | Jog: 26 minutes

CALORIE COMBOS

1 whole wheat roll: 76 cals

Gently Cooked Gazpacho (page 60): 87 cals

Quick Zucchini-Basil Soup (page 62): 99 cals

Gingery Squash Soup (page 63): 118 cals

7 whole wheat crackers: 120 cals

2 ounces (60 g) French baguette: 150 cals

Roasted Carrot and Fennel Soup (page 68): 159 cals

Cauliflower, Watercress, and Parmesan Soup (page 69): 159 cals

1 whole wheat pita bread: 165 cals

2 ounces (60 g) focaccia: 180 cals

4. Wipe out the skillet with paper towels if necessary, then add the remaining 1 tablespoon olive oil and heat over medium-high heat. Season the scallops and cook, turning once, for about 5 minutes (depending on the thickness), or until cooked through. Transfer the scallops and any juices to a separate bowl to cool. Once they are cool, cut them in half horizontally.

5. Add all of the cooked seafood and the mussels to the bowl of vegetables. Toss gently, adjust the seasoning, and add more lemon juice or herbs to taste. Set aside.

6. To serve, gently mix the greens and salad dressing in a bowl. Dress to taste, keeping in mind that the seafood salad also has a dressing. Place a bed of dressed greens on each serving plate and top with a portion of the seafood salad, or serve the seafood salad and greens separately. Serve promptly and refrigerate any leftovers.

ENDIVE, RADICCHIO, WHITE BEAN, AND BLUE CHEESE SALAD

This makes a great light lunch with whole wheat crackers or flatbread. The endive (white and/or purple varieties) and radicchio can be a bit bitter, especially for young eaters, so feel free to switch out those greens for other milder ones, such as spinach or mâche. The blue cheese can be replaced with your favorite cheese. Ideally, make the dressing a couple of hours before serving so the garlic flavor infuses it, or up to 3 days in advance; cover and refrigerate.

SERVES 5

Simple Dressing

2 tablespoons balsamic vinegar

3 tablespoons extra virgin olive oil

1 tablespoon water

1 small garlic clove, smashed and peeled

Salad

2 heads (4 ounces/120 g) Belgian endive, ends trimmed, rinsed, dried, and thinly sliced (about 2 cups, 500 ml)

½ small head radicchio (2 ounces/60 g), outer leaves removed, cored, quartered, and thinly sliced (about 2 cups, 500 ml)

2 cups (100 g) sliced romaine lettuce

1½ cups (180 g) canned white beans (such as great Northern, cannellini, or navy) rinsed and drained

1 ripe avocado, halved, pitted, and sliced

⅓ cup (50 g) crumbled blue cheese

¼ cup (25 g) coarsely chopped toasted walnuts

2 tablespoons chopped fresh dill

1. To make the dressing, in a small bowl, combine the ingredients and whisk; set aside. Remove the garlic clove before serving.
2. Divide the salad ingredients among 4 serving plates, or place them in a large salad bowl. Drizzle the dressing on top of the plated salads or, if using a salad bowl, add the dressing, toss, and adjust the seasoning. Serve promptly.

281 CALORIES IN

Protein: 10 g; Carbohydrates: 20 g; Fat: 19 g; Fiber: 7 g; Sodium: 156 mg; Carb Choices: 1; Diabetic Exchange: 1 Starch, 1 Vegetable, 1 High-Fat Meat, 2 Fat

281 CALORIES OUT

Women: Walk: 68 minutes | Jog: 32 minutes

Men: Walk: 57 minutes | Jog: 27 minutes

CALORIE COMBOS

Roasted Asparagus with Dill and Lemon Zest (page 88): 47 cals

1 whole wheat roll: 76 cals

Gingery Squash Soup (page 63): 118 cals

Crab Cakes with Super-Easy Tartar Sauce (page 119): 145 cals

2 ounces (60 g) French baguette: 150 cals

Roasted Carrot and Fennel Soup (page 68): 159 cals

Grilled Lemony Lamb Chops (page 130): 177 cals

Quick Herb-Coated Tilapia (page 120): 196 cals

Rosemary-and-Smoked-Paprika Chicken Kebabs (page 128): 199 cals

CALORIE CUTS

The delicious combination of avocados, walnuts, blue cheese, and beans is what makes this salad caloric. Cut back as you wish: per serving, the white beans have 75 calories and zero fat; the avocado has 45 calories and 4 grams of fat; the blue cheese has 36 calories and 3 grams of fat; and the walnuts have 38 calories and 4 grams of fat.

SIDES

MINTY BASMATI RICE AND POTATOES

Dried mint, cumin seeds, ginger, and green chile lift plain basmati rice to new heights here. The dried mint, which has infinitely more flavor than fresh, gives the dish a darkish green color. The basmati rice does not require soaking in this recipe, as it will be cooked with the potatoes. Just make sure to cut the potatoes into small dice, or the rice will be mushy by the time they are cooked. This dish does not freeze well. Reheat any leftovers in a microwave oven.

SERVES 6

1¼ cups (260 g) basmati rice

2 tablespoons vegetable oil

1 medium onion, thinly sliced

1 tablespoon cumin seeds

Pinch of cayenne

1 large potato, peeled and cut into ½-inch (1.25 cm) dice

2 tablespoons minced peeled fresh ginger

1 to 2 tablespoons minced green chile, to taste

1 tablespoon plus 1 teaspoon dried mint

2¼ cups (560 ml) boiling water

½ teaspoon salt, or to taste

1. Place the basmati rice in a bowl, cover it with water, and gently swish your fingers to remove the excess starch. Drain the rice in a sieve and rinse it with cold running water; set aside.

2. In a large saucepan, heat the vegetable oil over medium-high heat. Add the onions and sauté until light golden brown, 5 to 7 minutes. Add the cumin seeds, cayenne, potatoes, ginger, green chile, and dried mint and sauté for 2 minutes.

3. Add the rice and sauté for 3 minutes. Add the boiling water and salt and bring to a boil, then reduce the heat and simmer, covered, until the rice and potatoes are cooked, 15 to 20 minutes. Do not stir while the rice is cooking. Adjust the seasoning, fluff the rice, and serve promptly.

LEMONY BASMATI RICE

Delicious, beautiful, and easy to prepare. For truly authentic Indian flavors, I sizzle black mustard seeds and curry leaves, and add them to the rice before serving (I don't expect you to have these items on hand, but if you do, please read How to Make a Basic Indian Tarka, page 216). You can use brown basmati rice, but the white showcases the colors better. If you don't have cashews, peanuts are a good substitute. Reheat any leftovers in a microwave oven.

SERVES 5

1 cup (200 g) white basmati rice

1 tablespoon vegetable oil

2 tablespoons minced seeded green chiles

1 cup (100 g) grated carrots

½ teaspoon turmeric

1 teaspoon cumin seeds

1¾ cups (430 ml) boiling water

½ teaspoon salt, or to taste

2 to 3 tablespoons fresh lemon juice, or to taste

3 tablespoons chopped fresh cilantro

⅓ cup (35 g) chopped toasted cashews

1. Place the basmati rice in a bowl, cover it with water, and gently swish your fingers to remove the excess starch. Drain the rice though a sieve and rinse it with cold running water; set aside.

2. Heat the vegetable oil in a medium saucepan over medium heat until hot. Add the green chiles and carrots and sauté, stirring occasionally, for 2 minutes. Add the rice, turmeric, and cumin seeds and stir until all of the ingredients are well combined. Add the boiling water and salt and stir. Lower the heat to a gentle simmer, cover, and cook for 15 minutes, or until the rice is tender. Remove from the heat and allow the rice to sit, covered, undisturbed, for 10 minutes.

3. Using a fork, gently lift and separate the cooked grains of rice. Add the lemon juice and adjust the seasoning. Transfer to a serving bowl, garnish with the cilantro and cashews, and serve.

210 CALORIES IN

Protein: 4 g; Carbohydrates: 33 g; Fat: 8 g; Fiber: 2 g; Sodium: 251 mg; Carb Choices: 2; Diabetic Exchange: 2 Starch, 1 Fat

210 CALORIES OUT

Women: Walk:
51 minutes; Jog: 24 minutes

Men: Walk:
43 minutes; Jog: 20 minutes

CALORIE COMBOS

Paneer with Spinach, Tomatoes, and Spices (page 113): 143 cals

Grilled Chicken Tandoori (page 236): 212 cals

Minty Middle Eastern–Style Turkey Burgers (page 242): 231 cals

Classic Dal (page 217): 232 cals

Quinoa, Paneer, and Cabbage Patties (page 220): 235 cals

Indian-Spiced Broiled Salmon (page 226): 262 cals

Classic Chicken Curry with Coconut Milk (page 248): 266 cals

Chicken Thighs with Capers and Parsley (page 250): 273 cals

Butter Chicken Made Easy (page 251): 276 cals

Old Bay and Dill Salmon Patties (page 231): 283 cals

CALORIE CUTS

Skip the cashews and save 52 calories and 4 grams of fat per serving.

HOW TO MAKE A BASIC INDIAN TARKA

In Indian cooking, a *tarka* refers to a finishing touch of roasted spices, and sometimes onions and tomatoes, spooned on top of a dish just before serving. It adds an incredible depth of flavor, and heat if hot chiles are used. This is a basic tarka that can be dolloped onto rice, dals, soups, stews, or other dishes. If the recipe you are making lends itself to including diced tomatoes (use 1 medium tomato), and add them after the curry leaves. See Ingredients Notes and Recommended Brands (page 339) for more information on the spices and curry leaves.

BASIC TARKA

½ tablespoon vegetable oil
1 to 2 teaspoons black mustard seeds
Pinch of red pepper flakes or cayenne, optional
1 to 2 teaspoons cumin seeds, to taste
10 to 15 fresh or dried curry leaves

In a small saucepan, heat the oil over medium-low heat. Add the mustard seeds, then stand back, as they will start to pop and splatter. Add the red pepper flakes and cumin seeds and cook for 45 seconds. Add the curry leaves and please be careful again as they will splatter, too. If using tomatoes, add them now, and sauté 1 minute longer. Remove from the heat and spoon the tarka on top of your dish.

MEXICAN RICE

One thing to remember when cooking rice is that all grains are different: some absorb more water than others, some require a longer cooking time, and some just seem to get mushy no matter what you do (at least that's my honest experience). For this recipe, I call for long-grain white rice, but if you prefer another type, use it. Brown rice will require longer cooking—about 40 minutes. The squeeze of fresh lime and the cilantro brighten the flavor. To save time, I call for canned tomatoes as the first option here, but you can use diced ripe tomatoes.

SERVES 6

1½ tablespoons extra virgin olive oil

1 onion, chopped

2 garlic cloves, minced

1 tablespoon minced fresh or jarred serrano or jalapeño chiles

1 teaspoon roasted ground cumin

1 teaspoon dried oregano

1 teaspoon paprika

Pinch of red pepper flakes, optional

1½ cups (280 g) long-grain white rice

One 14.5-ounce (411 g) can diced tomatoes or 1½ cups (375 ml) diced ripe tomatoes

1½ cups (375 ml) water

½ teaspoon salt, or to taste

Grated zest and juice of 1 lime, or to taste

3 tablespoons chopped fresh cilantro

1. In a large saucepan, heat the olive oil over medium heat until hot. Add the onions, garlic, and chiles and sauté, stirring occasionally, for 3 minutes. Add the cumin, oregano, paprika, and red pepper flakes, if using, and sauté for 30 seconds longer, then add the rice and sauté, stirring, for 2 minutes.

2. Mix in the tomatoes, add the water and salt, stir, and bring to a boil. Reduce the heat and gently simmer, covered, for 15 minutes to 20 minutes, until the rice is tender and all of the water has been absorbed. Remove from the heat and let stand, covered, for 10 minutes.

3. Fluff the rice with a fork. Adjust the seasoning, then add the lime zest and lime juice. Sprinkle with the cilantro and serve.

222 CALORIES IN

Protein: 4 g; Carbohydrates: 42 g; Fat: 4 g; Fiber: 2 g; Sodium: 201 mg; Carb Choices: 2½; Diabetic Exchange: 2 Starch, 2 Vegetable

222 CALORIES OUT

Women: Walk: 54 minutes; Jog: 25 minutes

Men: Walk: 45 minutes; Jog: 21 minutes

CALORIE COMBOS

Grilled Vegetables (page 108): 89 cals

Quick Herb-Coasted Tilapia (page 120): 196 cals

Roasted Pork Tenderloin with Mustard-Tarragon Marinade (page 127): 198 cals

Rosemary-and-Smoked-Paprika Chicken Kebabs (page 128): 199 cals

Easy Lime-Cilantro Grilled Chicken (page 238): 215 cals

Memorable Meat Loaf (page 253): 233 cals

Grilled Chicken with Fresh Mango Salsa (page 243): 234 cals

Roasted Chicken with Rosemary-Lemon-Garlic Rub (page 244): 244 cals

Aussie-Style BBQ Chicken (page 252): 279 cals

Snapper with Olive-Artichoke-Tomato Tapenade (page 228): 279 cals

EVERYONE'S FAVORITE VEGGIE BURGERS

With this combination of brown rice, refried beans, corn, mushrooms, and red bell peppers, you can't go wrong. Serve for lunch or dinner with salsa, or another condiment from this book. I love them with the Yummy Guacamole. They are delicious on whole wheat buns or in pita pockets, but if you're cutting back on calories, bunless burgers with a simple side salad are just as satisfying. "Easy, delicious, better than frozen," was how one of my recipe testers described them. Keep a stash of them in your freezer, and you'll never buy store-bought burgers again. You can freeze them for up to 1 month; thaw when ready to cook.

SERVES 5

1½ cups (270 g) cooked brown rice

½ cup (30 g) frozen corn, thawed

¾ cup (190 g) canned refried beans

2 tablespoons chopped fresh cilantro

2 tablespoons thinly sliced scallions

1 large egg, lightly beaten

⅓ cup (20 g) panko bread crumbs, plus ½ cup (25 g) for coating

1½ tablespoons vegetable oil

1 cup (60 g) mushrooms, such as cremini, shiitake, or any other mushrooms you like, rinsed, stems trimmed, and finely sliced

½ cup (70 g) finely diced red bell peppers

½ teaspoon roasted ground cumin

¼ teaspoon salt, or to taste

Freshly ground pepper, to taste

1. In a large bowl, combine the brown rice, corn, refried beans, cilantro, scallions, egg, and ⅓ cup (20 g) of the bread crumbs. Mix gently and set aside.

2. Heat ½ tablespoon of the vegetable oil in a medium nonstick skillet over medium heat. Add the mushrooms and sauté, stirring occasionally, until they are light golden brown, about 5 minutes. Add the red bell peppers and cumin and cook 1 minute longer. Cool slightly.

3. Add the sautéed vegetables to the reserved brown rice mixture and stir until well combined. Chill in the refrigerator for at least 1 hour, or overnight.

4. Place the remaining ½ cup (25 g) bread crumbs in a pie plate. Using a ½-cup (125 ml) measuring cup, scoop up the burger mixture and form it into 5 patties. Coat each patty with the bread crumbs and refrigerate, covered, for at least 20 minutes and up to 12 hours before cooking.

5. Heat the remaining 1 tablespoon vegetable oil in a large nonstick skillet over medium heat. Add the patties and cook for 5 to 7 minutes on each side, until heated through. If they begin browning too fast, lower the heat a bit. Serve hot with or without buns.

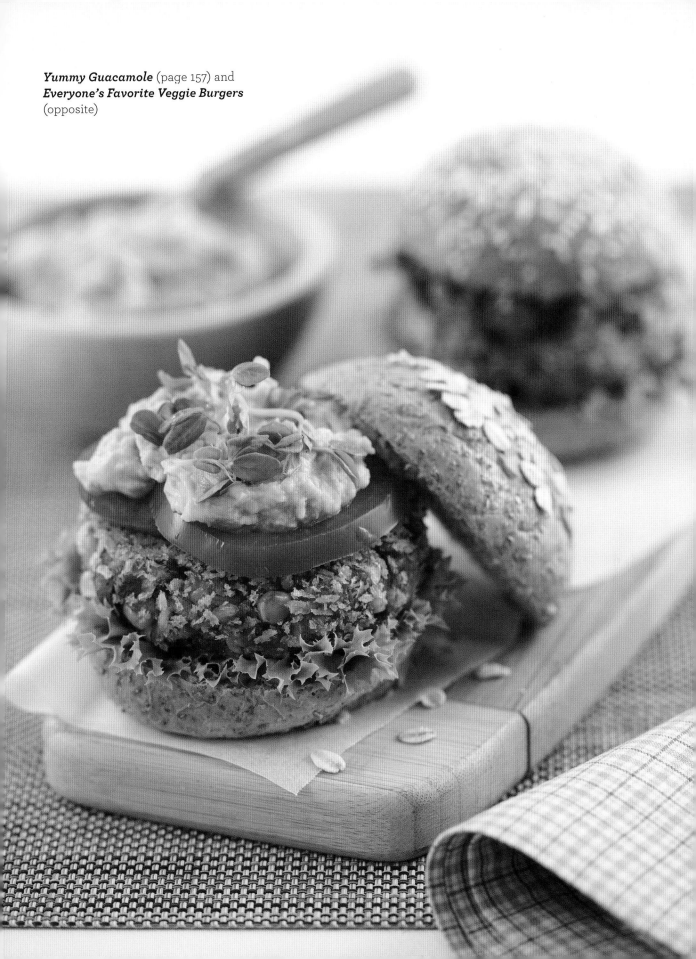

Yummy Guacamole (page 157) and
Everyone's Favorite Veggie Burgers
(opposite)

226 CALORIES IN

Protein: 14 g; Carbohydrates: 18 g; Fat: 13 g; Fiber: 5 g; Sodium: 521 mg; Carb Choices: 1; Diabetic Exchange: 3 Vegetable, 2 Medium-Fat Meat

226 CALORIES OUT

Women: Walk:
55 minutes | Jog: 26 minutes

Men: Walk:
46 minutes | Jog: 22 minutes

CALORIE COMBOS

Napa Cabbage with Ginger and Oyster Sauce (page 89): 48 cals

Hot-and-Sweet Cucumber, Carrot, and Red Bell Pepper Salad (page 77): 61 cals

Japanese Eggplant in Sweet Chili Sauce (page 94): 86 cals

2 cups (40 g) salad greens with 1 tablespoon Benihana-Style Ginger-Sesame Dressing (page 155): 89 cals

Broccolini with Sesame and Spice (page 96): 99 cals

½ cup (80 g) plain white rice: 103 cals

½ cup (90 g) plain brown rice: 108 cals

½ cup (65 g) plain quinoa: 111 cals

Miso Soup with Tofu, Shiitakes, Noodles, and Baby Spinach (page 64): 139 cals

1 cup (200 g) plain udon noodles: 210 cals

STIR-FRIED TOFU, SHIITAKES, AND BEAN SPROUTS

The fresh, crisp bean sprouts play off the earthy, soft shiitakes and delicate tofu in this dish. Include your favorite veggies, just keep in mind that different vegetables require different cooking times, and add them accordingly. Tempeh can stand in for the firm tofu. Fresh shiitake mushrooms work best in this recipe. If you can't find them, you can substitute sliced fresh oyster or cremini mushrooms. For a complete meal, serve with some brown rice or whole grains and a side salad. This dish does not freeze well.

SERVES 4

Stir-Fry Sauce

3 tablespoons lite soy sauce

1 tablespoon hoisin sauce

Pinch of sugar

3 tablespoons water

1 teaspoon cornstarch

Tofu and Vegetables

1½ tablespoons vegetable oil

14 ounces (420 g) firm tofu, drained, patted dry, sliced into 2-inch (5 cm) by ½-inch (1.25 cm) rectangles, and patted dry again

2 garlic cloves, minced

¼ cup (20 g) thinly sliced peeled fresh ginger

1 teaspoon minced seeded hot or mild green or red chile

8 ounces (240 g) shiitake mushrooms, rinsed, stems removed, and sliced

Salt and freshly ground pepper, to taste

½ red bell pepper, cored, seeded, and thinly sliced

8 ounces (240 g) fresh mung bean sprouts, trimmed (see How to Clean Fresh Mung Bean Sprouts, opposite)

½ cup (30 g) sliced scallions (white and green parts, cut into 1-inch/2.5 cm pieces)

3 tablespoons chopped toasted cashews, for garnish

1. For the sauce, in a small bowl, mix all of the ingredients until well combined; set aside.

2. Line a large plate with paper towels. In a large nonstick skillet, heat 1 tablespoon of the vegetable oil over medium-high heat. Add the tofu and sauté, turning frequently, until lightly browned, about 5 minutes. Transfer to the prepared plate and cover with foil to keep warm. (Do not rinse the skillet.)

3. Add the remaining ½ tablespoon vegetable oil to the skillet and heat over medium heat. Add the garlic, ginger, and chile and cook for 1 minute. Add the shiitakes, season with a tiny bit of salt and pepper, and cook for 2 minutes. Move the shiitakes to one side of the skillet, add the red bell peppers to the empty space, and sauté for 1 minute.

4. Add the bean sprouts and scallions to the peppers and sauté for 2 minutes. Add the reserved sauce and tofu and gently mix all of the ingredients together. Sauté just until the sauce slightly thickens, about 1 minute. Adjust the seasoning, garnish with the cashews, and serve promptly.

HOW TO CLEAN FRESH MUNG BEAN SPROUTS

I learned this method of cleaning fresh mung bean sprouts from my wonderful Chinese cook, Luan Wong, in Malaysia. In most grocery stores in the United States, the cleaning has already been done for you and your sprouts come neatly packaged in a plastic bag. But if your sprouts still have roots and green leaves intact (the leaves can be bitter), here's what to do: Snap off the root ends and then gently pull off any leaves from the top. Luan always blanched the sprouts in boiling water for 30 seconds after trimming them, which she claimed removed impurities and bitterness. She bought our fresh sprouts from the farmers' market, so maybe this was her way of being overly cautious (which I appreciate). If your sprouts have been cleaned and bagged, there is no need for blanching.

229 CALORIES IN

Protein: 15 g; Carbohydrates: 14 g; Fat: 13 g; Fiber: 2 g; Sodium: 468 mg; Carb Choices: 1; Diabetic Exchange: 1 Starch, 2 Medium-Fat Meat

229 CALORIES OUT

Women: Walk:
56 minutes | Jog: 26 minutes

Men: Walk:
47 minutes | Jog: 22 minutes

CALORIE COMBOS

2 cups (40 g) salad greens with 1 tablespoon Almost-Fat-Free Dieter's Lemony Dressing (page 140): 38 cals

Tomato, Cucumber, and Radish Salad (page 76): 55 cals

2 cups (40 g) salad greens with 1 tablespoon Balsamic Vinaigrette (page 150): 73 cals

Gently Cooked Gazpacho (page 60): 87 cals

Quick Zucchini-Basil Soup (page 62): 99 cals

Caesar Salad with a Light Touch (page 83): 163 cals

Tomato, Artichoke Heart, Feta, and White Bean Salad (page 84): 168 cals

Allie's Bruschetta (page 71): 172 cals

Endive, Radicchio, White Bean, and Blue Cheese Salad (page 207): 281 cals

BROCCOLI, MUSHROOM, CHEDDAR, AND CURRY FRITTATA

A frittata, which is like a crustless quiche, is a fantastic way to use your leftovers from roasted potatoes, hash browns, or grilled vegetables. Inspired by the delicious egg curries I sampled in Malaysia, I added curry powder (see ingredient note on page 344), which offers a uniquely Indian flavor. For a more Western flavor, use fresh or dried herbs such as Italian seasoning, tarragon, or oregano. Ideally, you should use a 10-inch (25 cm) ovenproof skillet; see the Baking Note below if using a Pyrex pie dish. The teaspoon of flour is added to prevent a watery texture.

SERVES 5

5 large eggs

1 cup (250 ml) whole milk or 2% milk

½ teaspoon salt

Freshly ground pepper, to taste

1 teaspoon unbleached all-purpose flour

2 tablespoons vegetable oil

1 cup (80 g) mushrooms (any kind), rinsed, stems trimmed, and thinly sliced

1 cup (160 g) finely diced cooked potatoes

1 cup (100 g) blanched broccoli florets, finely chopped

1 teaspoon red or yellow curry powder

⅓ cup (25 g) sliced scallions

2 to 3 tablespoons chopped fresh flat-leaf parsley

⅓ cup (50 g) finely diced sun-dried tomatoes packed in oil

1 cup (80 g) grated reduced-fat cheddar cheese

1. Center an oven rack and preheat the oven to 400°F (200°C).

2. Combine the eggs, milk, salt, pepper, and flour in a bowl and mix until well blended; set aside.

3. Heat the vegetable oil in a 10-inch (25 cm) ovenproof skillet over medium heat, swirling or brushing the oil up the sides of the skillet. Add the mushrooms and sauté for 2 minutes, then add the potatoes, broccoli, and curry powder and sauté, stirring, for 1 to 2 minutes, until the vegetables are heated through and there is almost no liquid in the pan. Turn off the heat and add the scallions, parsley, sun-dried tomatoes, and the reserved egg mixture. Stir gently to distribute the liquid. Sprinkle the top with the cheddar cheese.

4. Bake for about 15 minutes, or until set. The frittata will look a bit puffed like a soufflé, but it will fall as it cools. Remove from the oven and allow to cool for 5 minutes before slicing.

Cooking Note: Finely dicing the vegetables will facilitate cutting the baked frittata. Also, if you notice the vegetables sticking to the pan in Step 3, brush the bottom and sides with a bit more oil, or use canola oil cooking spray.

Baking Note: To bake this frittata in a 9-inch (23 cm) Pyrex pie dish, follow Steps 1 and 2, then cook the vegetables according to Step 3, but instead of adding the reserved egg mixture to the skillet, grease the pie dish and arrange the cooked vegetables, including the scallions, parsley, and sun-dried tomatoes in the bottom of it. Add the egg mixture and top with the cheese. Bake for about 25 minutes, or until the middle is set. You won't get the same puffed-up effect of baking it in a skillet, but it will still be delicious.

CLASSIC DAL

This simple, wholesome, and fabulous lentil stew (also spelled *dahl* or *daal*) goes with just about any menu. Red lentils turn a golden yellow when cooked, so don't be surprised. You'll notice the Indian cooking term *tarka* here; see How to Make a Basic Indian Tarka (page 210) for more information on tarkas. It refers to a final seasoning that often includes sautéed cumin seeds, black mustard seeds, fresh ginger, garlic, curry leaves, dried chile peppers, and, sometimes, diced fresh tomatoes. Don't panic! You don't need all of these ingredients. Use what you have on hand. For optimal flavor, add the tarka just before serving. Short on time? Skip soaking the lentils and increase the cooking time a bit. This dal can be refrigerated for up to 3 days or frozen for up to 1 month. Keep in mind that the lentils will absorb water as they sit in the fridge, so you may need to thin this with a small amount of water when reheating. Be sure to garnish the dal with some chopped cilantro, mint leaves, and thinly sliced scallions.

SERVES 6

Dal

1½ cups (300 g) red lentils

3¼ cups (810 ml) water

½ teaspoon turmeric

Tarka

2 tablespoons vegetable oil

1 tablespoon cumin seeds

2 teaspoons black mustard seeds

¼ teaspoon cayenne, or to taste

2 garlic cloves, minced

2 cups (320 g) diced ripe tomatoes

2 tablespoons minced seeded green chiles

Garnishes

1 tablespoon fresh lemon juice, or to taste

3 to 4 tablespoons chopped fresh cilantro leaves

1. To wash the lentils, place them in a bowl, cover with tepid water, and gently swish with your fingers. Drain the lentils in a sieve and repeat this procedure one more time. (Note: The lentils will foam as you wash them; this is normal.)

2. To soak the lentils, place them back in the bowl, add water to cover them by about 4 inches (13 cm), and let them soak for 15 minutes before cooking. Soaked red lentils cook very quickly.

3. Bring the water to a boil in a medium saucepan. Drain the lentils and add them, along with the turmeric. Return to a boil, then reduce the heat and simmer for about 20 minutes, or until the lentils are soft and most of the water has evaporated. (Note: The lentils should be the consistency of a thick pea soup, but if you prefer a thinner dal, add more water.) Remove the saucepan from the heat, cover, and set aside while you make the tarka.

4. Heat the vegetable oil in skillet over medium heat until hot. Add the cumin

232 CALORIES IN

Protein: 13 g; Carbohydrates: 33 g; Fat: 6 g; Fiber: 6 g; Sodium: 9 mg; Carb Choices: 2; Diabetic Exchange: 2 Starch, 2 Very Lean Meat

232 CALORIES OUT

Women: Walk:
56 minutes | Jog: 27 minutes

Men: Walk:
47 minutes | Jog: 22 minutes

CALORIE COMBOS

Radish-Tomato-Cucumber Salsa (page 135): 12 cals

Cucumber Yogurt Sauce (page 141): 19 cals

Indian-Style Cucumber Yogurt Salad (page 75): 45 cals

Tomato, Cucumber, and Radish Salad (page 76): 55 cals

Hot-and-Sweet Cucumber, Carrot, and Red Bell Pepper Salad (page 77): 61 cals

½ cup (80 g) plain boiled diced potatoes: 67 cals

½ cup (75 g) plain couscous: 88 cals

½ cup (80 g) plain white rice: 103 cals

½ cup (90 g) plain brown rice: 108 cals

½ cup (65 g) plain quinoa: 111 cals

1 whole wheat chapati (Indian flatbread): 137 cals

Paneer with Spinach, Tomatoes, and Spices (page 113): 143 cals

Aromatic Brown Basmati Rice (page 107): 184 cals

Beans and Rice Indian-Style (page 118): 189 cals

Minty Basmati Rice and Potatoes (page 208): 206 cals

Lemony Basmati Rice (page 209): 210 cals

Quinoa, Paneer, and Cabbage Patties (page 220): 235 cals

(RECIPE CONTINUES)

seeds and mustard seeds and cook for 30 seconds, or until they are fragrant. Add the cayenne, then add the garlic, followed by the tomatoes and chiles, and cook, stirring, for about 2 minutes, or until the tomatoes release

their juices. Remove from the heat and stir the tarka into the lentils.

5. Rewarm the lentils if needed, then stir in the cilantro and lemon juice. Adjust the seasoning, transfer to a serving dish, and serve promptly.

HOW TO COOK LENTILS

Lentils are a nutritional powerhouse and so easy to prepare. All they require is a good rinse and a quick soak (10 to 20 minutes), depending on how much time you have before boiling them. I like to flavor the water with turmeric, and I hold off on adding salt until later—some say adding salt during cooking makes the lentils tough. The cooking time varies greatly according to the type of lentil (red cook the most quickly, black require the longest time), their quality (bins versus commercially processed boxes), and their age. I did not really believe the age factor until I had a bunch of old yellow lentils that took forever to cook, and to be honest, they never really got soft. But what is "old"? You won't know unless the packaging has an expiration date. If the lentils have been in your cupboard, fridge, or freezer for more than 9 months, consider them old. I use a conventional saucepan to cook lentils, but many Indians use a pressure cooker.

HOW TO COOK AND FREEZE QUINOA

Cooking quinoa is a lot like cooking couscous, though it takes a little longer. But before we get to the cooking, if your grains come from a bin, I highly recommend rinsing them in a fine-mesh sieve under cold running water to remove any bitterness from the natural outer coating. Packaged quinoa is usually well cleaned. Use 2 cups water for every 1 cup quinoa, or follow the package directions. Bring the water to a boil, add the quinoa, return to a boil, and stir, then reduce the heat to low and cook, covered, for 14 to 18 minutes, until the water has been absorbed and the quinoa is tender; the germ will have separated from the seed. Fluff with a fork, and add anything you want. Cooked quinoa can be refrigerated for up to 3 days, and it can be frozen for up to 1 month. I keep meal-size portions in Ziploc bags in the freezer, ready for an easy side dish for almost any meal. Thaw or reheat in a microwave.

QUINOA, PANEER, AND CABBAGE PATTIES

Keep a stash of these quinoa patties in your freezer for an easy vegetarian lunch or dinner. If you don't have paneer, an equal amount of ricotta cheese works well. These patties have a delicate flavor, but if you want more oomph, simply increase the spices. For a true feast, combine them with the Fresh Mint, Cilantro, and Green Chile Chutney; the Cucumber Yogurt Sauce; store-bought tamarind chutney; or one of the salsas or salads in this book. If you're on the go, stuff 2 patties into a whole wheat pita pocket and add greens, tomatoes, and a touch of your favorite dressing. The patties can be formed, covered, and refrigerated for up for 24 hours. Cooked patties can be frozen for up to 1 month; reheat in a microwave or in a skillet with a tiny bit of oil over medium-low heat.

MAKES TWELVE 2½-INCH (7 CM) PATTIES; SERVES 6

¾ cup (125 g) uncooked quinoa

1¼ cups (75 g) panko bread crumbs (see Cooking Note, opposite)

3 large eggs, lightly beaten

1½ cups (7 ounces/210 g) crumbled paneer

⅓ cup (20 g) thinly sliced scallions

½ cup (15 g) chopped fresh cilantro

1 cup (100 g) finely diced green cabbage

2 tablespoons fresh lemon juice

2 tablespoons minced seeded green chiles

2 teaspoons roasted ground cumin

2 tablespoons Dijon mustard

½ teaspoon salt, or to taste

Pinch of cayenne, optional

Freshly ground pepper, to taste

1½ tablespoons vegetable oil

1. In a small saucepan, combine the quinoa and 1½ cups (375 ml) water and bring to a boil. Cover and cook over low heat until the water has been absorbed, about 15 minutes (see How to Cook and Freeze Quinoa, page 219). Fluff with a fork and set aside to cool a bit.

2. In a medium bowl, combine the cooked quinoa, ¾ cup (45 g) of the bread crumbs, and all the remaining ingredients except the vegetable oil and mix until well blended. Before you shape the patties, you may want to make a test patty to check the seasoning: form about 1 tablespoon of the mixture into a patty and cook it in a little oil, turning once, until golden brown and heated through. Adjust the seasoning in the remaining mixture if needed.

3. To form the patties, spread the remaining ½ cup (30 g) bread crumbs in a pie plate. Have a plate ready large enough to hold the finished patties. Divide the quinoa mixture evenly into 12 portions, about ⅓ cup (80 ml) each, and form each portion into a patty. (Note: At this point, the patties can be covered and refrigerated for up to 12 hours.)

4. To cook, heat the vegetable oil in a large nonstick skillet over medium-low heat. Add the patties and cook for 3 to 4 minutes on each side, until they are golden brown and heated through. If your skillet cannot hold all of the patties without crowding, cook them in two batches. Transfer to the cooked patties to a platter and serve hot, with any accompanying sauces of your choice.

Cooking Note: Brown and black quinoa grains are finer than golden quinoa, about the size of black mustard seeds. They make beautiful patties, but they do tend to fall apart more easily because the grains are so much smaller. So if you use brown, black, or a mixture of quinoa grains, add an extra 1/3 cup (20 g) bread crumbs to the patty mixture.

BROILED SOLE WITH LEMONY PARMESAN GLAZE

This lemony Parmesan glaze is the perfect accompaniment for the delicate flavor of sole or any other mild white fish, such as flounder. I like to serve this dish with the Roasted New Potatoes and a vegetable or green salad. Be sure to use a high-quality light mayonnaise, such as Hellman's, for the glaze.

SERVES 4

Lemony Parmesan Glaze

¼ cup (60 ml) high-quality light mayonnaise

⅓ cup (25 g) finely grated Parmesan cheese

2 tablespoons grated lemon zest

2 tablespoons fresh lemon juice

½ teaspoon Worcestershire sauce

1 teaspoon minced garlic

Freshly ground pepper, to taste

Sole Rolls

Canola oil cooking spray

4 sole fillets, about 6 ounces (180 g) each, rinsed and patted dry with paper towels

Sprinkle of salt and freshly ground pepper

3 tablespoons chopped fresh flat-leaf parsley, for garnish

Lemon wedges, for garnish

1. To make the glaze, combine all the ingredients in a small bowl and mix well. Set aside.

2. To make the sole rolls, line a baking sheet with foil and lightly grease it with cooking spray. Lightly season both sides of the fillets with salt and pepper and turn them skinned side up (note that the skinned side will appear darker). Starting at the narrow end of one fillet, fold it in three and turn seam side down on the baking sheet. Repeat with the remaining fillets.

3. Position an oven rack 4 to 5 inches from the heating element and preheat the broiler to high. Broil the sole rolls until the tops are a light golden and the fish is cooked through, 7 to 10 minutes. The cooking time will depend on the thickness of the fillets. You can check by inserting the tip of a paring knife into the center of one roll; the fish should flake easily all the way through and be white. *Alternatively,* you can bake the fish in a preheated 400°F (200°C) oven for about 15 minutes; however, cooking the glaze will still need to be done under a broiler.

4. Remove the fish from the broiler (keep the broiler on) and divide the reserved glaze evenly over the tops of the rolls. Broil until the glaze is browned and bubbling, about 2 minutes. Transfer the fish to a serving platter, garnish with the parsley and lemon wedges, and serve promptly.

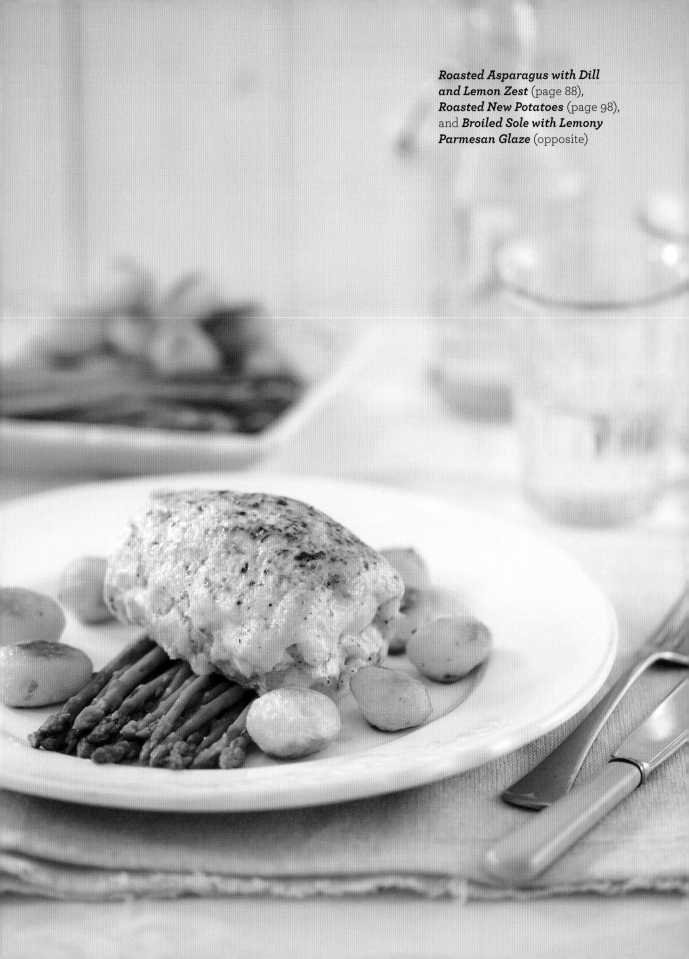

Roasted Asparagus with Dill and Lemon Zest (page 88), *Roasted New Potatoes* (page 98), and *Broiled Sole with Lemony Parmesan Glaze* (opposite)

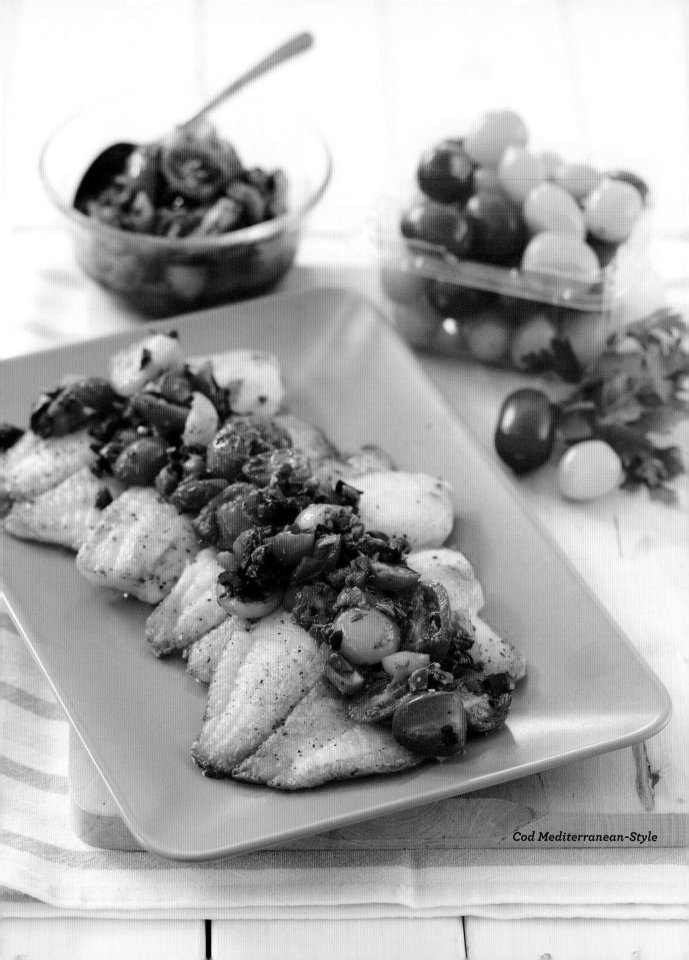

Cod Mediterranean-Style

COD MEDITERRANEAN-STYLE

"Mediterranean" here refers to the extra virgin olive oil, oregano, Kalamata olives, capers, tomatoes, and fresh herbs—some of my favorite ingredients to cook with. This sauce works with well any fish, shellfish, white meat, or even tofu. Any leftover sauce is scrumptious with pasta, rice, or whole grains.

SERVES 4

2 tablespoons extra virgin olive oil

1 garlic clove, minced

1 teaspoon dried oregano or Italian seasoning

½ cup (80 g) pitted Kalamata or other brine-cured black olives, coarsely chopped

15 ounces (about 3 cups, 450 g) cherry or grape tomatoes, halved

¼ cup (35 g) diced jarred roasted red bell peppers

2 tablespoons medium capers

¼ cup (10 g) chopped fresh flat-leaf parsley

¼ cup (10 g) chopped fresh basil

2 tablespoons fresh lemon juice, or to taste

Salt and freshly ground pepper, to taste

1½ pounds (720 g) cod fillets, rinsed and patted dry with paper towels

1. Heat 1 tablespoon of the olive oil in a large nonstick skillet over medium-high heat. Add the garlic and oregano and sauté for 30 seconds. Add the olives, tomatoes, red peppers, capers, parsley, basil, and lemon juice and cook for 2 minutes, or just until the tomatoes are soft and their skin begins to wrinkle. Do not overcook; the sauce will continue to cook off the heat. Adjust the seasoning, transfer to a heatproof bowl, cover, and set aside. (Do not rinse the skillet.)

2. Have a serving platter ready. Heat the remaining 1 tablespoon olive oil in the skillet over medium-high heat. (Note: If you can fit all of the fillets into the skillet without crowding them, cook them all at once. If not, cook them in batches.) Add half of the fish, lightly season it with salt and pepper, and cook for 3 minutes on each side, turning once. The fish should be cooked through and completely white when flaked with the tip of a knife in the thickest part of the flesh. Transfer the cooked fish to a serving platter or individual plates and cover with aluminum foil. Repeat with the remaining fish, making sure to reheat the skillet before adding the second batch.

3. Spoon the sauce over the fillets, and serve promptly.

247 CALORIES IN

Protein: 32 g; Carbohydrates: 6 g; Fat: 10 g; Fiber: 2 g; Sodium: 797 mg; Carb Choices: ½; Diabetic Exchange: 4½ Lean Meat

247 CALORIES OUT

Women: Walk: 60 minutes | Jog: 28 minutes

Men: Walk: 50 minutes | Jog: 24 minutes

CALORIE COMBOS

Roasted Asparagus with Dill and Lemon Zest (page 88): 47 cals

Broiled Zucchini with Parmesan (page 90): 49 cals

½ cup (80 g) plain boiled diced potatoes: 67 cals

Greek-Style Broccoli (page 91): 71 cals

½ cup (75 g) plain couscous: 88 cals

½ cup (80 g) plain white rice: 103 cals

½ cup (90 g) plain brown rice: 108 cals

½ cup (65 g) plain quinoa: 111 cals

Roasted New Potatoes (page 98): 118 cals

Brussels Sprouts with Parmesan and Pine Nuts (page 99): 118 cals

Smashed Potatoes with Herbs (page 102): 144 cals

Polenta with Herbs and Cheese (page 103): 146 cals

Caesar Salad with a Light Touch (page 83): 163 cals

Spinach Salad with Mushrooms, Fennel, and Avocado (page 201): 251 cals

CALORIE COMBOS

Cucumber Yogurt Sauce (page 141): 19 cals

Fresh Mint, Cilantro, and Green Chile Chutney (page 143): 30 cals

Roasted Asparagus with Dill and Lemon Zest (page 88): 47 cals

Tomato, Cucumber, and Radish Salad (page 76): 55 cals

Roasted Cauliflower and Mushrooms with Pine Nuts (page 93): 85 cals

½ cup (75 g) plain couscous: 88 cals

Grilled Vegetables (page 108): 89 cals

Maple-Glazed Carrots (page 95): 98 cals

½ cup (80 g) plain white rice: 103 cals

½ cup (90 g) plain brown rice: 108 cals

½ cup (65 g) plain quinoa: 111 cals

Roasted New Potatoes (page 98): 118 cals

Paneer with Spinach, Tomatoes, and Spices (page 113): 143 cals

Aromatic Basmati Rice (page 107): 184 cals

Minty Basmati Rice and Potatoes (page 208): 206 cals

Lemony Basmati Rice (page 209): 210 cals

INDIAN-SPICED BROILED SALMON

This delicious marinade can be used for almost anything. The salmon is one of my favorite dishes for entertaining. One of my recipe testers tried it out for a dinner party. In her notes, she wrote: "Tell readers not to be overwhelmed by the number of unfamiliar spices. It's easy to handle. Just mix them all, and the sauce is ready in 10 minutes. Thank you for opening my eyes to the world of spices. This was delicious." My pleasure! I like to serve this dish with Minty Basmati Rice and Potatoes or Aromatic Brown Basmati Rice. For more information on the Indian spices, see Ingredient Notes (page 339).

SERVES 4

Indian-Spiced Marinade

1 teaspoon roasted ground coriander

1 teaspoon roasted ground cumin

¼ teaspoon ground cinnamon

1 teaspoon garam masala

2 teaspoons paprika

½ teaspoon turmeric

¼ teaspoon cayenne, or to taste

1 teaspoon sugar

½ teaspoon salt

1 teaspoon garlic powder

3 tablespoons low-fat plain Greek-style yogurt

1 tablespoon fresh lemon juice

Salmon

4 skinless center-cut salmon fillets, about 6 ounces (180 g) each, rinsed and patted dry with paper towels

Canola oil cooking spray

Coarsely chopped fresh cilantro, for garnish, optional

Sliced scallions, for garnish, optional

Lemon or lime wedges, for garnish, optional

1. To make the marinade, combine all of the ingredients in a small bowl and mix until smooth.

2. To marinate the salmon, place the salmon fillets in a Pyrex baking dish. Cover each with some of marinade, then gently turn them until all sides are well coated. Cover with plastic wrap and refrigerate for at least 2 hours, and up to 8 hours.

3. To broil the salmon, adjust an oven rack one or two rungs down from the heating element and preheat the broiler to high. Line a baking sheet with sides with foil, grease it with cooking spray, and arrange the fillets on it, skinned side down. Place the fish under the broiler and cook for 10 to 12 minutes, depending on the thickness. (There is no need to turn the fish.) Check every 5 minutes: the fish should be cooked through when flaked with the tip of a knife in the thickest part of the flesh.

4. Transfer the salmon to a serving platter or individual plates and garnish with the optional garnishes, if using, and serve promptly.

TUNA WITH TOMATO-BASIL-BALSAMIC DRESSING

This light balsamic-tomato dressing works for any fish. Here I pair it with pan-seared tuna, but you could also cook the tuna on the grill. If you want to avoid the brown hue of regular balsamic vinegar, use white balsamic. I like to serve the fillets on small mounds of baby greens or arugula. The amount of garlic can be adjusted to suit your taste. This dressing is best served promptly, as the tomatoes tend to get soggy and the basil will brown if left in the refrigerator. But if you do have any left over, it can be added to a salad or used for Allie's Bruschetta (page 71).

SERVES 4

Tomato-Basil-Balsamic Dressing

2 tablespoons balsamic vinegar, or to taste

2 tablespoons extra virgin olive oil

1 garlic clove, minced, or to taste

Salt and freshly ground pepper, to taste

12 ounces (360 g) ripe tomatoes (about 3 large), seeded, finely diced, and drained (1½ cups, 375 ml), or 12 ounces (360 g) cherry tomatoes, diced

2 tablespoons chopped fresh basil, or to taste

Tuna

4 tuna steaks, about 4 ounces (120 g) each, rinsed and patted dry with paper towels

Sprinkle of salt and freshly ground pepper

1 tablespoon extra virgin olive oil

1. To make the dressing, in a bowl, whisk the balsamic vinegar, olive oil, garlic, salt, and pepper. Add the tomatoes and basil and gently mix with a spoon. Adjust the seasoning and set aside at room temperature while you cook the fish.

2. Season both sides of the tuna steaks with salt and pepper. In a large nonstick skillet, heat the olive oil over medium-high heat. Add the tuna steaks and cook for 3 to 5 minutes on each side, depending on the thickness. The steaks should be light golden brown on the outside and cooked to your desired doneness; some people prefer tuna on the rare side, while others like it well done.

3. Transfer the fish to a serving platter. Spoon some of the dressing over each steak, or pass it in a bowl at the table.

263 CALORIES IN

Protein: 27 g; Carbohydrates: 5 g; Fat: 14 g; Fiber: 1 g; Sodium: 196 mg; Carb Choices: 0; Diabetic Exchange: 4 Lean Meat, 1 Vegetable

263 CALORIES OUT

Women: Walk: 64 minutes | Jog: 30 minutes

Men: Walk: 54 minutes | Jog: 25 minutes

CALORIE COMBOS

Roasted Asparagus with Dill and Lemon Zest (page 88): 47 cals

Broiled Zucchini with Parmesan (page 90): 49 cals

Lemony Dill Cabbage Slaw (page 78): 63 cals

Greek-Style Broccoli (page 91): 71 cals

Roasted Cauliflower and Mushrooms with Pine Nuts (page 93): 85 cals

½ cup (80 g) plain white rice: 103 cals

½ cup (90 g) plain brown rice: 108 cals

½ cup (65 g) plain quinoa: 111 cals

Roasted New Potatoes (page 98): 118 cals

Brussels Sprouts with Parmesan and Pine Nuts (page 99): 118 cals

Smashed Potatoes with Herbs (page 102): 144 cals

Polenta with Herbs and Cheese (page 103): 146 cals

Caesar Salad with a Light Touch (page 83): 163 cals

Spinach Salad with Mushrooms, Fennel, and Avocado (page 201): 251 cals

CALORIE CUTS

The dressing has 85 calories and almost 7 grams of fat per serving, so maybe use less of it if you're trying to cut back on calories.

279 CALORIES IN

Protein: 36 g; Carbohydrates: 5 g; Fat: 12 g; Fiber: 2 g; Sodium: 444 mg; Carb Choices: 0; Diabetic Exchange: 5 Lean Meat

279 CALORIES OUT

Women: Walk: 68 minutes | Jog: 32 minutes

Men: Walk: 57 minutes | Jog: 27 minutes

CALORIE COMBOS

Broiled Portobello Mushrooms with Herbs (page 86): 23 cals

Roasted Asparagus with Dill and Lemon Zest (page 88): 47 cals

Broiled Zucchini with Parmesan (page 90): 49 cals

½ cup (80 g) plain boiled diced potatoes: 67 cals

Greek-Style Broccoli (page 91): 71 cals

½ cup (75 g) plain couscous: 88 cals

½ cup (80 g) plain white rice: 103 cals

½ cup (90 g) plain brown rice: 108 cals

½ cup (65 g) plain quinoa: 111 cals

Roasted New Potatoes (page 98): 118 cals

Smashed Potatoes with Herbs (page 102): 144 cals

1 medium baked potato: 161 cals

Caesar Salad with a Light Touch (page 83): 163 cals

1 cup (100 g) plain whole wheat pasta: 174 cals

CALORIE CUTS

The tapenade has 94 calories and almost 8 grams of fat per serving, so use less of it if you're trying to cut back on calories.

SNAPPER WITH OLIVE-ARTICHOKE-TOMATO TAPENADE

Don't be surprised if you find yourself eating spoonfuls of this tapenade before you serve it. I love it with whole wheat crackers, and I often serve it as a topping for Allie's Bruschetta (page 71). To save time, you can put the whole artichoke hearts in a food processor and pulse into dice, then add the chopped olives and dill and process a bit more. The tomatoes should be sliced by hand. Do not process to a puree. Any extra artichoke hearts can be used in salads.

SERVES 4

Olive-Artichoke-Tomato Tapenade

⅓ cup (40 g) chopped green olives with pimientos

½ cup (130 g) finely chopped drained canned artichoke hearts

½ cup (80 g) finely diced red and/or yellow cherry or grape tomatoes, or a mix of both

1 tablespoon grated lemon zest, or to taste

2 tablespoons extra virgin olive oil

2 tablespoons fresh lemon juice, or to taste

3 tablespoons chopped fresh dill

Pinch of red pepper flakes or cayenne, optional

Snapper

4 skin-on snapper fillets, about 6 ounces (180 g) each, rinsed and patted dry with paper towels

Salt and freshly ground pepper

1 tablespoon extra virgin olive oil

1. To make the tapenade, in a small bowl, mix all of the ingredients until well combined. Adjust the seasoning and set aside.

2. Season both sides of each fillet with salt and pepper. Heat the olive oil in a large nonstick skillet over medium-high heat. When it is hot, add the snapper fillets, flesh side down, and cook until light golden, about 4 minutes. Flip the fillets and cook the other side for about 4 minutes, depending on the thickness. The fish should be cooked through and white when flaked with the tip of a knife in the thickest part of the flesh.

3. Transfer the fish to a platter or individual plates and serve with the tapenade spooned on the fish, or on the side.

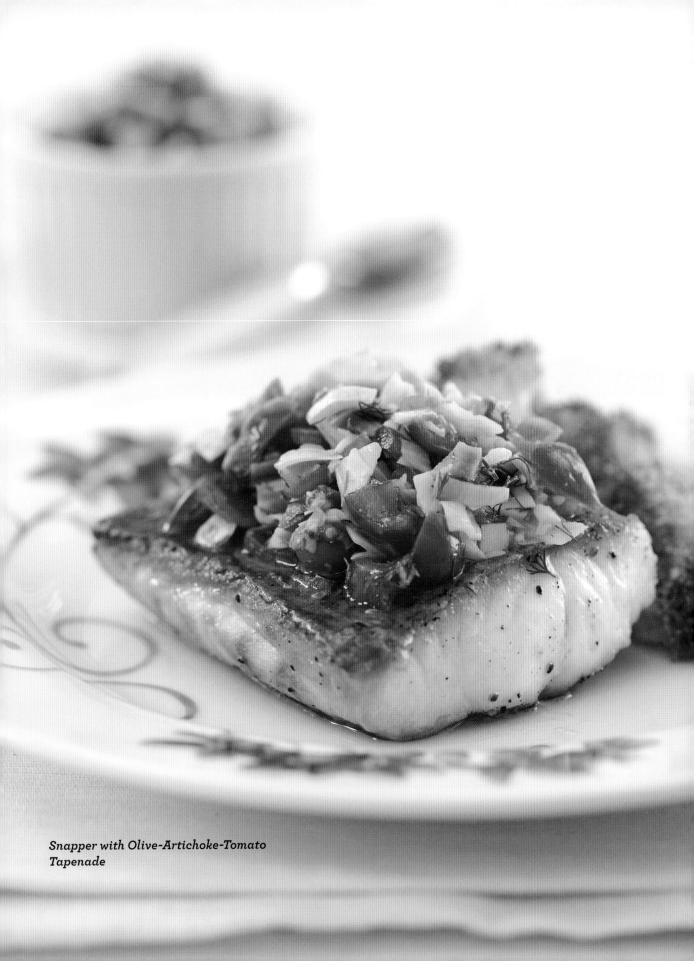

Snapper with Olive-Artichoke-Tomato Tapenade

FISH STICKS FOR HALE

These fish sticks are for my son, Hale, because this is his favorite way to eat fish, and for me, that's okay for a teenager. Truth be told, I like these too, especially with a squeeze of lemon or lime and some of my Super-Easy Tartar Sauce or Creamy Cocktail Sauce. (Hale prefers ketchup.) The tempura-like batter, which I learned to make in Asia, absorbs less oil than a traditional thicker one made with egg, and it produces crispy, very light fish sticks. This batter also works well with calamari and shrimp. You may need to adjust the batter to get the right consistency: if it's too thin, the bread crumbs won't adhere well; too thick, and it becomes a bit like glue.

SERVES 3

½ cup (about 50 g) cornstarch

About ¼ cup (60 ml) warm water

12 ounces (360 g) skinless white fish fillets, such as tilapia, rinsed, patted dry with paper towels, and sliced into 2½ by 1-inch (7 by 3 cm) strips

Sprinkle of salt and freshly ground pepper

About 1 cup (50 g) panko bread crumbs

5 tablespoons vegetable oil

Lemon or lime wedges, for garnish

1. To make the batter, in a medium bowl, combine the cornstarch and water and mix until smooth. The batter should be the consistency of heavy cream. Add more water to thin, or cornstarch to thicken, a couple of teaspoons at time, if needed.

2. Season the fish with the salt and pepper. Add it to the batter and gently mix until well coated. Place the bread crumbs in a pie dish. Have another pie dish or large plate ready for the breaded fish. Lift one piece of fish at a time from the batter, coat it with the bread crumbs, and place it in the second pie dish. (Note: The fish can be breaded up to 8 hours in advance; cover and refrigerate.)

3. Line a serving platter with paper towels. Heat the vegetable oil in a medium nonstick skillet over medium-high heat. When the oil is hot, add the fish sticks in batches (avoid crowding) and fry, turning as needed, until they are golden and cooked through, about 5 minutes. Drain on the paper towels and serve with the lemon wedges.

OLD BAY AND DILL SALMON PATTIES (📷 page 232)

It's easy to get hooked on these salmon cakes. The serving options are endless: two classics are the Super-Easy Tartar Sauce and the Creamy Cocktail Sauce. For a fantastic appetizer, make bite-size patties or balls. One of my recipe testers wrote, "This was an unexpected hit with everyone. My family is not super keen on seafood, but they all enjoyed this dish. My son suggested serving the patties with buns next time so that he could eat his as a burger." Kids liking fish—music to my ears.

SERVES 4

1 pound (480 g) skinless center-cut salmon fillets (2½ cups/625 ml loosely packed minced salmon)

3 tablespoons panko bread crumbs, plus ½ cup (35 g) for breading the patties

1 large egg, lightly beaten

2 tablespoons chopped fresh dill

1 tablespoon finely sliced fresh chives or scallions

1 tablespoon drained and chopped medium capers

2 teaspoons grated lemon zest

2 teaspoons fresh lemon juice

2 teaspoons Dijon mustard

2 tablespoons nonfat mayonnaise

1 teaspoon Old Bay seasoning, or to taste

¼ teaspoon salt, or to taste

2 tablespoons vegetable oil, for cooking

Lemon or lime wedges, for garnish

1. To make the salmon cakes, remove any pin bones from the salmon. Using a sharp chef's knife, finely chop the salmon. Put the salmon in a pile and give it a few more chops to give it a minced texture. (Note: Do not use a food processor, or the salmon will become pasty and the cakes will be very dry.)

2. Place the salmon in a bowl and add the 3 tablespoons bread crumbs and all of the remaining ingredients except the vegetable oil and lemon wedges. Mix gently until well incorporated.

3. Place the remaining ½ cup (125 ml) bread crumbs in a pie dish. Form the patties into the desired size, then dip them in the bread crumbs, pressing gently so the crumbs adhere. Place the patties on a plate, cover with plastic wrap, and refrigerate until ready to cook (Note: The patties can be made up to 8 hours in advance; cover, refrigerate, and cook straight from the fridge.)

4. To cook, heat the vegetable oil in a large nonstick skillet over medium-high heat. Add 3 or 4 patties, to avoid overcrowding, and cook the first side for 3 to 5 minutes, until golden brown. Carefully flip and cook the other side for 3 to 5 minutes, until golden brown and thoroughly heated. You may need to adjust the heat if the patties begin browning too quickly. Transfer the cooked patties to a serving platter and cover loosely with foil to keep warm. Cook the remaining salmon patties, and serve promptly, with your preferred sauce, if desired, and lemon wedges.

---

283 CALORIES IN

Protein: 25 g; Carbohydrates: 8 g; Fat: 16 g; Fiber: 0 g; Sodium: 428 mg; Carb Choices: ½; Diabetic Exchange: 3 Medium-Fat Meat, ½ Starch

283 CALORIES OUT

Women: Walk:
69 minutes | Jog: 32 minutes

Men: Walk:
58 minutes | Jog: 27 minutes

CALORIE COMBOS

1 tablespoon jarred salsa: 5 cals

1 tablespoon Super-Easy Tartar Sauce (page 119): 14 cals

1 tablespoon Creamy Cocktail Sauce (page 136): 14 cals

Roasted Asparagus with Dill and Lemon Zest (page 88): 47 cals

Broiled Zucchini with Parmesan (page 90): 49 cals

Lemony Dill Cabbage Slaw (page 78): 63 cals

½ cup (75 g) plain couscous: 88 cals

2 cups (40 g) salad greens with 1 tablespoon Benihana-Style Ginger-Sesame Dressing (page 155): 89 cals

½ cup (80 g) plain white rice: 103 cals

½ cup (90 g) plain brown rice: 108 cals

1 whole wheat hamburger bun: 110 cals

Roasted New Potatoes (page 98): 118 cals

Creamy All-American Potato Salad (page 80): 121 cals

Caesar Salad with a Light Touch (page 83): 163 cals

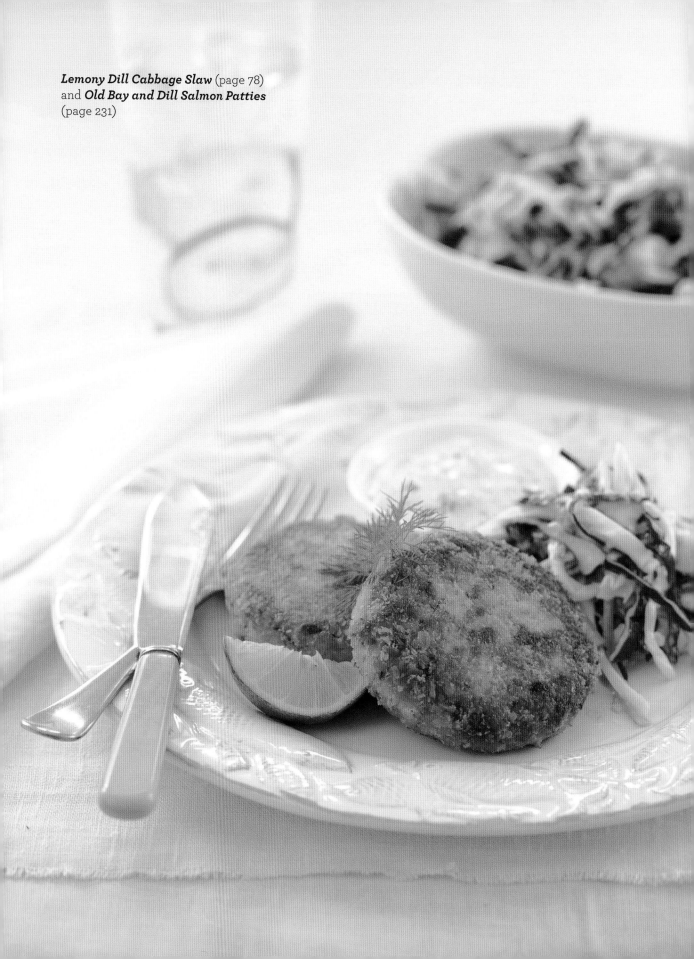

Lemony Dill Cabbage Slaw (page 78) and *Old Bay and Dill Salmon Patties* (page 231)

SWORDFISH WITH CILANTRO-MINT SAUCE

This light, supremely satisfying cilantro-mint sauce is a brilliant addition to any fish or shellfish, or just about any main course. It can be made up to 12 hours in advance; cover with plastic wrap (pressing it flush with the surface of the sauce), and refrigerate. I often make extra sauce and freeze it to have on hand. The swordfish is grilled in this recipe, but it can also be pan-seared for about 8 minutes over medium-high heat, or broiled under high heat. The timing will depend on the intensity of your broiler and the thickness of the swordfish steaks.

SERVES 4

Swordfish

4 swordfish steaks, about 4 ounces (120 g) each, rinsed and patted dry with paper towels

2 tablespoons balsamic vinegar

1 tablespoon extra virgin olive oil

Sprinkle of salt and freshly ground pepper

Cilantro-Mint Sauce

1 cup (40 g) tightly packed fresh cilantro leaves

⅓ cup (15 g) tightly packed fresh mint leaves

2 tablespoons fresh lime juice, or to taste

2 teaspoons toasted sesame oil

2 tablespoons canola oil

Salt and freshly ground pepper, to taste

1. Place the swordfish steaks in a Pyrex baking dish, add the balsamic vinegar, olive oil, salt, and pepper, and turn to coat all sides. Cover with plastic wrap and refrigerate for at least 30 minutes, and up to 6 hours.

2. To make the sauce, combine all of the ingredients in a food processor and process until fairly smooth. If you need more liquid, add 1 tablespoon water. Adjust the seasoning, transfer to a small bowl, and set aside. Refrigerate if not using right away.

3. For a charcoal grill: Light a chimney starter filled with charcoal briquettes. When the coals are hot, spread them evenly over the bottom of the grill and set the cooking grate in place. Cover and heat until hot, about 5 minutes. For a gas grill: Turn all the burners to medium, cover, and heat until hot, about 10 minutes.

4. Have a serving platter ready for the cooked swordfish. Oil the grill grate. Grill the steaks over medium heat, closing the lid and adjusting the heat as necessary, for 4 to 5 minutes per side, depending on the thickness. The fish should be cooked through when checked with the tip of a knife in the thickest part of the flesh. Transfer the swordfish to the platter and serve with the sauce on top or on the side.

284 CALORIES IN

Protein: 23 g; Carbohydrates: 2 g; Fat: 20 g; Fiber: 0 g; Sodium: 96 mg; Carb Choices: 0; Diabetic Exchange: 3 High-Fat Meat

284 CALORIES OUT

Women: Walk:
69 minutes | Jog: 33 minutes

Men: Walk:
58 minutes | Jog: 27 minutes

CALORIE COMBOS

Broiled Portobello Mushrooms with Herbs (page 86): 23 cals

Roasted Asparagus with Dill and Lemon Zest (page 88): 47 cals

Broiled Zucchini with Parmesan (page 90): 49 cals

2 cups (40 g) salad greens with 1 tablespoon Classic Red Wine Vinaigrette (page 146): 62 cals

Lemony Dill Cabbage Slaw (page 78): 63 cals

Greek-Style Broccoli (page 91): 71 cals

½ cup (75 g) plain couscous: 88 cals

½ cup (80 g) plain white rice: 103 cals

½ cup (90 g) plain brown rice: 108 cals

½ cup (65 g) plain quinoa: 111 cals

CALORIE CUTS

You could skip the sauce (a sad thought) and save 84 calories and almost 7 grams of fat per serving.

WHITE MEATS

CHICKEN TERIYAKI WITH VEGETABLES

Chicken teriyaki is a favorite recipe among all ages. There are numerous bottled teriyaki sauces on grocery store shelves and some of them are excellent. If you're short on time, substitute one of them for my sauce. One great thing about this dish is that the sauce can be made up in advance and refrigerated for up to 3 days or frozen for up to a month. If your skillet is not large enough to accommodate all of the vegetables, sauté them in two batches; overcrowding a stir-fry is never a good idea. Shrimp, tofu, or beef can be used in place of the chicken. Also, feel free to replace the vegetables with your favorite ones.

SERVES 6

Teriyaki Sauce

¾ cup (185 ml) water

3 tablespoons lite soy sauce

1 teaspoon Worcestershire sauce

¼ cup (40 g) brown sugar

2 tablespoons seasoned rice vinegar

2 teaspoons cornstarch

Stir-Fry

1¼ pounds (600 g) chicken tenders, cut into 1½-inch (4 cm) strips

Freshly ground pepper

2 teaspoons cornstarch

2 teaspoons toasted sesame oil

1 tablespoon lite soy sauce

1 tablespoon plus 1 teaspoon vegetable oil

1 large sweet onion, halved and sliced into thin strips

1 medium red bell pepper, cored, seeded, and sliced into thin strips

1 medium zucchini, halved lengthwise and sliced into thin strips on the diagonal

1 large garlic clove, minced

1. To make the sauce, in a small saucepan, combine all of the ingredients, stir, and bring to a boil. Reduce the heat and simmer for about 10 minutes, or until the sauce becomes a bit syrupy and reduces to about 1 cup. Set aside.

2. Combine the chicken with the pepper, cornstarch, sesame oil, and soy sauce in a bowl, turning to coat; set aside.

3. Have a large serving platter ready for the finished dish. In a very large nonstick skillet, heat ½ tablespoon of the vegetable oil over high heat. Add half the vegetables and garlic and sauté, stirring constantly, for 2 to 3 minutes, until crisp-tender; do not overcook. If the vegetables stick, add 1 tablespoon water to the skillet. Transfer the vegetables to the middle of the serving platter. Cover with foil.

4. Add ½ tablespoon of the vegetable oil to the skillet and heat over high heat. Sauté the remaining vegetables in the same way, then add them to the platter. (Do not rinse the skillet.)

5. Add the remaining 1 teaspoon vegetable oil to the skillet and heat over high heat. Add half of the reserved chicken and cook until golden brown on both sides and cooked through, about 7 minutes. Transfer the chicken to the platter with the vegetables, arranging it around or on top of the vegetables. Cook the remaining chicken in the same way, adding 1 teaspoon more oil if needed, and transfer to the platter.

6. While the chicken is cooking, reheat the teriyaki sauce over low heat. Adjust the seasoning and pour the sauce over the chicken and vegetables. Serve promptly.

212 CALORIES IN

Protein: 37 g; Carbohydrates: 3 g;
Fat: 5 g; Fiber: 0 g; Sodium: 447
mg; Carb Choices: 0; Diabetic
Exchange: 6 Very Lean Meat

212 CALORIES OUT

Women: Walk:
52 minutes | Jog: 24 minutes

Men: Walk:
43 minutes | Jog: 20 minutes

CALORIE COMBOS

Fresh Mint, Cilantro, and Green
Chile Chutney (page 143): 30 cals

Indian-Style Cucumber Yogurt
Salad (page 75): 45 cals

Tomato, Cucumber, and Radish
Salad (page 76): 55 cals

Grilled Vegetables (page 108):
89 cals

½ cup (80 g) plain white rice:
103 cals

½ cup (90 g) plain brown rice:
108 cals

½ cup (75 g) plain quinoa: 111 cals

Roasted New Potatoes (page 98):
118 cals

1 whole wheat chapati (Indian
flatbread): 137 cals

Aromatic Brown Basmati Rice
(page 107): 184 cals

Minty Basmati Rice and Potatoes
(page 208): 206 cals

Lemony Basmati Rice (page 209):
210 cals

Classic Dal (page 217): 232 cals

Spinach Salad with Mushrooms,
Fennel, and Avocado (page 201):
251 cal

1 naan (Indian bread): 234 cals

GRILLED CHICKEN TANDOORI

There is no doubt that the delicious cuisine of India is becoming increasingly popular and accessible around the globe. Spices are the key to Indian food, and lucky for cooks in the West, high-quality spices are becoming more readily available, too. One particularly good all-natural tandoori mix is Sukhi's Tandoori Marinade. To save time, you can mince the garlic and ginger in a mini food processor. If you have the time and you want to make your marinade using a homemade spice blend, see How to Make a Tandoori Yogurt Marinade, opposite, and use it in place of the simpler marinade in this recipe. Traditional garnishes for chicken tandoori include fresh lemon wedges, onion slices (see How to Take the Edge off Raw Onions, page 192), tomato slices, and cilantro sprigs. Serve with the Fresh Mint, Cilantro, and Green Chile Chutney or Cucumber Yogurt Sauce, if you like.

SERVES 5

Tandoori Marinade

**½ cup (120 g) nonfat plain
Greek-style yogurt**

2 teaspoons minced garlic

**2 teaspoons minced peeled
fresh ginger**

**1 tablespoon fresh lemon
juice**

**2 tablespoons tandoori spice
mix (see headnote)**

½ teaspoon paprika

**2½ pounds (1.25 kg) skinless
bone-in chicken parts**

1. For the marinade, in a medium bowl, combine all of the ingredients and mix well; set aside.

2. Using the tip of a sharp knife, score each piece of chicken 2 or 3 times in the thickest part (see How To Score Bone-In Chicken Parts, page 245). Add the chicken to the bowl, mix until it is well coated with the marinade, cover, and refrigerate for at least 2 hours, and up to 24 hours.

3. For a charcoal grill: Light a chimney starter filled with charcoal briquettes. When the coals are hot, spread them evenly over the bottom of the grill and set the cooking grate in place. Cover and heat until hot, about 5 minutes. For a gas grill: Turn all the burners to medium, cover, and heat until hot, about 10 minutes.

4. Have a serving platter ready for the cooked chicken. Oil the grill grate. Grill the chicken over medium heat, turning and moving the pieces and adjusting the heat as needed, and moving the lid off and on, until the meat is completely cooked, 6 to 8 minutes per side. Pierce the meat in the thickest parts to make sure the juices run clear. (Note: An instant-read thermometer should read 165°F [74°C].) Transfer to the serving platter and serve promptly.

HOW TO MAKE A TANDOORI YOGURT MARINADE

There is nothing like homemade spice mixes, and all serious Indian cooks have their own secret recipes. Here is my own delicious recipe. You can use this in place of the marinade in the recipe opposite, or as a marinade for chicken, seafood, tofu, or anything you like.

MAKES ABOUT I CUP (250 ML)

⅓ cup (80 ml) chopped onion

2 garlic cloves, halved

2 tablespoons coarsely chopped peeled fresh ginger

2 tablespoons fresh lemon juice

½ cup (120 g) nonfat plain Greek-style yogurt

2 teaspoons roasted ground coriander

1 teaspoon roasted ground cumin

½ teaspoon salt

½ teaspoon turmeric

¼ teaspoon cayenne

½ teaspoon garam masala

¼ teaspoon ground cinnamon

½ teaspoon sugar

Combine the onions, garlic, ginger, and lemon juice in a food processor and process to a paste. Add the remaining ingredients and pulse until combined. Proceed with your recipe. If not using immediately, cover and refrigerate for up to 2 days.

HOW TO ROAST AND GRIND SPICES

The key to bringing out the flavors and aromas of whole spices, such as cumin and coriander, is to dry-roast the whole seeds before grinding. Roasting small amounts of seeds is most easily done in a very small skillet; use a larger one for bigger batches. Heat the skillet over medium-low heat (never use high heat, or the spices may burn). When it's hot, add the seeds and shake the skillet, adjusting the heat if needed, until they begin to smell fragrant, 1 to 2 minutes. Keep an eye on them and try not to brown them. Seeds tend to burn very easily, and if burned, they turn bitter so you will have to toss them. Cool, then grind in a spice grinder, or use a mortar and pestle.

EASY LIME-CILANTRO GRILLED CHICKEN

A simple marinade that takes Asian-inspired chicken to a delicious new level. The best way to get the most flavor in the meat, as well as to speed up the cooking process, is to score the bone-in chicken parts. I give detailed instructions in the box on page 245. This marinade is also perfect for meaty seafood, such as salmon, swordfish, halibut, or tuna steaks. Feel free to add more lime juice to the marinade if you like.

SERVES 5

Marinade

½ cup (20 g) lightly packed chopped fresh cilantro leaves and stems

3 tablespoons lite soy sauce

3 tablespoons fresh lime juice, or to taste

½ teaspoon garlic powder

¼ teaspoon red pepper flakes, or to taste, optional

Pinch of sugar

2 pounds (1 kg) skinless bone-in chicken parts, scored

Lime wedges, for garnish

3 tablespoons chopped fresh cilantro leaves, for garnish

1. To make the marinade, in a medium bowl, combine all of the ingredients and mix well. Add the scored chicken, mix well, cover, and refrigerate for at least 6 hours, and up to 12 hours.

2. For a charcoal grill: Light a chimney starter filled with charcoal briquettes. When the coals are hot, spread them evenly over the bottom of the grill and set the cooking grate in place. Cover and heat until hot, about 5 minutes. For a gas grill: Turn all the burners to medium, cover, and heat until hot, about 10 minutes.

3. Have a serving platter ready for the cooked chicken. Oil the grill grate. Grill the chicken over medium heat, turning and moving the pieces and adjusting the heat as needed, and closing the lid off and on, until the meat is completely cooked, 6 to 8 minutes per side. Pierce the meat in the thickest parts to make sure the juices run clear. (Note: An instant-read thermometer should read 165°F [74°C].) Transfer to the serving platter, garnish with the lime wedges, sprinkle with the cilantro, and serve promptly.

CHICKEN, MUSHROOM, RED BELL PEPPER, AND PINEAPPLE KEBABS (📷 page 241)

Dijon mustard, white wine, fresh basil, garlic, and Italian seasoning can make any chicken dish taste great. Add mushrooms, onions, red bell peppers, and sweet pineapple, and you have a spectacular kebab. Vary the amounts of the ingredients as you wish. This marinade is also delicious with grilled seafood or roasted chicken (see Cooking Note). Don't grill over a high flame, as that could singe the vegetables and fruit.

MAKES ABOUT 12 SKEWERS; SERVES 6

Dijon-Basil Marinade

⅓ cup (80 ml) white wine

1 tablespoon extra virgin olive oil

1 tablespoon Dijon mustard

3 tablespoons chopped fresh basil

1 teaspoon garlic powder

½ teaspoon cayenne, or to taste, optional

1 tablespoon Italian seasoning

½ teaspoon salt

1 teaspoon sugar

Freshly ground pepper, to taste

Skewers

1½ pounds (720 g) skinless, boneless chicken breasts or tenders, cut into 1½-inch (4 cm) pieces

2 to 3 small onions, cut into cubes

About 10 ounces (300 g) fresh pineapple, cut into 1-inch (2.5 cm) pieces

1 large red bell pepper, cored, seeded, and cut into 1-inch (2.5-cm) pieces

About 8 ounces (240 g) cremini or button mushrooms, rinsed, stems trimmed, and cut in half if large

Canola oil cooking spray

1. To make the marinade, in a medium bowl, whisk together all of the ingredients. Add the chicken, stir until well coated, and then, using a fork, prick the chicken to allow the marinade to seep in. Cover with plastic wrap and refrigerate for at least 3 hours, and up to 12 hours.

2. To make the skewers, thread the chicken, onions, pineapple, red bell peppers, and mushrooms, alternating them, onto twelve 12-inch (30 cm) metal or soaked bamboo skewers. Leave enough room at the ends of the skewers so you can hold them comfortably during grilling. Keep the extra marinade for basting the skewers as they cook.

3. For a charcoal grill: Light a chimney starter filled with charcoal briquettes. When the coals are hot, spread them evenly over the bottom of the grill and set the cooking grate in place. Cover and heat until hot, about 5 minutes. For a gas grill: Turn all the burners to high, cover, and heat until hot, about 10 minutes.

4. Have a serving platter ready for the cooked kebabs. Oil the grill grate with the cooking spray, then reduce the heat to medium. Grill the kebabs, uncovered, basting them occasionally in the first few minutes of

224 CALORIES IN

Protein: 26 g; Carbohydrates: 15 g; Fat: 5 g; Fiber: 2 g; Sodium: 394 mg; Carb Choices: 1; Diabetic Exchange: 4 Very Lean Meat, 1 Fruit, 1 Vegetable

224 CALORIES OUT

Women: Walk:
55 minutes | Jog: 26 minutes

Men: Walk:
46 minutes | Jog: 22 minutes

CALORIE COMBOS

Broiled Portobello Mushrooms with Herbs (page 86): 23 cals

Lemony Dill Cabbage Slaw (page 78): 63 cals

Grilled Vegetables (page 108): 89 cals

½ cup (80 g) plain white rice: 103 cals

½ cup (90 g) plain brown rice: 108 cals

½ cup (65 g) plain quinoa: 111 cals

Sautéed Kale with Beans and Balsamic Vinegar (page 97): 116 cals

Roasted New Potatoes (page 98): 118 cals

Polenta with Herbs and Cheese (page 103): 146 cals

Great Green Couscous (page 105): 152 cals

Austrian-Style Potato Salad (page 82): 156 cals

Caesar Salad with a Light Touch (page 83): 163 cals

Tomato, Artichoke Heart, Feta, and White Bean Salad (page 84): 168 cals

Couscous Salad with Harissa Dressing (page 198): 241 cals

Pasta Salad with Sun-Dried Tomato Pesto and Mozzarella Cheese (page 202): 264 cals

(RECIPE CONTINUES)

cooking with the reserved marinade. Turn and move the pieces and adjust the heat as needed, until the vegetables and chicken are nicely browned and the chicken is cooked through, 5 to 7 minutes. Cut a piece of chicken in half to check for doneness. Transfer the kebabs to the platter and serve promptly.

Cooking Note: This marinade is wonderful on roasted bone-in chicken parts. To serve 4, use about 2½ pounds (1.25 kg) of chicken parts and marinate, covered and refrigerated, for at least 6 hours, and up to 24 hours. Be sure to score the chicken and prick it with a fork before marinating; see How to Score Bone-In Chicken Parts, page 245.

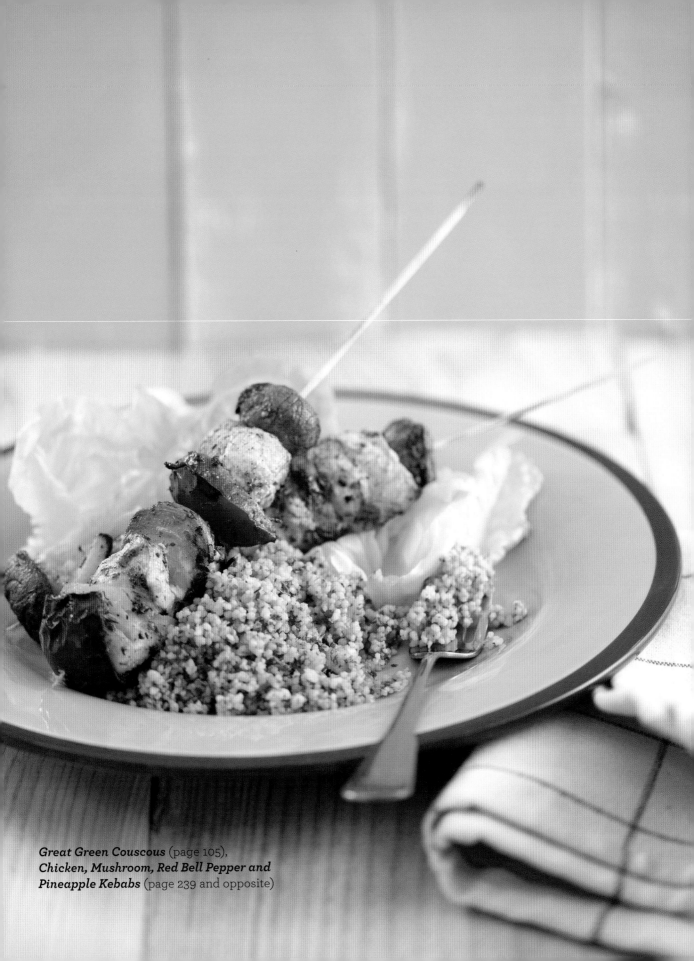

Great Green Couscous (page 105),
*Chicken, Mushroom, Red Bell Pepper and
Pineapple Kebabs* (page 239 and opposite)

MINTY MIDDLE EASTERN–STYLE TURKEY BURGERS

Fresh herbs and spices make these pan-fried burgers exceptional. One of my recipe testers commented that she added even more spice than called for, and that her family "absolutely loved" the burgers, especially the addition of the feta cheese. Skip the traditional bun and serve them in a whole wheat pita pocket or flatbread, with baby greens, tomatoes, sliced raw onions (see How to Take the Edge off Raw Onions, page 192), and tahini dressing, a dollop of hummus, or a spoonful of Cucumber Yogurt Sauce. For delicious and festive appetizers, make small, single-bite-size balls.

SERVES 4

1 pound (480 g) ground turkey or chicken

⅓ cup (60 g) crumbled reduced-fat feta cheese

1 large egg

¼ cup (15 g) panko bread crumbs

1 tablespoon dried mint

2 teaspoons roasted ground cumin

1 teaspoon roasted ground coriander

2 teaspoons minced garlic

3 tablespoons thinly sliced scallions

3 tablespoons chopped fresh flat-leaf parsley

2 tablespoons chopped fresh mint

¼ teaspoon cayenne, or to taste

½ teaspoon salt, or to taste

Freshly ground pepper, to taste

1 tablespoon canola oil

1. Combine all of the ingredients except the canola oil in a bowl and mix until well blended. If the mixture is too sticky or pasty, add 1 tablespoon water. The consistency should be slightly softer than a burger made with ground beef, but firm enough to hold its shape. Before you shape the burgers, you may want to make a test patty to check the seasoning: form about 1 tablespoon of the mixture into a patty and cook in a little oil until well done. Taste, and adjust the seasoning in rest of the mixture if needed.

2. Divide the mixture into 4 portions (or more, if you prefer smaller burgers), form each portion into a patty, and place them a large plate. Refrigerate, covered, for at least 30 minutes, and up to 6 hours.

3. When ready to cook, heat the canola oil in a large nonstick skillet over medium-high heat. Add the burgers and cook for 5 minutes, or until the underside is golden. Flip the burgers and cook for 4 to 5 minutes, until the burgers are completely cooked through. Remove from the skillet and serve hot.

GRILLED CHICKEN WITH FRESH MANGO SALSA

Here's a light chicken dish bursting with the sweetness of ripe mangoes, the tang of red onions, and the freshness of cilantro, with a jolt of jalapeños. If you can't get fresh mangoes in your area, or they are not in season, use finely diced fresh pineapple or peaches. The chicken can be grilled, broiled, or pan-fried. The mango salsa is best on the same day it is made. It is also great on grilled salmon.

SERVES 4

Lime Marinade

1 tablespoon grated lime zest

3 tablespoons fresh lime juice

1 tablespoon white wine vinegar

2 teaspoons extra virgin olive oil

1 teaspoon roasted ground coriander

½ teaspoon roasted ground cumin

½ teaspoon salt

Sprinkle of red pepper flakes

Four 4-ounce (120 g) boneless, skinless chicken breasts

Fresh Mango Salsa

1 ripe mango, peeled, pitted, and diced (about 1½ cups, 375 ml)

¼ cup (40 g) minced red onion

3 tablespoons chopped fresh cilantro

1 tablespoon minced jalapeño chiles

1 tablespoon Thai-style sweet chili sauce

1 tablespoon fresh lime juice, or to taste

2 tablespoons chopped fresh cilantro or sliced fresh mint leaves

1. To make the marinade, in a bowl large enough to hold the chicken, combine all of the marinade ingredients except the chicken and mix well. Prick the chicken with a fork and then, using a sharp paring knife, make two ¼-inch (6 mm) deep slashes in each breast. Add the chicken to the bowl and turn to cover with the marinade. Cover the bowl with plastic wrap and refrigerate for at least 2 hours and up to 24 hours.

2. To make the salsa, in a small bowl, combine all of the ingredients and gently mix until well blended. Adjust the seasoning and set aside. (The salsa can be made up to 6 hours in advance; cover with plastic wrap pressed flush against the surface and refrigerate.)

3. For a charcoal grill: Light a chimney starter filled with charcoal briquettes. When the coals are hot, spread them evenly over the bottom of the grill and set the cooking grate in place. Cover and heat until hot, about 5 minutes. For a gas grill: Turn all the burners to medium, cover, and heat until hot, about 10 minutes.

4. Have a serving platter ready for the cooked chicken. Oil the grill grate. Grill the chicken over medium heat, turning and moving the pieces and adjusting the heat as needed, and closing the lid off and on, until completely cooked through, 6 to 8 minutes per side. (Note: An instant-read thermometer inserted in the center of a breast should read 165° F [74°C].) Transfer to the platter and serve with the salsa.

234 CALORIES IN

Protein: 31 g; Carbohydrates: 12 g; Fat: 6 g; Fiber: 1 g; Sodium: 495 mg; Carb Choices: 1; Diabetic Exchange: 4 Very Lean Meat, 1 Fruit, 1 Fat

234 CALORIES OUT

Women: Walk: 57 minutes | Jog: 27 minutes

Men: Walk: 48 minutes | Jog: 22 minutes

CALORIE COMBOS

Roasted Asparagus with Dill and Lemon Zest (page 88): 47 cals

2 cups (40 g) salad greens with 1 tablespoon Benihana-Style Ginger-Sesame Dressing (page 155): 89 cals

½ cup (80 g) plain white rice: 103 cals

½ cup (90 g) plain brown rice: 108 cals

½ cup (65 g) plain quinoa: 111 cals

Sweet Potato Oven Fries (page 104): 147 cals

Great Green Couscous (page 105): 152 cals

Caesar Salad with a Light Touch (page 83): 163 cals

Lemony Basmati Rice (page 209): 210 cals

Couscous Salad with Harissa Dressing (page 198): 241 cals

CALORIE CUTS

The only real way to save calories in this dish is to skip the mango salsa. You will save about 45 calories per serving.

ROASTED CHICKEN WITH ROSEMARY-LEMON-GARLIC RUB

This roasted chicken, which is dry-brined in the marinating process, comes out of the oven incredibly juicy and bursting with flavor. Feel free to substitute your favorite fresh or dried herbs for the ones I've called for. (Note: Your hands will get garlicky, so if you don't want your hands to smell, wear gloves to rub the spice mix onto the chicken.) "The meat is so moist and tender," wrote one of my recipe testers. "I loved the fresh garlic, tastier than powder. Served it with mashed potatoes and stir-fried vegetables. Really love this!"

SERVES 5

Rosemary-Lemon-Garlic Rub

1 tablespoon chopped fresh rosemary

2 teaspoons salt

1 teaspoon dried thyme

½ teaspoon dried oregano

1 tablespoon minced garlic or 1 teaspoon garlic powder

½ teaspoon freshly ground pepper

1 tablespoon grated lemon zest

1 tablespoon extra virgin olive oil

One 3½- to 4-pound (1.5 to 2 kg) whole roaster chicken, rinsed and patted dry with paper towels

1. To make the rub, in a small bowl, mix together all of the ingredients; set aside.

2. Using your fingers, loosen the skin from the chicken breast and thigh areas as much as possible. Spread the rub under the skin, over the skin, and in the cavities of the bird. Place the chicken in a very large Ziploc bag, or put in a large bowl and cover with plastic wrap. Refrigerate for at least 3 hours, and up to 24 hours, the longer the better.

3. Center an oven rack and preheat the oven to 450°F (230°C).

4. Place the chicken in a roasting pan, ideally on an elevated roasting rack. If using a rack, add a bit of water to the bottom of the pan to prevent the pan drippings from burning and/or splattering. Roast for 30 minutes, then reduce the heat to 350°F (180°C) and continue cooking for 1 hour, or until an instant-read thermometer inserted into the center of the breast meat reads 165°F (74°C) and the juices run clear when the chicken is pierced with a knife in the breast and thigh areas. Remove the chicken from the oven, transfer to a carving board, and cover loosely with foil for 5 minutes before carving.

5. Meanwhile, strain the juices from the pan and remove as much of the grease as possible. Carve and plate the chicken, drizzle some of the juices over the meat to keep it moist, and serve.

HOW TO PERFECTLY ROAST A CHICKEN

First, start with the best-quality chicken you can find. Ideally, this means an organic, antibiotic-free, hormone-free, humanely raised bird. Next, to keep the meat as juicy as possible, use a brine. This can be a liquid brine infused with herbs and other seasonings, or a salt-herb rub, as in the recipe above. When you are ready to roast, start with a high temperature (at least 400°F, 200°C), then lower it to finish cooking the meat through. If the skin is browning too fast, tent a piece of aluminum foil over the chicken; do not tuck it in. You may want to remove the foil during the last 10 minutes of roasting to allow the skin to crisp.

HOW TO SCORE BONE-IN CHICKEN PARTS

Scoring bone-in chicken helps ensure that the marinade penetrates the meat and that it cooks quickly and evenly, with less chance of burning. Using a sharp knife, make 3 slashes, each about ⅛ inch (3 mm) deep, in the thickest part of chicken breasts, 2 slashes in the thighs, and 1 in each side of drumsticks. You can also prick the meat with a fork to infuse it with even more flavor.

HOW TO MINCE RAW CHICKEN OR TURKEY

If you are a stickler for using only the best products, including ground chicken or turkey, the ideal solution is to grind the meat yourself. This way, you are guaranteed lean, organic, hormone and antibiotic-free breast meat without the addition of inferior cuts, fillers, salt, and/or water. If you do have a meat grinder or meat grinder attachment, use it. If not, you can mince chicken or turkey by hand using a chef's knife or Chinese-style cleaver; it's not hard, but it does take a bit of muscle. First, slice the meat into small cubes, then start chopping it. After a few chops, pick up the meat with the side of your knife, or with your hands, return it to the board, and continue to chop until it is uniformly minced but not pasty.

CHICKEN WITH ZUCCHINI, MUSHROOMS, CELERY, AND CASHEWS

Simple to make, this light chicken stir-fry is a staple in my home. Add your favorite vegetables in place of the zucchini, mushrooms, and celery. Tofu, shrimp, or scallops can be substituted for the chicken. As with all stir-fries, it is critical to have all of the ingredients, including sides, ready before you begin cooking.

SERVES 5

1 pound (480 g) chicken tenderloins, cut into 1½-inch (4 cm) pieces

Basic Stir-Fry Marinade

1 tablespoon cornstarch

1 tablespoon lite soy sauce

1 teaspoon toasted sesame oil

¼ teaspoon salt

¼ teaspoon sugar

Freshly ground pepper, to taste

Stir-Fry Sauce

½ teaspoon sugar

2 teaspoons cornstarch

¼ teaspoon freshly ground pepper

1 tablespoon lite soy sauce

2 tablespoons oyster sauce

1 teaspoon toasted sesame oil

½ cup (125 ml) water or low-sodium fat-free chicken stock

Stir-Fry

1½ tablespoons vegetable oil

3 tablespoons very thin matchsticks fresh ginger

1 large garlic clove, minced

4 ounces (120 g) button or shiitake mushrooms, rinsed, stems trimmed, and sliced

Sprinkle of salt

1 cup (120 g) zucchini matchsticks (about 2 inches, 5 cm)

1 cup (100 g) celery matchsticks (about 2 inches, 5 cm)

1 cup (45 g) sliced scallions (about 2 inches, 5 cm)

⅓ cup (45 g) roasted salted cashews, for garnish

1. To marinate the chicken, place it in a bowl, add all of the marinade ingredients, and mix well. Cover and refrigerate for at least 6 hours, and up to 24 hours.

2. Just before cooking, in a small bowl, mix the sauce ingredients; set aside.

3. In a large nonstick skillet or wok, heat 1 tablespoon of the vegetable oil over high heat. Add half of the ginger and half of the garlic and cook for 30 seconds. Add the mushrooms and sauté, stirring occasionally, for 2 minutes. Add the zucchini and celery and sauté, stirring, for 2 minutes longer; do not overcook. Transfer the vegetables to a serving platter. (Do not rinse the skillet.)

4. Reheat the skillet over high heat and add the remaining ½ tablespoon vegetable oil. Add the remaining garlic and ginger and the marinated chicken. Sauté, stirring, for 3 minutes, or until the chicken is lightly browned. Return the reserved vegetables to the skillet, add the scallions and the sauce, and cook, stirring constantly, over medium heat until the sauce thickens slightly and the chicken is cooked through, 3 to 5 minutes. Add a sprinkle of salt, adjust the seasoning, transfer to a serving dish, sprinkle with the scallions and cashews, and serve promptly.

CHICKEN-ZUCCHINI BURGERS WITH RICOTTA AND SUN-DRIED TOMATOES

With or without buns, these moist and flavorful chicken burgers rock! The ricotta cheese keeps the lean ground chicken from getting dry during cooking. I like to serve them with a green salad and one of the chutneys, sauces, salsas, or dressings in this book, without buns. For an incredible appetizer, make small, single-bite-size balls and serve them skewered with toothpicks, accompanied by the Fresh Mint, Cilantro, and Green Chile Chutney. Chicken sliders are also fun for social gatherings. Optional garnishes include salad greens, sliced fresh tomatoes, sliced raw onions, and assorted condiments. (See How to Mince Raw Chicken or Turkey, page 245).

SERVES 4

1 pound (480 g) ground chicken

½ cup (50 g) grated zucchini (use the large holes of a box grater)

⅓ cup (90 g) part-skim ricotta cheese

1 teaspoon minced garlic

1 teaspoon Dijon mustard

1 teaspoon Worcestershire sauce

2 tablespoons chopped fresh basil, flat-leaf parsley, or cilantro

3 tablespoons thinly sliced scallions

3 tablespoons chopped sun-dried tomatoes in oil, drained

½ teaspoon salt, or to taste

Freshly ground pepper, to taste

¼ cup (12 g) panko bread crumbs, plus about ½ cup (25 g) for breading the burgers

1 tablespoon vegetable oil

1. In a large bowl, combine all of the ingredients except the bread crumbs for breading the burgers and the vegetable oil. Mix until well blended. If the mixture is too sticky or pasty, add 1 tablespoon water. Before you shape the burgers, you may want to make a test patty to check the seasoning: form about 1 tablespoon of the chicken mixture into a patty and cook in a little oil until well done. Taste, and adjust the seasoning in the rest of the mixture if needed.

2. Divide the chicken mixture into 4 portions. Form each portion into a patty, then coat with the remaining ½ cup (25 g) of bread crumbs. Place the finished patties on a large plate and refrigerate, covered, for at least 30 minutes, and up to 6 hours.

3. When ready to cook, heat the vegetable oil in a large nonstick skillet over medium-high heat. Add the burgers and cook for 6 minutes, or until the underside is golden. Flip the burgers and cook for 4 to 5 minutes, until they are completely cooked through. Remove from the skillet and serve hot.

261 CALORIES IN

Protein: 24 g; Carbohydrates: 11 g; Fat: 14 g; Fiber: 1 g; Sodium: 478 mg; Carb Choices: 1; Diabetic Exchange: 3 Medium-Fat Meat, 2 Vegetable

261 CALORIES OUT

Women: Walk: 64 minutes | Jog: 30 minutes

Men: Walk: 53 minutes | Jog: 25 minutes

CALORIE COMBOS

1 slice tomato: 4 cals

1 slice red onion: 5 cals

1 teaspoon Dijon mustard: 5 cals

1 tablespoon light mayonnaise: 49 cals

Lemony Dill Cabbage Slaw (page 78): 63 cals

2 cups (40 g) salad greens with 1 tablespoon Balsamic Vinaigrette (page 150): 73 cals

1 whole wheat hamburger bun: 110 cals

The Best Roasted Ratatouille (page 112): 130 cals

Sweet Potato Oven Fries (page 104): 147 cals

Great Green Couscous (page 105): 152 cals

1 pita bread: 165 cals

Tomato, Artichoke Heart, Feta, and White Bean Salad (page 84): 168 cals

Glorious Greek Salad (page 192): 210 cals

Couscous Salad with Harissa Dressing (page 198): 241 cals

CALORIE CUTS

Skip the buns and save 110 calories per serving.

CLASSIC CHICKEN CURRY WITH COCONUT MILK

For this fabulous South Indian–style curry, featuring coconut milk and red curry powder, I like to use a mix of chicken thighs on the bone and chicken tenderloins, which I add toward the end of cooking so they stay moist. In India, fresh curry leaves would be added with the tomatoes in Step 4. If you have them, add about 15 fresh or dried leaves. They impart a heavenly taste and aroma. See page 344 for more information on red curry powder. This dish freezes well. You may need to add a bit of water to thin the sauce as you reheat it.

SERVES 8

Curry Marinade

1½ teaspoons red curry powder

½ teaspoon cayenne, optional

1 tablespoon water

2 pounds (1 kg) skinless bone-in chicken thighs,

1½ pounds (720 g) chicken tenderloins, cut into 1½-inch (6 cm) pieces

Curry

2 tablespoons vegetable oil

1 cinnamon stick

3 star anise pods, optional

5 whole green cardamom pods or 1 teaspoon ground cardamom

1 large onion, chopped

2 tablespoons minced garlic

3 tablespoons minced fresh peeled ginger

One 14.5-ounce (411 g) can diced tomatoes, with their juices (1½ cups, 375 ml)

2 tablespoons red curry powder

½ teaspoon salt

½ cup (125 ml) boiling water

Scant 1 cup (200 ml) coconut milk or evaporated milk

1 tablespoon fresh lemon juice, or to taste

1. To marinate the chicken, in a large bowl, mix the curry powder, cayenne, if using, and water to make a paste. Prick the chicken tenderloins and thighs with a fork and then, using a sharp paring knife, make two ¼-inch (6 mm) deep slashes in each thigh. Add the chicken to the bowl, cover, and refrigerate for at least 1 hour and up to 24 hours.

2. To make the curry, in a large saucepan or deep skillet, heat 1 tablespoon of the vegetable oil over medium heat. Add the cinnamon stick, star anise, if using, and cardamom and cook for 30 seconds. Add the onions and sauté for 5 minutes, or until light golden. Add the garlic and ginger and sauté for 1 minute more, then transfer the contents of the saucepan to a large heatproof bowl. (Do not rinse the saucepan.)

3. Return the saucepan to the stove, add ½ tablespoon of the remaining vegetable oil, and sauté the chicken thighs over medium-high heat for 5 minutes, or until they pick up a bit of color. Transfer them to the bowl with the onions. Repeat the procedure with the remaining ½ tablespoon vegetable oil and the chicken tenderloins, cooking them for 3 minutes (they will be cooked again later). Transfer the tenderloins to a separate bowl and set aside.

4. Return the saucepan to the stove and add the reserved thighs and onions, then add the diced tomatoes, curry powder, salt, and boiling water. Stir and bring to a boil, then reduce the heat to low and simmer for 15 minutes.

5. Add the reserved chicken tenderloins and the coconut milk to the pan and simmer for 7 minutes, or until the tenderloins and thighs are cooked through. Adjust the seasoning, add the lemon juice, and serve.

HOW TO FREEZE GINGER AND GARLIC PASTE

If you ask me what slows me down when I cook, it's all the chopping, mincing, slicing, and other prep work that goes into a meal. I'm sure many of you will agree. During my Indian cooking classes in Malaysia, I learned to keep a supply of frozen garlic and ginger paste in my freezer, and I have been doing so ever since. To make the paste, place equal amounts by weight of peeled garlic and ginger in the bowl of a food processor and process until fairly smooth. (You can adjust the ratio of garlic and ginger depending on which flavor you like best.) If the paste is too dry while you are processing, add a couple of tablespoons of water. Transfer the puree to a small container and freeze, then scoop out spoonfuls as needed. Some grocery stores carry very good ready-made pastes including ginger, garlic, lemongrass, and fresh red chili. Gourmet Garden is one such brand. They are all great time savers.

CHICKEN THIGHS WITH CAPERS AND PARSLEY

Capers, garlic, sun-dried tomatoes, parsley, wine, and lemon are a natural combo for flavoring chicken. In this dish, I use boneless chicken thighs, but you can also use chicken tenderloins; just decrease the cooking time. A touch of chopped fresh rosemary is a wonderful addition. This dish freezes well.

SERVES 4

1¼ pounds (600 g) boneless, skinless chicken thighs, cut in half or into quarters, or chicken tenderloins, cut in half

Freshly ground pepper, to taste

1 tablespoon cornstarch

1½ tablespoons vegetable oil

1 onion, chopped

1 large garlic clove, minced

2 tablespoons medium capers, or to taste, drained

¼ cup (35 g) sun-dried tomatoes in oil, drained

2 teaspoons dried oregano, thyme, or Italian seasoning

¼ cup (60 ml) white wine

1 cup (250 ml) low-sodium fat-free chicken stock

⅓ cup (10 g) chopped fresh flat-leaf parsley

2 tablespoons fresh lemon juice, or to taste

1. In a medium bowl, toss the chicken with the pepper and 2 teaspoons of the cornstarch.

2. In a large nonstick skillet, heat 1 tablespoon of the vegetable oil over medium-high heat. Add half of the chicken and cook until golden brown, about 3 minutes on each side. (Note: The chicken will be cooked again later, so don't overcook it at this stage. If you are using chicken tenderloins, they should be cooked for a total of 5 minutes, so reduce the time in this step to about 1 minute per side.) Transfer the chicken to a platter and cover to keep warm. Return the skillet to the stove and cook the remaining chicken in the same way. Add the chicken to the platter. (Do not rinse the skillet.)

3. Return the skillet to the stove, add the remaining ½ tablespoon vegetable oil, and heat over medium-high heat. Add the onions and sauté, stirring occasionally, until lightly browned, about 3 minutes. Add the garlic and cook for 30 seconds. Add the capers, sun-dried tomatoes, and oregano and cook for 1 minute, then add the white wine and cook for 3 minutes.

4. In a measuring cup or small bowl, mix the remaining 1 teaspoon cornstarch with the stock, and add it to the skillet. Add the reserved chicken and the parsley and gently simmer, stirring occasionally, for 10 minutes, or until the chicken is completely cooked and the sauce has slightly thickened. Add the lemon juice, adjust the seasoning, and serve promptly.

BUTTER CHICKEN MADE EASY

In an authentic Indian kitchen, leftover tandoori chicken and home-ground spices are used to make ever-popular butter chicken, and boy, oh boy, is it good. If you don't have time to roast and grind spices (see How to Roast and Grind Spices, page 237), McCormick carries a good line of roasted ground cumin, coriander, ginger, cinnamon, and other spices. I have tried packaged butter chicken spice mixes, and they are not as good as homemade, but if you're in a hurry, go for it. Despite the name, I do not add butter to this dish. I achieve the creamy consistency with a touch of coconut milk (freeze what you don't use). Like many Indian dishes, this chicken is even better the second or third day, if it lasts that long. It can also be frozen. This is one of my son's favorite chicken dishes, so I dedicate the recipe to him.

SERVES 5

2 teaspoons garam masala

2 teaspoons roasted ground coriander

2 teaspoons roasted ground cumin

2 teaspoons paprika

½ teaspoon cayenne

2 teaspoons minced garlic

½ cup (135 g) nonfat plain Greek-style yogurt

2 pounds (1 kg) chicken tenderloins, cut into 1½-inch (4 cm) pieces

1 tablespoon vegetable oil

3 tablespoons tomato paste

½ cup (125 ml) tomato puree

¾ cup (180 ml) low-sodium fat-free chicken stock

1 cinnamon stick or ½ teaspoon ground cinnamon, optional

3 whole green cardamom pods, optional

⅓ cup (80 ml) lite or regular coconut milk

3 tablespoons chopped fresh cilantro, for garnish

1. In a large bowl, combine the garam masala, coriander, cumin, paprika, cayenne, garlic, and yogurt and mix until well blended. Add the chicken and mix to thoroughly coat, then cover and refrigerate for at least 3 hours, and up to 24 hours.

2. In a large saucepan, heat ½ tablespoon of the vegetable oil over medium-high heat. Add half the chicken and sauté, stirring occasionally, for 2 minutes, or until light golden. Transfer the chicken to a heatproof bowl. (Note: The chicken will not be fully cooked at this point.) Return the saucepan to the heat, add the remaining ½ tablespoon oil, and sauté the remaining chicken in the same way. Return all the chicken to the pan.

3. Add the tomato paste, tomato puree, chicken stock, and cinnamon and cardamom pods, if using, and bring to a boil, then reduce the heat and simmer, uncovered for 15 minutes, or until the chicken is cooked through. Add the coconut milk, stir, and adjust the seasoning. Garnish with the cilantro and serve promptly.

276 CALORIES IN

Protein: 41 g; Carbohydrates: 7 g; Fat: 9 g; Fiber: 1 g; Sodium: 483 mg; Carb Choices: ½; Diabetic Exchange: 6 Very Lean Meat, 1 Vegetable, 1 Fat

276 CALORIES OUT

Women: Walk: 67 minutes | Jog: 32 minutes

Men: Walk: 56 minutes | Jog: 27 minutes

CALORIE COMBOS

Fresh Mint, Cilantro, and Green Chile Chutney (page 143): 30 cals

Indian-Style Cucumber Yogurt Salad (page 75): 45 cals

Tomato, Cucumber, and Radish Salad (page 76): 55 cals

Hot-and-Sweet Cucumber, Carrot, and Red Bell Pepper Salad (page 77): 61 cals

½ cup (80 g) plain white rice: 103 cals

½ cup (90 g) plain brown rice: 108 cals

½ cup (65 g) plain quinoa: 111 cals

1 whole wheat chapati (Indian flatbread): 137 cals

Paneer with Spinach, Tomatoes, and Spices (page 113): 143 cals

Aromatic Brown Basmati Rice (page 107): 184 cals

Minty Basmati Rice and Potatoes (page 208): 206 cals

Lemony Basmati Rice (page 209): 210 cals

AUSSIE-STYLE BBQ CHICKEN (📷 page 81)

I love the quintessential Australian weekend tradition of "firing up the barbie" to share a feast with family and friends. Lamb, done a million different ways, is almost always on the Australian menu, but I find their chicken dishes truly sublime. In this easy and delicious recipe, the chicken is cooked in advance, then marinated, reheated, and browned on the grill before serving. Fantastic, mate!

SERVES 6

Tomato-Beer Marinade

1 tablespoon vegetable oil

1 small onion, finely chopped

1 teaspoon minced fresh ginger

1 teaspoon minced garlic or ½ teaspoon garlic powder

1 cup (250 ml) tomato puree

1 cup (250 ml) beer (any kind)

1 tablespoon cider vinegar

2 tablespoons Worcestershire sauce

2 tablespoons ketchup

¼ cup (40 g) packed brown sugar

1 teaspoon salt

3½ to 4 pounds (1.6 to 2 kg) skinless bone-in chicken parts, such as breasts, thighs, and drumsticks

1. To make the marinade, heat the vegetable oil in a saucepan over medium heat. Add the onions, ginger, and garlic and cook for 3 minutes, stirring. Add the remaining ingredients, mix well, and bring to a boil. Reduce the heat and simmer for 15 minutes, or until slightly thickened. Set aside.

2. Place the chicken in a saucepan and add enough water to cover it by about 1 inch (2.5 cm). Bring to a boil, then reduce the heat and simmer for 45 minutes, or until the chicken is fully cooked. Transfer the chicken to a bowl and save the stock for another use, or discard it.

3. Add the reserved marinade to the chicken, mix well, and let cool, then cover and refrigerate for at least 6 hours and up to 24 hours. Turn at least once.

4. For a charcoal grill: Light a chimney starter filled with charcoal briquettes. When the coals are hot, spread them evenly over the bottom of the grill and set the cooking grate in place. Cover and heat until hot, about 5 minutes. For a gas grill: Turn all the burners to medium, cover, and preheat until hot, about 10 minutes.

5. Oil the grill grate. Grill the chicken over medium heat, uncovered, until heated through and nicely browned, about 20 minutes. Baste the chicken with the marinade as it cooks and move it around the grill. Adjust the heat as needed to prevent scorching. Transfer to a serving platter and serve promptly.

MEMORABLE MEAT LOAF

If you like meat loaf, you're going to love this version. I like to serve it with the Smashed Potatoes with Fresh Herbs, Roasted New Potatoes, or simple baked Idaho potatoes with fat-free sour cream and chives. Leftovers are great in a sandwich with Dijon mustard and cornichons, or served alongside a salad. Ideally, for the juiciest results, meat loaf should be made with a mix of pork and beef.

SERVES 8

Canola oil cooking spray

Ketchup Glaze

½ cup (125 ml) ketchup

2 tablespoons molasses or honey

2 teaspoons seasoned rice vinegar

Meat Loaf

1 pound (480 g) lean ground pork

1 pound (480 g) lean ground beef

2 large eggs, lightly beaten

¾ cup (45 g) thinly sliced scallions

¼ cup (10 g) chopped fresh flat-leaf parsley

¼ cup (7 g) chopped fresh dill

1 cup (50 g) panko bread crumbs

2 teaspoons dried oregano

1 teaspoon garlic powder

1 tablespoon Worcestershire sauce

1 tablespoon Dijon mustard

1½ teaspoons salt

½ teaspoon freshly ground pepper

½ cup (120 g) low-fat plain yogurt or whole milk

1. Center an oven rack and preheat the oven to 350°F (180°C). Line a large baking pan with foil and lightly grease it with cooking spray.

2. To make the glaze, mix all of the ingredients in a small bowl or measuring cup; set aside.

3. To make the meat loaf, combine all of the ingredients in a large bowl and mix with a spoon or your hands (wet your hands first to prevent sticking) until well blended. It is advisable to check the seasoning before baking: make a small patty of the meat loaf mixture and cook in a very lightly greased small skillet until well done. Taste, and adjust the seasoning in the remaining mixture if necessary.

4. Form the meat loaf mixture into a ball and transfer to the prepared baking pan. Using your hands, form it into an oval-shaped loaf approximately 10 inches (25 cm) long and 2½ inches (6 cm) high. Using the back of a spoon, spread the glaze evenly over the surface of the meat loaf.

5. Bake for 1 hour and 25 to 30 minutes, until completely cooked through: an instant-read thermometer inserted in the center should read 160°F (71°C), and the juices should run clear when the center is pierced with a knife or skewer. Remove the meat loaf from the oven and allow it to rest for 5 minutes before slicing.

233 CALORIES IN

Protein: 28 g; Carbohydrates: 15 g; Fat: 7 g; Fiber: 1 g; Sodium: 801 mg; Carb Choices: 1; Diabetic Exchange: 1 Starch, 3 Lean Meat

233 CALORIES OUT

Women: Walk: 57 minutes; Jog: 27 minutes

Men: Walk: 48 minutes; Jog: 22 minutes

CALORIE COMBOS

1 tablespoon fat-free sour cream: 11 cals

Greek-Style Broccoli (page 91): 71 cals

2 cups (40 g) salad greens with 1 tablespoon Balsamic Vinaigrette (page 150): 73 cals

Maple-Glazed Carrots (page 95): 98 cals

Roasted New Potatoes (page 98): 118 cals

Brussels Sprouts with Parmesan and Pine Nuts (page 99): 118 cals

Cheesy Southern-Style Spoon Bread (page 100): 127 cals

Smashed Potatoes with Fresh Herbs (page 102): 144 cals

Polenta with Herbs and Cheese (page 103): 146 cals

1 medium baked potato: 161 cals

CALORIE CUTS

Skip the ketchup glaze and save 29 calories per serving.

BEEF WITH BROCCOLI, SHIITAKES, AND SNOW PEAS

Although the five-step instructions may seem somewhat daunting, this beef and broccoli dish is very easy to make. Basically, it's a simple stir-fry, and once you start cooking, things move quickly, so make sure all of your ingredients are lined up and ready to go. I cook the broccoli and snow peas separately from the meat and then arrange them around the meat. This is how the Chinese do it, because it results in a more attractive look and also allows the flavors of the vegetables to stand on their own. Be sure to use the leanest beef you can find; tenderloin is best, though admittedly expensive. The beef can be substituted with an equal amount of boneless chicken breasts or chicken tenderloins cut into small strips.

SERVES 6

Marinade

¼ cup (60 ml) lite soy sauce

2 teaspoons toasted sesame oil

2 tablespoons seasoned rice wine

Freshly ground pepper, to taste

1 tablespoon sugar

2 teaspoons cornstarch

1¼ pounds (600 g) beef tenderloin, visible fat trimmed and sliced into very thin 1-inch (2.5 cm) long strips

6 ounces (180 g) broccoli, trimmed and cut into small florets

4 ounces (125 g) snow peas, ends trimmed

1½ tablespoons plus 1 teaspoon vegetable oil

8 ounces (240 g) shiitake mushrooms, rinsed, stems removed, and cut into quarters

Salt and freshly ground pepper, to taste

1 tablespoon thinly sliced peeled fresh ginger

½ cup (30 g) sliced scallions (1-inch/2.5 cm pieces)

1 tablespoon oyster sauce

½ teaspoon cornstarch, dissolved in 3 tablespoons water

1. To marinate the beef, in a large bowl, mix the marinade ingredients until well combined. Add the beef and mix well. Cover and refrigerate for at least 30 minutes, and up to 2 hours.

2. Cook the broccoli and snow peas in a large saucepan of boiling water for 3 minutes, or until crisp-tender; do not overcook. Drain and set aside, covered with foil, to keep warm.

3. Heat ½ tablespoon of the vegetable oil in a large nonstick skillet over medium-high heat. Add the shiitake mushrooms, season with salt and pepper, and sauté, stirring constantly, for 3 minutes. Transfer the mushrooms and any juices to a large heatproof bowl; set aside. (Do not rinse the skillet.)

4. Add ½ tablespoon of the vegetable oil to the skillet and heat it over medium-high heat. Add half the reserved beef, leaving behind any marinade, and sauté, stirring, until the meat is just cooked, about 2 minutes. Transfer to the bowl with the mushrooms. Cook the remaining meat in the same way with another ½ tablespoon of the vegetable oil and transfer to the bowl. (Do not rinse the skillet.)

5. Add the remaining 1 teaspoon vegetable oil to the skillet and heat over medium-high heat. Add the ginger and scallions and sauté for 30 seconds. Add the cooked beef and mushrooms, with any juices, the oyster sauce, and dissolved cornstarch and bring to a simmer. Cook until the sauce slightly thickens, about 2 minutes. Adjust the seasoning, transfer to a serving platter, and arrange the reserved broccoli and snow peas around the beef. Serve promptly.

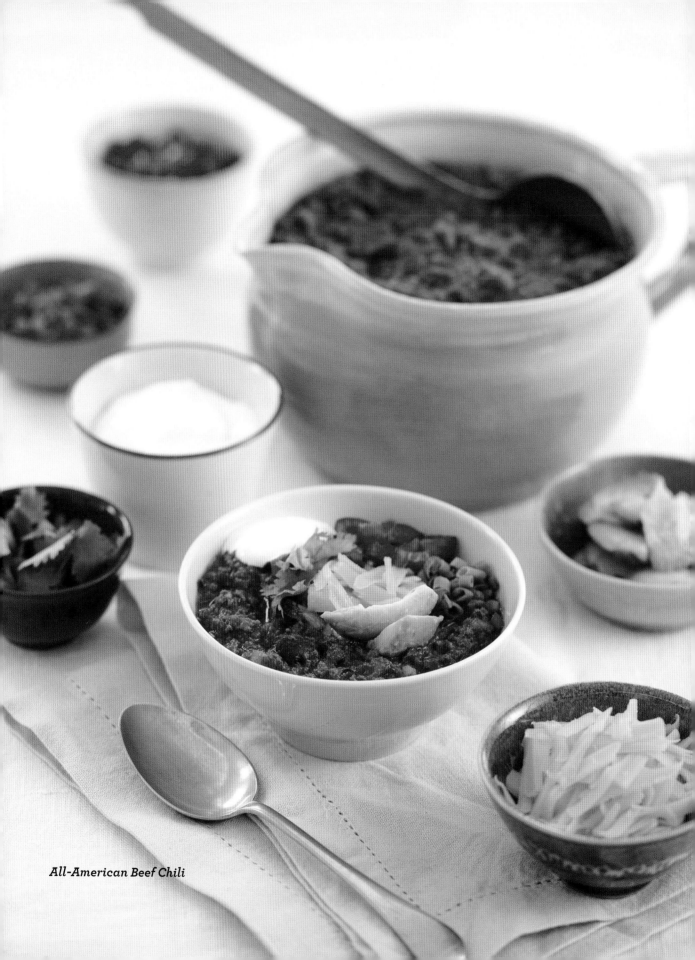

All-American Beef Chili

ALL-AMERICAN BEEF CHILI

A delicious fix-it-and-forget-it recipe, which I've made even easier by using canned beans, tomatoes, tomato sauce, tomato paste, and tomato juice. The chili is best made a day in advance to allow the flavors to meld. It can also be frozen in single-serving portions for easy weeknight dinners. Serve over brown rice, quinoa, or your favorite grain. Possible garnishes include diced avocados, grated reduced-fat cheddar cheese, fat-free sour cream, diced ripe tomatoes, sliced scallions, and chopped cilantro. They are all listed in the Calorie Combos.

SERVES 8

Two 15.25-ounce (432 g) cans kidney beans, rinsed and drained (about 3 cups, 375 ml)

One 14.5-ounce (411 g) can diced tomatoes, with their juices

2 tablespoons vegetable oil

1½ pounds (720 g) lean ground beef

1 large onion, chopped

1 red bell pepper, cored, seeded, and cut into small dice

1½ tablespoons chili powder

1 teaspoon roasted ground cumin

1 teaspoon dried oregano or Italian seasoning

1 teaspoon paprika

2 teaspoons garlic powder

1 teaspoon salt

2 teaspoons brown sugar

One 8-ounce (227 g) can tomato sauce

One 5.5-ounce (163 ml) can low-sodium V8 juice or tomato juice

3 tablespoons tomato paste

1. Place the kidney beans in a bowl, then transfer one third of them to the bowl of a food processor. Add the diced tomatoes and their juices and process until fairly smooth; set aside.

2. Heat 1 tablespoon of the vegetable oil in a Dutch oven or large heavy-bottomed saucepan over medium-high heat. Add the beef and sauté, breaking it up with a wooden spoon, until it loses its raw color, about 5 minutes. Transfer to a heatproof bowl and set aside. (Do not rinse the pot.)

3. Add the remaining 1 tablespoon vegetable oil to the pot and heat over medium heat. Add the onions and red bell peppers and sauté, stirring, for 3 minutes. Add the chili powder, cumin, oregano, paprika, garlic powder, salt, and brown sugar and cook for 2 minutes. Add the whole kidney beans, the pureed kidney bean–tomato mixture, and the cooked beef and stir until well combined. Add the tomato sauce, V8, and tomato paste, bring to a boil, then reduce the heat and gently simmer for 30 to 40 minutes, until the meat is very tender. If the chili becomes too thick, add some water, about ¼ cup (60 ml) at a time.

4. Adjust the seasoning and serve with any of the optional garnishes.

---

276 CALORIES IN

Protein: 25 g; Carbohydrates: 26 g; Fat: 9 g; Fiber: 8 g; Sodium: 967 mg; Carb Choices: 2; Diabetic Exchange: 2 Lean Meat, 2 Starch

276 CALORIES OUT

Women: Walk: 67 minutes; Jog: 32 minutes

Men: Walk: 56 minutes; Jog: 27 minutes

CALORIE COMBOS

1 tablespoon chopped fresh cilantro: 1 cal

1 tablespoon thinly sliced scallions: 2 cals

2 tablespoons chopped tomatoes: 4 cals

1 tablespoon fat-free sour cream: 11 cals

1 ounce reduced-fat cheddar cheese, grated: 49 cals

¼ avocado, diced: 56 cal

2 cups (40 g) salad greens with 1 tablespoon Balsamic Vinaigrette (page 150): 73 cals

½ cup (80 g) plain white rice: 103 cals

½ cup (90 g) plain brown rice: 108 cals

½ cup (65 g) plain quinoa: 111 cals

Caesar Salad with a Light Touch (page 83): 163 cals

1 piece (3 ounces/90 g) corn bread: 173 cals

CALORIE CUTS

Reduce the kidney beans to 1½ cups and save 38 calories per serving. Skip the optional avocado and cheese garnishes.

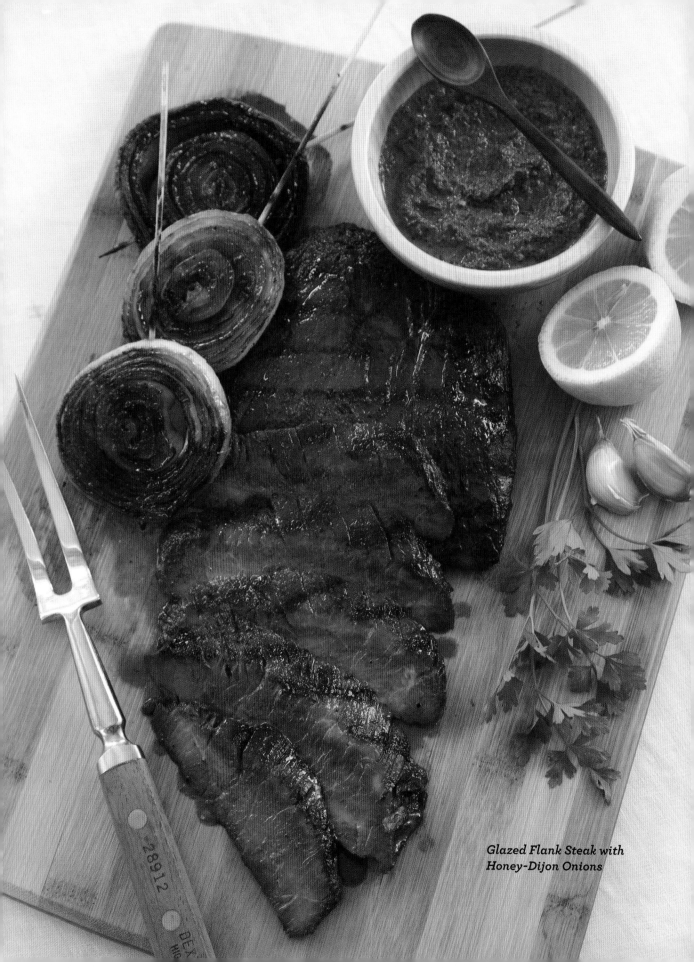

Glazed Flank Steak with Honey-Dijon Onions

GLAZED FLANK STEAK WITH HONEY-DIJON ONIONS

There are three components of a perfect grilled flank steak: 1) The marinade. Use your favorite or try mine below. 2) The cooking temperature. You don't want the grill to be too high, lest you burn the marinade, which can make it bitter; nor too low, or the meat will dry out. Start with high heat and then, after a few minutes, drop the heat to medium. 3) Basting. It takes a bit of energy and sweat, but it's worth the effort. Any leftover steak can be used in salads, fajitas, tacos, or sandwiches. The grilled sweet onions are a lovely add-on, but if you don't have the time, skip them. By the way, the onions go with grilled chicken or just about anything else.

SERVES 8

Glazed Flank Steak Marinade

3 tablespoons lite soy sauce

1 tablespoon hoisin sauce

1 tablespoon water

2 tablespoons honey

1 teaspoon garlic powder

1 teaspoon toasted sesame oil

Freshly ground pepper, to taste

One 2- to 3-pound (1 to 1.5 kg) flank steak, trimmed of all visible fat

Honey-Dijon Onions

2 large sweet onions, cut crosswise into ½-inch (1.25 cm) slices, keeping the slices intact

Canola oil cooking spray

1 tablespoon Dijon mustard

2 tablespoons honey

1 tablespoon Worcestershire sauce

Salt and freshly ground pepper, to taste

1. To make the marinade, in a Pyrex baking dish, combine all of the ingredients and whisk until blended.

2. With a sharp knife, lightly score both sides of the flank steak, only about ⅛-inch (3 mm) deep, in a crisscross pattern. Then poke the steak all over with a fork to allow the marinade to seep in. Place the steak in the baking dish and turn to coat both sides. Cover with plastic wrap and refrigerate for at least 1 hour and up to 24 hours.

3. To prepare the onions for grilling, run 1 or 2 soaked bamboo skewers through each onion slice to keep it intact as it cooks. Spray both sides of the onions with cooking spray, and place the onions on a baking sheet. Combine the Dijon mustard, honey, and Worcestershire sauce in a small bowl, mix well, and set aside.

4. For a charcoal grill: Light a chimney starter filled with charcoal briquettes. When the coals are hot, spread them evenly over the bottom of the grill and set the cooking grate in place. Cover and heat until hot, about 5 minutes. For a gas grill: Turn all the burners to high, cover, and heat until hot, about 10 minutes.

282 CALORIES IN | 4 OUNCES COOKED STEAK

Protein: 26 g; Carbohydrates: 21 g; Fat: 10 g; Fiber: 1 g; Sodium: 453 mg; Carb Choices: 1½; Diabetic Exchange: 3 Lean Meat, 1 Starch, 1 Vegetable

282 CALORIES OUT

Women: Walk: 69 minutes; Jog: 32 minutes

Men: Walk: 58 minutes; Jog: 27 minutes

CALORIE COMBOS

1 tablespoon fat-free sour cream: 11 cals

2 cups (40 g) salad greens with 1 tablespoon Balsamic Vinaigrette (page 150): 73 cals

½ cup (80 g) plain white rice: 103 cals

½ cup (90 g) plain brown rice: 108 cals

½ cup (65 g) plain quinoa: 111 cals

Roasted New Potatoes (page 98): 118 cals

Creamy All-American Potato Salad (page 80): 121 cals

1 medium baked potato: 161 cals

Caesar Salad with a Light Touch (page 83): 163 cals

Tomato, Artichoke Heart, Feta, and White Bean Salad (page 84): 168 cals

Minty Basmati Rice and Potatoes (page 208): 206 cals

Glorious Greek Salad (page 192): 210 cals

(RECIPE CONTINUES)

5. Have a platter ready for the cooked steaks. Oil the grill grate and grill the steak for 2 minutes on each side (reserve the marinade). Then reduce the heat to medium and continue to cook to the desired doneness, basting at the start of grilling with the marinade, and closing the lid as necessary, about 5 minutes per side, depending on the thickness. Transfer the steak to a carving board, cover it with foil, and allow it to rest for at least 5 minutes.

6. While the steak rests, place the onions on the grill and cook until they begin to pick up grill marks, turn light golden, and soften a bit, about 5 minutes on each side. As the onions cook, brush them with the mustard mixture and allow the glaze to bubble but not burn. Transfer the onions to a plate and cover with foil to keep warm.

7. To serve, using a very sharp knife, cut the steak across the grain into the desired thickness (see box, below). Serve promptly.

HOW TO SLICE FLANK AND SKIRT STEAK OR BRISKET

A good slicing knife and a little bit of technique will make all the difference when slicing meat. The first thing to do is determine the meat's grain, the direction the fibers run across the meat. Brisket and flank and skirt steaks need to be cut across (or against) the grain to achieve the most tender slices. Using a large fork, hold the meat in place on a chopping board or surface. (If your meat is juicy, you may want to surround the board with a paper towel or two.) Hold the knife at a 45-degree angle and cut the meat into thin slices, or the desired thickness.

FRENCH-STYLE BEEF STEW

Like many other stews, this is best prepared a day in advance, which gives the flavors a chance to meld overnight, adding to their depth. I've made this stew with fresh chanterelles and porcini, which were heavenly; the more flavorful your mushrooms, the better. This stew freezes well.

SERVES 8

2 pounds (1 kg) lean stewing beef, cut into ½-inch (1.25 cm) cubes and patted dry with paper towels

1 teaspoon salt

½ teaspoon freshly ground pepper

2 tablespoons unbleached all-purpose flour

3 tablespoons vegetable oil

2 carrots, cut into ½-inch (1.25 cm) slices

2 onions, halved and sliced

2 garlic cloves, minced

3 cups (750 ml) full-bodied young red wine, such as Chianti

2 to 3 cups (500 to 750 ml) low-sodium fat-free stock

2 tablespoons tomato paste

1 tablespoon dried thyme

3 bay leaves

10 ounces (300 g) shiitake or cremini mushrooms, rinsed, stems trimmed, and quartered

1 to 2 teaspoons cornstarch

¼ cup (60 ml) water

3 tablespoons chopped fresh flat-leaf parsley, for garnish

1. Place the beef in a bowl, add the salt, pepper, and flour, and toss until the cubes are evenly coated with the flour. Heat 1 tablespoon of the vegetable oil in a large Dutch oven or large heavy-bottomed saucepan over medium-high heat. Add half of the beef and sauté, turning the meat occasionally, until most sides are nicely browned. Transfer the browned beef to a pie dish or heatproof bowl. Don't worry about any bits sticking to the pot; scrape them up as much as possible (do not rinse the pot). Add 1 tablespoon of the vegetable oil to the pot and brown the rest of the meat the same way. Transfer the meat to the pie dish. (Again, do not rinse the pot.)

2. Add ½ tablespoon of the vegetable oil to the pot and sauté the carrots, onions, and garlic for 3 minutes. Add the wine and cook for 2 minutes, then return the reserved meat to the pot. Add enough stock, about 3 cups (750 ml), to cover the meat completely. Add the tomato paste, thyme, and bay leaves, stir, and bring to a boil, then reduce the heat to as low as possible and cook for 2 hours, or until the meat is fork-tender.

3. When the stew is close to finished, prepare the mushrooms: in a medium nonstick skillet, heat the remaining ½ tablespoon oil over medium-high heat. Add the mushrooms and sauté until light golden. Add them and any juices to the stew.

4. When the beef is tender, dissolve the cornstarch in the water and add to the stew. Mix well and then bring to a full boil. Turn off the heat, adjust the seasoning, and transfer to a serving dish. Garnish with the parsley and serve promptly.

286 CALORIES IN

Protein: 27 g; Carbohydrates: 12 g; Fat: 11 g; Fiber: 2 g; Sodium: 613 mg; Carb Choices: 1; Diabetic Exchange: 4 Lean Meat, 2 Vegetable

286 CALORIES OUT

Women: Walk: 70 minutes; Jog: 33 minutes

Men: Walk: 58 minutes; Jog: 27 minutes

CALORIE COMBOS

Roasted Asparagus with Dill and Lemon Zest (page 88): 47 cals

½ cup (80 g) plain boiled diced potatoes: 67 cals

Greek-Style Broccoli (page 91): 71 cals

2 cups (40 g) salad greens with 1 tablespoon Balsamic Vinaigrette (page 150): 73 cals

Grilled Vegetables (page 108): 89 cals

½ cup (80 g) plain white rice: 103 cals

½ cup (90 g) plain brown rice: 108 cals

½ cup (100 g) plain egg noodles: 110 cals

Cheesy Southern-Style Spoon Bread (page 100): 127 cals

Smashed Potatoes with Fresh Herbs (page 102): 144 cals

Caesar Salad with a Light Touch (page 83): 163 cals

DESSERTS

219 CALORIES IN

Protein: 4 g; Carbohydrates: 32 g;
Fat: 9 g; Fiber: 1 g; Sodium: 181
mg; Carb Choices: 2; Diabetic
Exchange: 2 Starch, 1 Fat

219 CALORIES OUT

Women: Walk:
53 minutes; Jog: 25 minutes

Men: Walk:
45 minutes; Jog: 21 minutes

SUPER-EASY APPLE CAKE

Super easy, super delicious. You'll find this apple cake has a surprisingly moist and light crumb, even without butter. Feel free to use 1 cup of either brown or white sugar, and use your favorite spices as well: ground cloves and allspice are naturals with apples; and, if you'd like, add 1 to 2 teaspoons vanilla extract in Step 3. This cake will keep, covered, at room temperature for 2 days, and it can be refrigerated for up to 5 days. It can also be frozen for up to 1 month.

SERVES 15

Canola oil cooking spray

2¼ cups (300 g) unbleached all-purpose flour, plus extra for the baking pan

1½ teaspoons baking powder

½ teaspoon baking soda

½ teaspoon salt

2 teaspoons ground cinnamon

½ teaspoon ground nutmeg

½ teaspoon ground ginger

½ cup (115 g) granulated sugar

½ cup (75 g) packed brown sugar

3 large eggs

½ cup (125 ml) canola oil

¾ cup (180 g) low-fat plain Greek-style yogurt

1¼ pounds (600 g) Granny Smith apples, peeled, cored, and thinly sliced (about 4 cups, 1 liter)

2 tablespoons confectioners' sugar, for dusting the cake, optional

1. Center an oven rack and preheat the oven to 350°F (180°C). Grease a 13 x 9 x 2-inch (33 x 23 x 5 cm) baking pan with cooking spray and lightly flour; set aside.

2. In a bowl, combine the flour, baking powder, baking soda, salt, cinnamon, nutmeg, and ginger and whisk together; set aside.

3. In the bowl of an electric mixer, combine the sugars with the eggs and beat on medium speed for about 4 minutes, or until light and fluffy. Add the canola oil and yogurt and beat for 30 seconds more.

4. Add the dry ingredients and beat on low speed just until blended, about 30 seconds. Then, using a rubber spatula, fold in the apples until well incorporated. Transfer the batter to the prepared baking pan and spread it evenly.

5. Bake for 45 minutes, or until a cake tester inserted into the center of the cake comes out clean and the apples feel soft. Remove the cake from the oven and cool for 5 minutes. To unmold, run a knife around the sides of the pan and invert the cake onto a cooling rack. When cooled, invert it again onto a serving platter. Dust the cake with confectioners' sugar, if using, before serving.

HOW TO MAKE HOMEMADE APPLESAUCE

This recipe for plain applesauce can be doctored up with dried apricots (about 15 pieces) and a small handful of dried cranberries. If using dried fruit, add it in Step 1, and increase the water a bit. Adjust the sugar to taste, depending on the tartness of the type of apples you use. Some of the best apples for applesauce are Jonagold, Jonathan, Macoun, Empire, and McIntosh.

1½ pounds (720 g) red or green apples, peeled, cored, and chopped
1 cup (250 ml) water
3 to 4 tablespoons sugar, to taste

1. Combine the apples and water in a medium saucepan and bring to a boil, then reduce the heat and simmer, stirring occasionally, for 10 to 15 minutes, until the fruit is soft. Remove from the heat, add the sugar, stir, and cool.
2. Puree the mixture in a blender or food processor to the desired consistency.

PERFECT PUMPKIN BREAD

222 CALORIES IN | 1 SLICE OF 1 LARGE LOAF

Protein: 4 g; Carbohydrates: 36 g; Fat: 8 g; Fiber: 2 g; Sodium: 173 mg; Carb Choices: 2½; Diabetic Exchange: 1 Starch, 1 Fruit, 2 Fat

222 CALORIES OUT

Women: Walk: 54 minutes; Jog: 25 minutes

Men: Walk: 45 minutes; Jog: 21 minutes

CALORIE CUTS

Skip the walnuts and save 48 calories and 5 grams of fat per slice. Skip the cranberries and save 23 calories per slice.

No mixer needed for these pumpkin loaves. I like to give away small loaves during the holidays for a healthy and delicious gift. One of my recipe testers took this bread to her church for fellowship time and said she overheard people talking about how delicious and amazing it was. That made me very happy. An equal amount of all-purpose flour can be substituted for the whole wheat flour. Also, feel free to add your favorite dried fruit and nuts in place of the ones I call for. For special occasions, I add chocolate chips. To freeze, wrap the cooled loaves in aluminum foil and freeze for up to 1 month. Store leftovers in an airtight container in a cool, dry place for up to 3 days.

MAKES 2 LARGE LOAVES OR 5 SMALL LOAVES; EACH LARGE LOAF SERVES 12, EACH SMALL LOAF SERVES 5

Canola oil cooking spray

2 cups (260 g) unbleached all-purpose flour

1½ cups (195 g) whole wheat flour

2¼ cups (514 g) sugar

2 teaspoons baking soda

½ teaspoon baking powder

½ teaspoon salt

2 teaspoons ground cinnamon

1 teaspoon ground nutmeg

½ teaspoon ground ginger

½ cup (125 ml) canola oil

½ cup (125 ml) unsweetened applesauce

2 large eggs plus 2 large egg whites

⅔ cup (160 ml) water

One 15-ounce (425 g) can solid-pack pumpkin (not pumpkin pie mix)

1 cup (140 g) dried cranberries or cherries, optional

1 cup (100 g) chopped toasted walnuts, optional

1. Center an oven rack and preheat the oven to 375°F (190°C). Spray two 8½ x 4½ x 2½-inch (21.5 x 11 x 6 cm) or five 5¾ x 3 x 2⅛-inch (14.5 x 7.5 x 5 cm) loaf pans with cooking spray; set aside.

2. In a large bowl, combine all the dry ingredients and whisk until well blended; set aside.

3. In another large bowl, combine the canola oil, applesauce, eggs, egg whites, and water and whisk to mix. Add to the dry ingredients and mix until combined. Add the pumpkin and the cranberries and walnuts, if using, and mix until well combined.

4. Divide the batter evenly among the prepared loaf pans. Bake for about 70 minutes for large loaves, about 40 minutes for smaller loaves, or until a cake tester inserted in the center comes out clean. If the loaves are browning too quickly on top, cover them loosely with a piece of foil. Let sit for 5 minutes, then remove from the pans and cool completely before slicing.

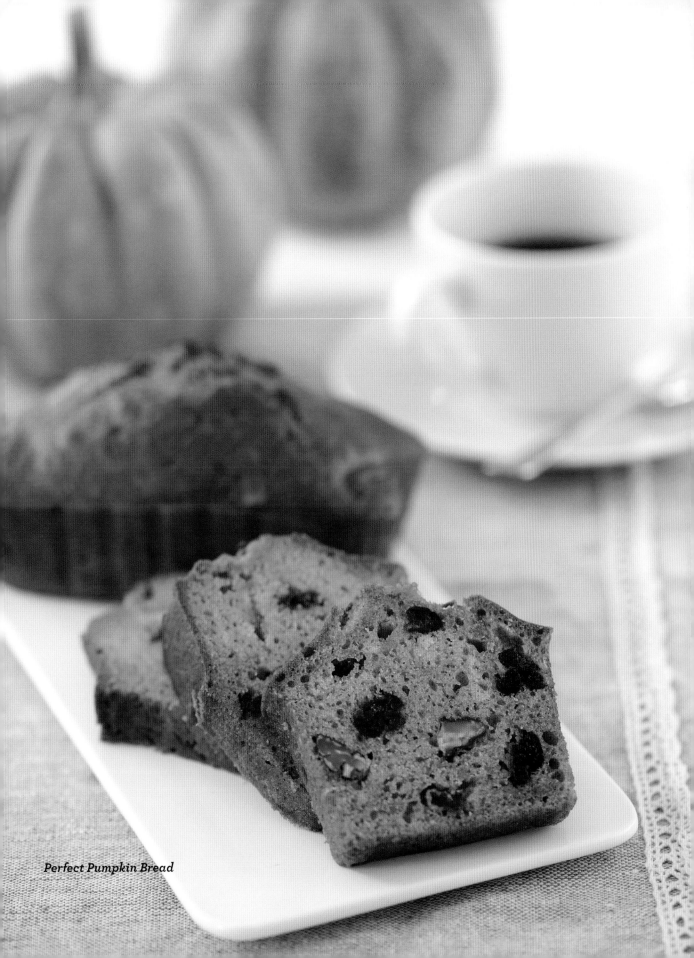

Perfect Pumpkin Bread

HOW TO PREVENT APPLES FROM BROWNING WHILE SLICING

If a recipe calls for slicing lots of apples, it can be tricky to keep them from browning in the time it takes to peel and slice them all. To prevent this natural oxidation, caused by an enzyme contained in the flesh of the apples, mix the sliced apples with some of the sugar called for in the recipe. The sugar will melt and coat the apples to prevent browning. Lemon or orange juice can also be used. This applies to other fruits that oxidize quickly, such as pears.

PLUM DELICIOUS CAKE

I whip up this lovely cake whenever plums are in season. Use Italian plums or any small ripe purple plums. This dessert is wonderful by itself and sublime when paired with a scoop of nonfat frozen vanilla yogurt or nonfat Greek-style yogurt. It is best served on the same day it is made. A dusting of confectioners' sugar, with the juicy plums poking through the white surface, is a gorgeous touch.

SERVES 8

Canola oil cooking spray

1 cup (130 g) unbleached all-purpose flour, plus extra for the baking pan

1 teaspoon baking powder

1 teaspoon ground cinnamon, or to taste

Pinch of salt

2 tablespoons canola oil

2 tablespoons unsalted butter, at room temperature

½ cup (115 g) sugar, plus about 3 tablespoons for sprinkling, depending on the sweetness of the plums

2 large eggs

1 teaspoon vanilla extract

1½ pounds (720 g) purple plums, halved, pitted, sliced, and each slice halved widthwise (about 4 cups, 1 liter)

1 to 2 tablespoons confectioners' sugar, for dusting the cake

1. Center an oven rack and preheat the oven to 350°F (180°C). Grease a 9-inch (23 cm) springform pan or a 9-inch (23 cm) round cake pan with cooking spray and lightly flour it; set aside.

2. Sift together the flour, baking powder, ½ teaspoon of the cinnamon, and the salt; set aside.

3. In a large bowl, combine the canola oil, butter, and ½ cup (115 g) of the sugar and beat with an electric mixer on medium speed for 2 minutes. Add the eggs and vanilla extract and beat for 1 minute, scraping down the sides of the bowl as needed. Add the sifted flour mixture and beat on low speed for 30 seconds, or just until the batter comes together.

4. Spoon the batter into the prepared pan. Arrange the plums on top of the batter; overlapping them is fine. Sprinkle the remaining 3 tablespoons sugar and the remaining ½ teaspoon cinnamon over the plums. Bake the cake for 50 to 55 minutes, until a cake tester comes out clean (it will show some juice from the plums). Remove from the oven and cool for 15 minutes.

5. Run a knife around the edges of the cake and remove the sides of the springform pan. Or, if using a regular cake pan, run a knife around the edges, invert the cake onto a plate, and invert it again onto a serving plate. Cool to room temperature. Dust the cake with confectioners' sugar before serving. Any leftovers can be covered and stored at room temperature for up to 2 days or refrigerated in an airtight container.

---

227 CALORIES IN

Protein: 4 g; Carbohydrates: 36 g; Fat: 8 g; Fiber: 2 g; Sodium: 64 mg; Carb Choices: 2½; Diabetic Exchange: 2 Starch, 1 Fat

227 CALORIES OUT

Women: Walk: 55 minutes; Jog: 26 minutes

Men: Walk: 46 minutes; Jog: 22 minutes

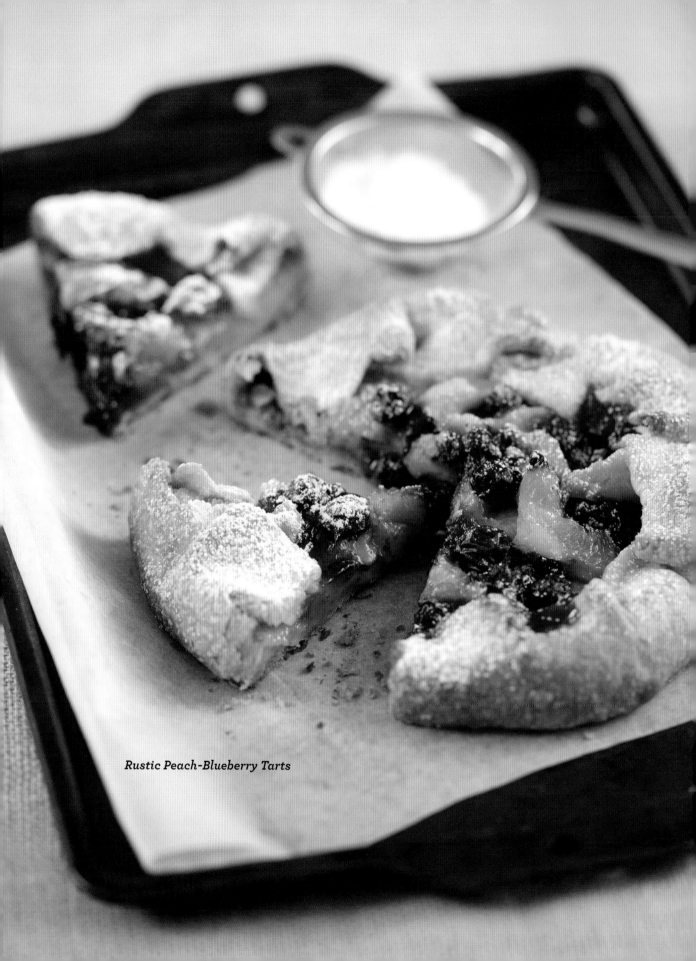

Rustic Peach-Blueberry Tarts

RUSTIC PEACH-BLUEBERRY TARTS

This beautiful free-form tart, dusted with confectioners' sugar, is an end-of-meal stunner. It might seem complicated, but it's not; in fact, I think it's easier than making a traditional pie. The recipe makes 2 tarts, each one serving 4. If you prefer, you can make one very large tart. Feel free to substitute your favorite berries and fruits for the peaches and blueberries; I also give you a recipe for an apple-blueberry filling below. Depending on how juicy the fruits are, you may need to use slightly more flour to thicken the filling. Serve with a scoop of nonfat frozen yogurt, if desired. The tarts can be stored, covered, at room temperature for up to 2 days.

MAKES TWO 9-INCH (23 CM) TARTS; EACH TART SERVES 4

242 CALORIES IN

Protein: 3 g; Carbohydrates: 42 g; Fat: 7 g; Fiber: 2 g; Sodium: 11 mg; Carb Choices: 2½; Diabetic Exchange: 1 Starch, 2 Fruit, 1 Fat

242 CALORIES OUT

Women: Walk: 59 minutes; Jog: 28 minutes

Men: Walk: 49 minutes; Jog: 23 minutes

Dough

1 cup (130 g) unbleached all-purpose flour

2 tablespoons cornmeal

2 tablespoons sugar

Pinch of salt

5 tablespoons (75 g) chilled unsalted butter, cut into pieces

1½ tablespoons nonfat plain Greek-style yogurt

2 to 3 tablespoons very cold water

Peach-Blueberry Filling

1½ cups (225 g) fresh blueberries

Two 15-ounce (425 g) cans "extra firm" yellow cling peaches in light syrup, drained and cut into ½-inch (1.25 cm) slices, or 3 cups (375 ml) sliced fresh peaches

¼ cup (54 g) sugar, or to taste, depending on the sweetness of the fruit

1 teaspoon ground cinnamon

1 teaspoon vanilla extract

2 to 3 tablespoons unbleached all-purpose flour

1 teaspoon grated lemon zest, optional

2 tablespoons confectioners' sugar, for dusting

1. To make the dough, in the bowl of a food processor, pulse the flour, cornmeal, sugar, and salt to combine. Add the butter and pulse until it is the size of small pebbles. Add the yogurt and 2 tablespoons water and pulse just until the dough forms a ball; do not overmix. The dough should stick together when pinched; if it's too dry, add up to 1 tablespoon more water. Turn the dough out onto a piece of plastic wrap, divide it in two, press each half into a disk, and refrigerate for at least 30 minutes or up to 3 days. If the dough is very cold, let it sit at room temperature for 10 minutes to become more pliable before rolling out.

2. To make the filling, combine all of the ingredients in a bowl and mix gently until well combined; set aside at room temperature.

3. Center an oven rack and preheat the oven to 400°F (200°C). Line two baking sheets (or one very large one), with baking paper or Silpats; set aside. On a separate piece of baking paper, roll out one piece of the dough into a thin 11-inch (28 cm) round. Transfer the round to a baking sheet (an easy way to do this is to flip the round of dough onto the prepared sheet). Repeat with the remaining piece of dough. If your dough gets too soft, place it with the baking paper in the freezer to firm up.

(RECIPE CONTINUES)

4. Mound half the filling in the center of one round of dough, then spread it out to within 3 inches (7.5 cm) of the edges. Carefully fold over the edges to create a 2-inch (5 cm) rim around the tart, pleating the dough as you fold it. Repeat with the remaining filling and the second dough round. Brush the dough with a little bit of cold water and sprinkle with a bit of sugar (about ½ teaspoon per tart).

5. Bake for 35 to 40 minutes, until the dough is light golden and the fruit filling is bubbling. If you use two baking sheets you will need to bake them one at a time. Transfer to a rack and cool slightly before slicing.

Cooking Note: To make an apple-blueberry tart, use the following recipe for the filling. The baking time for the apple tarts will be about 40 minutes, or until the apples feel soft when pierced with a cake tester.

APPLE-BLUEBERRY FILLING FOR TARTS

1½ cups (225 g) fresh blueberries

12 ounces (360 g) Granny Smith apples, peeled, cored, and thinly sliced

½ cup (115 g) sugar

¾ teaspoon ground cinnamon

3 tablespoons unbleached all-purpose flour

LIGHT ORANGE CHIFFON CAKE WITH ORANGE GLAZE (📷 page 273)

This deliciously moist orange chiffon cake is for anyone who loves to bake light and airy cakes but fears the risk of a fallen angel cake. The cake rises high and keeps its height once cool. The orange glaze is a lovely crowning touch. Serve with assorted fresh berries. The cake is best eaten on the day it is made. Store any leftovers in an airtight container at room temperature for up to 2 days.

SERVES 15

2 cups (260 g) unbleached all-purpose flour

1 tablespoon plus 1 teaspoon baking powder

¼ teaspoon salt

1 cup (230 g) sugar

½ cup (125 ml) canola oil

6 large eggs, separated

2 tablespoons finely grated orange zest

½ cup (125 ml) fresh orange juice

¼ cup (60 ml) cold water

¼ teaspoon cream of tartar

Orange Glaze
(makes about ¾ cup/180 ml)

1½ cups (180 g) confectioners' sugar

2 teaspoons grated orange zest, or to taste

3 tablespoons fresh orange juice

1 teaspoon hot water

1. Position an oven rack in the lower third of the oven and preheat the oven to 325°F (160°C). Have ready a 10-inch (25 cm) angel food cake pan with a removable bottom.

2. In a large bowl, combine the flour, baking powder, salt, and ¾ cup (180 ml) of the sugar and whisk together. Make a well in the center of the flour mixture. Add the canola oil, egg yolks, orange zest, orange juice, and cold water to the well and whisk until blended, then whisk the wet ingredients into the surrounding flour until smooth; set aside.

3. In the bowl of an electric mixer, combine the egg whites and cream of tartar and beat on low speed for 30 seconds. Increase the speed to medium and add the remaining ¼ cup (60 ml) sugar, then increase the speed to high and continue beating until stiff glossy peaks form, 2 to 3 minutes.

4. Using a rubber spatula, gently fold half of the beaten egg whites into the batter. When fairly well incorporated, fold in the remaining half, just until combined. Try not to overmix, as you risk deflating the egg whites, but make sure you mix in all of the flour.

5. Transfer the batter to the cake pan and bake for 55 to 60 minutes, until a cake

252 CALORIES IN

Protein: 4 g; Carbohydrates: 38 g; Fat: 9 g; Fiber: 0 g; Sodium: 162 mg; Carb Choices: 2½; Diabetic Exchange: 2 Starch, 2 Fat

252 CALORIES OUT

Women: Walk: 61 minutes; Jog: 29 minutes

Men: Walk: 51 minutes; Jog: 24 minutes

(RECIPE CONTINUES)

tester inserted in the center comes out clean. Remove from the oven and invert the cake. Some angel food cake pans have legs for this purpose; if not, suspend the cake pan over the top of a bottle (the old-fashioned way). Don't worry, the cake will stay in the pan as it hangs upside down. Cool completely, then turn the pan right side up, run a knife around the edges of the pan and the center tube to release the cake, and invert onto a large serving plate.

6. To make the orange glaze, mix all of the ingredients in a bowl until smooth. (The glaze can be made a day ahead; cover and refrigerate.) Pour the glaze over the top of the cooled cake, allowing it to drip down the sides.

HOW TO WHIP PERFECT EGG WHITES

There is definitely an art to whipping egg whites perfectly every time. To begin, your bowl and beaters should be impeccably clean; no grease, please. Ideally, you should use a standing mixer (especially for large volumes of whites), but a handheld mixer will work, too; you might have to beat a little longer. You will need a bit of acid to stabilize the whites, which can come from a couple drops of fresh lemon juice, or cream of tartar. Combine the egg whites and lemon juice or cream of tartar in a large bowl and beat on low speed for 30 seconds. Once small bubbles begin to form, increase the speed to medium and beat for 30 seconds, or until large, frothy bubbles begin to appear. If the recipe calls for sugar, add it at this stage, then increase the speed to high and continue beating until soft, glossy peaks form, about 2 minutes. Voilà, mountains of perfect whites!

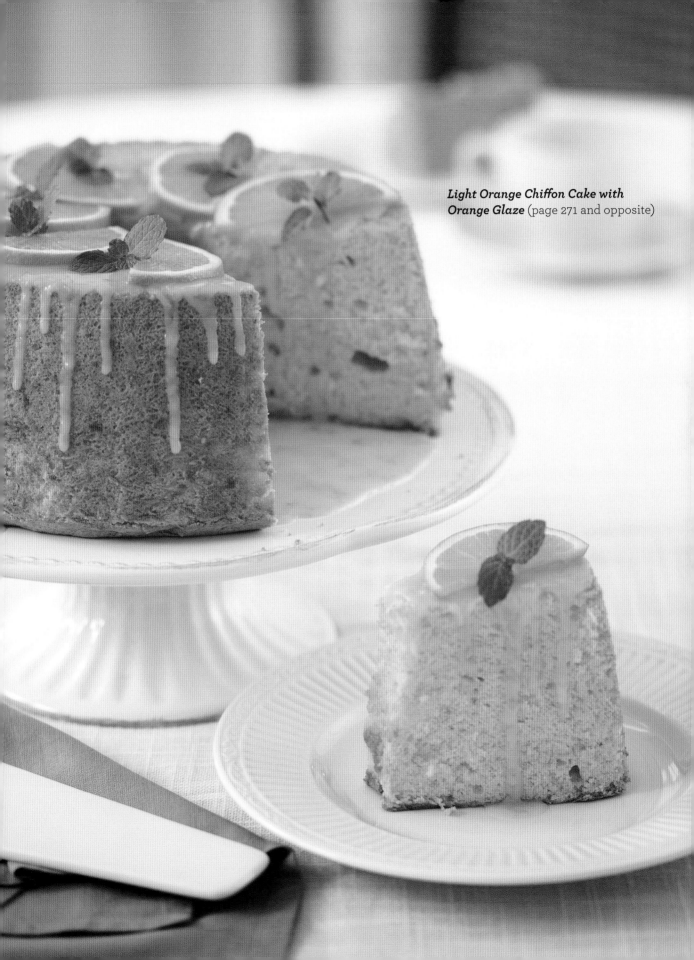

Light Orange Chiffon Cake with Orange Glaze (page 271 and opposite)

THE BEST ICE BOX BERRY PIE

In this no-bake stunner, raspberries are cooked with sugar, water, and cornstarch to make a sauce that binds the sliced fresh strawberries for the filling. The result is an intense berry flavor that is light and rich at the same time. My recipe testers and I have made this pie countless times, so I have some helpful tips to share: the pie can be made up to 1 day in advance; more than that, and the strawberries tend to weep and get too soft. Cover and refrigerate any leftovers.

SERVES 8

Graham Cracker Crust

1 cup (100 g) graham cracker crumbs

¼ cup (25 g) very finely chopped walnuts

4 tablespoons (60 g) unsalted butter, melted

Berry Filling

12 ounces (360 g) fresh or frozen unsweetened raspberries

¾ cup (162 g) sugar, or to taste

¼ cup (25 g) cornstarch (see Cooking Notes)

⅓ cup (80 ml) water

2 teaspoons vanilla extract

1½ tablespoons fresh lemon juice

1 pound (480 g) fresh strawberries, hulled and quartered, or cut smaller if the berries are large (about 3 cups, 750 ml)

Canola oil cooking spray

1. To make the crust, center an oven rack and preheat the oven to 350°F (180°C). Combine all of the crust ingredients in a bowl and mix until well blended and the crumbs are moist. Transfer the mixture to a 9-inch (23 cm) pie plate and press it evenly over the bottom and up the sides. Bake for 10 minutes, or until the crust is slightly firm to the touch. Remove from the oven and let cool before filling.

2. To make the filling, puree the raspberries in a food processor or blender until smooth. (Note: The pureed berries should yield about 2 cups/500 ml.) Combine the puree, sugar, cornstarch, water, vanilla extract, and lemon juice in a medium saucepan. Bring to simmer over medium heat and cook, stirring constantly, for 2 minutes, or until the sauce becomes thick and shiny. Remove from the heat.

3. Distribute half of the sliced strawberries evenly in the pie shell. Pour half of the hot sauce over them. Make another layer with the remaining strawberries, and top with the remaining sauce. Using a spoon, gently move the strawberries until all of them are covered and the sauce reaches the edges of the pie crust.

4. Cool the pie to room temperature, then take a piece of plastic wrap and very (very!) lightly grease it with cooking spray. Lay it directly on top of the pie, flush with the surface, and refrigerate for at least 4 hours, or until firmly set.

Cooking Notes: 1) Taste the raspberries and add more sugar in Step 2 if needed; don't risk a too-tart pie. If the strawberries are not sweet, just before assembling the pie, place the slices in a bowl and toss with an extra tablespoon of sugar. 2) The amount of juice in the berries will vary, so you may need to make a small adjustment to the amount of cornstarch: as a test, take a spoonful of the cooked raspberry sauce and place it on a plate in the refrigerator until it is cool. If it is too runny, increase the cornstarch by ½ tablespoon at a time, dissolving it in a little bit of water before adding it. 3) Allow at least 4 hours of refrigeration for the pie to set.

BLUEBERRY BUCKLE WITH ALMOND CRISP TOPPING

A buckle, defined as fruit mixed with a simple cake batter, is an easy dessert that doesn't require a mixer. Simply whisk the ingredients together in a bowl, transfer to a cake pan or baking dish, and pop in the oven. The result is a moist, bread pudding–like dessert that takes some serious willpower not to consume in large amounts. The crisp topping adds a sweet nutty almond flavor, but if you're cutting back on calories, skip it. Serve with a scoop of nonfat frozen yogurt, if desired. This buckle is best eaten on the day it is baked.

SERVES 8

Almond Crisp Topping

¼ cup (40 g) packed brown sugar

¼ cup (35 g) unbleached all-purpose flour

1 teaspoon ground cinnamon

3 tablespoons unsalted butter

¼ cup (25 g) sliced almonds

Cake

Canola oil cooking spray

2 cups (300 g) fresh blueberries

¾ cup (105 g) plus 1 tablespoon unbleached all-purpose flour

⅓ cup (70 g) sugar

2 teaspoons baking powder

1 teaspoon ground cinnamon

¼ cup (60 ml) canola oil

1 large egg

½ cup (125 ml) low-fat buttermilk

½ teaspoon grated lemon zest, optional

1. To make the topping, combine all of the ingredients except the almonds in a small bowl and quickly mix with your fingers to the consistency of coarse cornmeal. Add the almonds, mix again, and refrigerate until ready to use.

2. Center an oven rack and preheat the oven to 350°F (180°C). Grease an 8-inch (20 cm) cake pan or Pyrex baking dish with cooking spray and set aside.

3. To make the cake, mix the blueberries with 1 tablespoon of the flour and set aside. In a large bowl, whisk the remaining ¾ cup (105 g) of flour, the sugar, baking powder, and cinnamon; set aside.

4. In a small bowl, combine the canola oil, egg, buttermilk, and lemon zest, if using, and whisk until well blended. Add to the bowl of dry ingredients and mix until combined. Using a spatula, gently fold in the reserved blueberries.

5. Transfer the batter to the prepared cake pan. Distribute the crumble topping evenly over the batter. Bake for 45 minutes, or until the topping is golden and a cake tester inserted into the cake comes out clean (except for the blueberry juices). Remove from the oven and allow to cool slightly before serving. Refrigerate any leftovers.

268 CALORIES IN

Protein: 5 g; Carbohydrates: 36 g; Fat: 13 g; Fiber: 4 g; Sodium: 120 mg; Carb Choices: 2½; Diabetic Exchange: 2 Starch, 2 Fat

268 CALORIES OUT

Women: Walk: 65 minutes; Jog: 31 minutes

Men: Walk: 55 minutes; Jog: 26 minutes

CALORIE CUTS

Skip the almond crisp topping and save 87 calories and 6 grams of fat per serving.

279 CALORIES IN

Protein: 4 g; Carbohydrates: 51 g; Fat: 7 g; Fiber: 3 g; Sodium: 61 mg; Carb Choices: 3; Diabetic Exchange: 3 Starch, 1 Fat

279 CALORIES OUT

Women: Walk: 68 minutes; Jog: 32 minutes

Men: Walk: 57 minutes; Jog: 27 minutes

PLUM-BLUEBERRY DROP BISCUIT COBBLER

The classic American cobbler consists of fruit, most often apples, peaches, plums, and/or berries, covered with a biscuit or pastry dough that is either rolled out, stamped out, or simply dropped, which is the easiest way. Play around with the fruit: come up with your own fruit combinations and adjust the flour to the amount of juices the fruits will likely release. If your fruits are juicy, add another tablespoon of flour. The biscuit dough takes on a new dimension if you add spices such as ground ginger and minced candied ginger, cinnamon, or allspice. The most important thing is to leave the cobbler in the oven long enough to make sure the biscuit dough is fully cooked; undercooked dough is no fun. But fear not, I've made this mistake before; if necessary, you can return the cobbler to the oven to finish baking. My recipes testers loved this cobbler, saying that it was super easy to make and that people asked for seconds. The cobbler is best eaten on the day it is baked, though I admit I also like leftovers cold for breakfast.

SERVES 8

Cobbler Dough

1 cup plus 2 tablespoons (150 g) unbleached all-purpose flour

1 teaspoon baking powder

⅓ cup (60 g) packed brown sugar

Pinch of salt

4 tablespoons (60 g) chilled unsalted butter, cut into small pieces

1 large egg, lightly beaten

2 tablespoons nonfat plain Greek-style yogurt

1½ teaspoons vanilla extract

Cobbler Filling

About 2 pounds (1 kg) purple plums, pitted and quartered (5 cups/1.25 l)

2 cups (300 g) fresh blueberries

⅓ cup plus 2 tablespoons (80 g) sugar

¼ cup (35 g) unbleached all-purpose flour

1 teaspoon ground cinnamon

1 teaspoon vanilla extract

2 tablespoons fresh lemon juice

1. Center an oven rack and preheat the oven to 425°F (220°C). Have ready an ungreased 9-inch (23 cm) baking dish.

2. To make the dough, combine the flour, baking powder, brown sugar, and salt in a large bowl and stir to mix. Add the butter and using a pastry blender or your fingers, rub the mixture until it resembles a coarse meal. Stir in the egg, yogurt, and vanilla extract and mix just until the dough comes together; it will be sticky. Set aside.

3. To prepare the filling, combine all of the ingredients in a large bowl and mix until well blended. Transfer the filling to the baking dish, then drop heaping tablespoonfuls of the cobbler dough over the fruit, leaving some spaces for the fruit to show through.

4. Bake for 12 minutes, then reduce the heat to 400°F (200°C) and continue to bake for 30 to 35 minutes, until the dough is cooked and the juices are bubbling. Remove the cobbler from the oven and allow to cool slightly before serving. Refrigerate any leftovers.

LEMON DROP

A refreshing lemony twist on a vodka martini. Please note that 1 tablespoon of lite agave syrup is 60 calories.

SERVES 1

Ice

2 ounces (¼ cup, 60 ml) lemon vodka

2 tablespoons fresh lemon juice, or to taste

1 to 2 tablespoons lite agave syrup or simple syrup (see How to Make Simple Syrup, page 175), to taste

Splash of Cointreau

Fill a cocktail shaker with ice. Add all of the remaining ingredients and shake well. Strain into a chilled martini glass.

213 CALORIES IN | 1 SERVING WITH 1 TABLESPOON LITE AGAVE SYRUP

Protein: 0 g; Carbohydrates: 18 g; Fat: 0 g; Fiber: 0 g; Sodium: 1 mg; Carb Choices: 1; Diabetic Exchange: 1 Starch, 3 Fat*

*Note to diabetics: Alcohol can cause problems with blood sugar control; it should be consumed in moderation with meals or snacks.

213 CALORIES OUT

Women: Walk: 52 minutes; Jog: 24 minutes

Men: Walk: 43 minutes; Jog: 20 minutes

FESTIVE MARGARITA PUNCH (page 178)

A fantastic punch for entertaining, especially when the mood calls for casual fun. Elaine's brother-in-law, Ernie Renda, has spent time in Texas, which is where he perfected this margarita recipe. For a stunning presentation, garnish the pitcher with citrus slices and fresh mint sprigs.

SERVES 14

215 CALORIES IN | 1 SERVING

Protein: 0 g; Carbohydrates: 16 g; Fat: 0 g; Fiber: 0 g; Sodium: 1 mg; Carb Choices: 1; Diabetic Exchange: 2 Starch, 1 Fat*

*Note to diabetics: Alcohol can cause problems with blood sugar control; it should be consumed in moderation with meals or snacks.

215 CALORIES OUT

Women: Walk: 52 minutes; Jog: 25 minutes

Men: Walk: 44 minutes; Jog: 21minutes

One 12-ounce (360 ml) can limeade, plus 3 cans of water (do not follow the can instructions for the water amount)

3 cups (750 ml) tequila, preferably Cuervo Gold

1 cup (250 ml) Cointreau

⅓ cup (80 ml) fresh orange juice (preferably from Valencia oranges)

2 to 3 tablespoons fresh lime juice, to taste

Ice

In a very large pitcher, mix all of the ingredients except the ice. Adjust the flavor if necessary and then add ice to the pitcher. Serve cold.

POMETINI (page 178)

This pomegranate twist on a martini is as tasty as it is beautiful. Fresh pomegranate seeds make the perfect garnish.

SERVES 1

226 CALORIES IN

Protein: 0 g; Carbohydrates: 7 g; Fat: 0 g; Fiber: 0 g; Sodium: 2 mg; Carb Choices: ½; Diabetic Exchange: ½ Fruit, 4 Fat*

*Note to diabetics: Alcohol can cause problems with blood sugar control. It should be consumed in moderation with meals or snacks.

226 CALORIES OUT

Women: Walk: 55 minutes; Jog: 26 minutes

Men: Walk: 46 minutes; Jog: 22 minutes

Ice

2 ounces (¼ cup, 60 ml) vodka

1 tablespoon Cointreau, or to taste

1 tablespoon pomegranate liqueur, such as Pama

2 tablespoons Pom Wonderful 100% pomegranate juice

1 tablespoon fresh lime juice, or to taste

Fill a cocktail shaker with ice. Add all of the remaining ingredients and shake well. Strain into a chilled martini glass and serve.

PART THREE

300 to 399

CALORIES PER SERVING

BREAKFAST

OAT FLOUR–BUTTERMILK WAFFLES

I love a good waffle, preferably hot off the waffle iron, drizzled with warm pure maple syrup and sprinkled with fresh blueberries. These crisp, light waffles are ideal for leisurely weekend breakfasts, and they can also be made in advance, frozen, and reheated in a toaster for quick and easy weekday breakfasts. If you love nuts and can afford a calorie splurge, add ⅓ cup (30 g) finely chopped pecans (which will add 50 calories per serving) to the batter. To freeze, place the cooled waffles in a plastic container, ideally separated by baking paper, and freeze.

MAKES ABOUT 20 REGULAR-SIZE WAFFLES; SERVES 5

1 cup (130 g) oat flour

1 cup (130 g) unbleached all-purpose flour

1 tablespoon baking powder

1 tablespoon sugar

¼ teaspoon salt

2 large eggs, separated, plus 1 large egg white

3 tablespoons canola oil

2 cups (500 ml) reduced-fat buttermilk

Canola oil cooking spray

1. Place the dry ingredients in a large bowl and whisk together.
2. In a small bowl or large measuring cup, whisk together the egg yolks, canola oil, and buttermilk. Add this mixture to the dry ingredients and whisk until well blended; set aside.
3. Place the 3 egg whites in a large bowl and beat with an electric mixer on medium speed for about 30 seconds, or until frothy bubbles begin to appear. Increase the speed to high and beat until stiff, glossy peaks form, 2 to 3 minutes. Gently fold the whites into the reserved batter.
4. Preheat your waffle iron on high heat. Spray the hot waffle grids with cooking spray or brush with oil. Spoon some batter onto the hot grids and spread it almost to the edges. Close the lid and cook until the waffles are golden brown. Serve immediately. Repeat with the remaining batter.

Cooking Note: To prevent cooked waffles from getting soggy, place them on a cake rack, or lean them against each other in a tentlike formation, to allow the steam to escape. If they do get soggy or cold, reheat them in a toaster or a preheated 350°F (180°C) oven; place them directly on an oven rack for a few minutes.

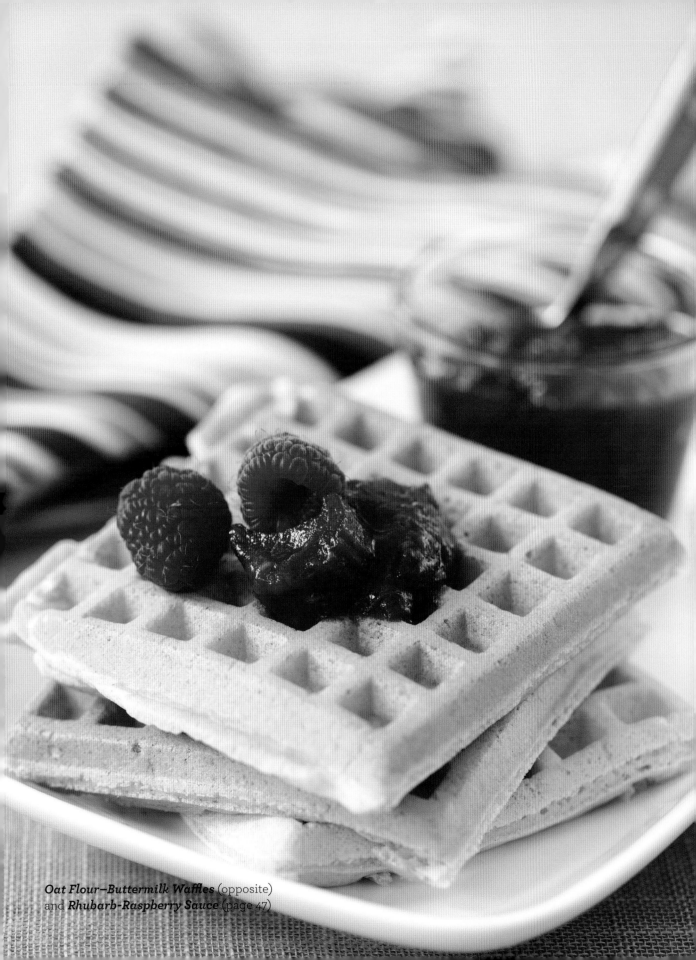

Oat Flour–Buttermilk Waffles (opposite)
and *Rhubarb-Raspberry Sauce* (page 47)

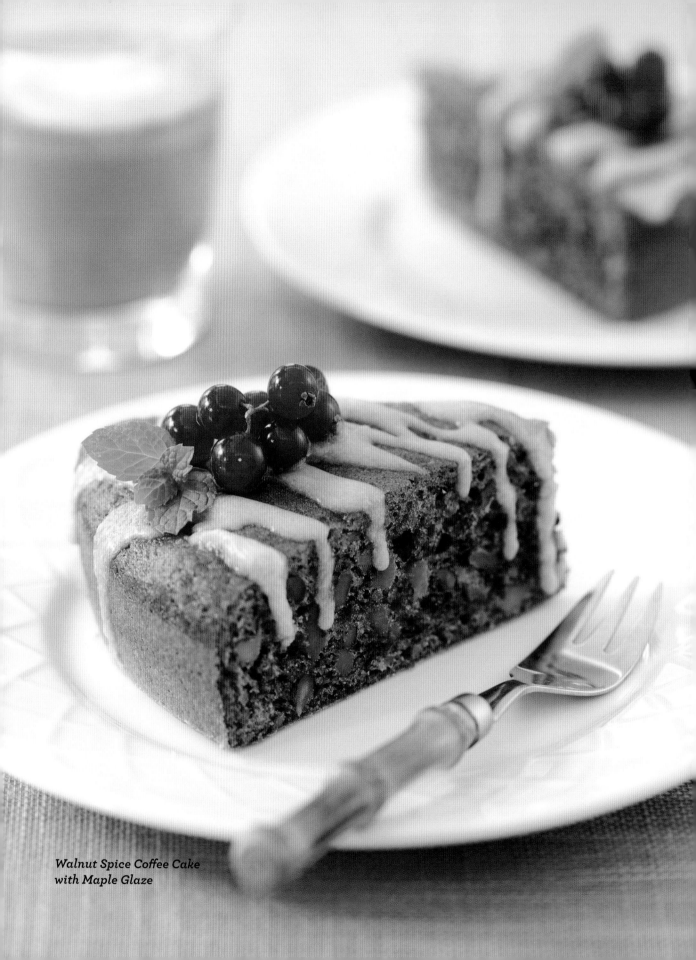

Walnut Spice Coffee Cake with Maple Glaze

WALNUT SPICE COFFEE CAKE WITH MAPLE GLAZE

Easy, quick, and loaded with nutty flavor, this coffee cake is a joy any time of day, including dessert. I've given you a recipe for a decadent maple glaze, which takes the cake to a new level. Store leftovers in an airtight container for up to 3 days; if keeping longer, cover and refrigerate or freeze.

SERVES 12

Canola oil cooking spray

1 cup (130 g) unbleached all-purpose flour, plus extra for the cake pan

1⅓ cups (130 g) chopped toasted walnuts

1 teaspoon baking powder

½ teaspoon baking soda

1 teaspoon ground ginger

2½ teaspoons ground cinnamon

½ teaspoon ground nutmeg

¼ teaspoon salt

¾ cup (120 g) packed brown sugar

2 large eggs

⅓ cup (60 ml) canola oil

1 teaspoon vanilla extract

½ cup (125 ml) plus 2 tablespoons reduced-fat sour cream

1 tablespoon confectioners' sugar, for dusting, if you are not using the maple glaze

Optional Maple Glaze

2 tablespoons unsalted butter

¼ cup (40 g) packed brown sugar

3 tablespoons 2% milk

1 cup (120 g) confectioners' sugar

1. Center an oven rack and preheat the oven to 350°F (180°C). Grease a 9-inch (23 cm) round cake pan with cooking spray and dust with flour; set aside.

2. Place the walnuts in the bowl of a food processor and pulse until finely ground; do not process to a paste. Transfer the ground walnuts to a medium bowl and add the flour, baking powder, baking soda, ginger, cinnamon, nutmeg, and salt. Mix until well combined; set aside.

3. In a large bowl, using an electric mixer, beat the brown sugar and eggs on medium speed for about 4 minutes, or until light and fluffy. Add the canola oil, vanilla extract, and sour cream and beat 30 seconds more. Using a rubber spatula, fold the egg mixture into the reserved flour mixture until well incorporated. Pour the batter into the prepared cake pan. Bake for 30 minutes, or until a cake tester inserted into the center of the cake comes out clean.

4. Remove the cake from the oven and let cool for 5 minutes, then run a knife around the sides of the pan and invert the cake onto a serving platter.

5. To make the optional maple glaze, combine the butter, brown sugar, and milk in a small saucepan and heat over medium heat, stirring constantly, until it reaches a full boil. Remove from the heat and cool to room temperature. Whisk in the confectioners' sugar until smooth.

6. Spread the glaze on the cooled cake and allow to set for 1 hour before serving, or dust with the 1 tablespoon of confectioners' sugar.

247 CALORIES IN | I SERVING WITHOUT MAPLE GLAZE

Protein: 5 g; Carbohydrates: 21 g; Fat: 17 g; Fiber: 1 g; Sodium: 155 mg; Carb Choices: 1; Diabetic Exchange: 1½ Starch, 3 Fat

247 CALORIES OUT

Women: Walk: 60 minutes | Jog: 28 minutes

Men: Walk: 50 minutes | Jog: 24 minutes

307 CALORIES IN | I SERVING WITH MAPLE GLAZE

Protein: 5 g; Carbohydrates: 31 g; Fat: 19 g; Fiber: 1 g; Sodium: 158 mg; Carb Choices: 2; Diabetic Exchange: 1½ Starch, 3 Fat

307 CALORIES OUT

Women: Walk: 75 minutes | Jog: 35 minutes

Men: Walk: 63 minutes | Jog: 30 minutes

CALORIE COMBOS

Customized Fruit Salad (page 44): 23 to 57 cals

½ cup (125 ml) orange juice: 56 cals

Three Delicious Fruit Smoothies (page 173): 62 to 89 cals

Five-a-Day Green Power Drink (page 176): 145 cals

Five-a-Day Pink Power Drink (page 177): 157 cals

CALORIE CUTS

Omit the maple glaze, which adds 63 calories per serving. Reduce the walnuts to 1 cup and save 21 calories and about 2 grams of fat per serving.

BAKED OATMEAL-WALNUT CRISP WITH PEACHES AND BLACKBERRIES

244 CALORIES IN | I SERVING WITHOUT THE CRISP TOPPING

Protein: 10 g; Carbohydrates: 41 g; Fat: 5 g; Fiber: 6 g; Sodium: 66 mg; Carb Choices: 2½; Diabetic Exchange: 3 Starch

244 CALORIES OUT

Women: Walk:
59 minutes | Jog: 28 minutes

Men: Walk:
50 minutes | Jog: 23 minutes

318 CALORIES IN | I SERVING WITH CRISP TOPPING

Protein: 11 g; Carbohydrates: 50 g; Fat: 9 g; Fiber: 7 g; Sodium: 68 mg; Carb Choices: 3; Diabetic Exchange: 3 Starch, 2 Fat

318 CALORIES OUT

Women: Walk:
77 minutes | Jog: 36 minutes

Men: Walk:
65 minutes | Jog: 31 minutes

CALORIE COMBOS

Customized Fruit Salad (page 44): 23 to 57 cals

½ cup (125 ml) orange juice: 56 cals

Three Delicious Fruit Smoothies (page 173): 62 to 89 cals

4 ounces (120 g) nonfat plain yogurt: 72 cals

4 ounces (120 g) low-fat plain yogurt: 77 cals

Five-a-Day Green Power Drink (page 176): 145 cals

Five-a-Day Pink Power Drink (page 177): 157 cals

This oatmeal crisp is enough to get anyone out of bed in the morning. I use canned or jarred peaches for convenience; sliced frozen ones are delicious, too. Feel free to swap in your favorite fruits. This recipe calls for rolled oats. Quick-cooking oats get too mushy, and steel-cut oats require a long time to cook (see page 347). The crisp topping is optional, but it does keep the top layer of oats moist during baking. Leftovers can be refrigerated or frozen and reheated in a microwave oven.

SERVES 8

Optional Crisp Topping

⅓ cup (45 g) unbleached all-purpose flour

¼ cup (40 g) packed brown sugar

2 tablespoons unsalted butter, cut into pieces

2 tablespoons chopped walnuts or pecans, or sliced almonds, for sprinkling on top

Oatmeal Crisp

Canola oil cooking spray

One 15-ounce (425 g) can or jar of peaches in light syrup, drained and thinly sliced (1⅓ cups/325 ml), or 10 ounces (284 g) frozen sliced peaches, thawed

1½ cups (6 ounces/180 g) fresh blackberries

2 cups (200 g) old-fashioned rolled oats

¼ cup (40 g) packed brown sugar, plus 3 tablespoons if you are not making the crisp topping

½ teaspoon baking powder

2 teaspoons ground cinnamon

Pinch of salt

2 cups (500 ml) 2% milk

1 large egg

2 teaspoons vanilla extract

1. If making the optional topping, combine the flour and brown sugar in a small bowl. Add the butter and, using your fingers, rub the mix until it resembles coarse cornmeal. Refrigerate until ready to use.
2. Center an oven rack and preheat the oven to 375°F (190°C). Grease a 9-inch (20 cm) baking dish with cooking spray.
3. Arrange the peaches in a single layer in the bottom of the baking dish and arrange the blackberries on top; set aside.
4. In a medium bowl, mix together the rolled oats, brown sugar, baking powder, cinnamon, and salt. Set aside.
5. In a small bowl or large measuring cup, whisk together the milk, egg, and vanilla extract.
6. Cover the fruit with the reserved oat mixture, then pour the milk mixture evenly over the oats. Use a spoon to move the liquid through the oats to make sure it is evenly distributed. Sprinkle the reserved crisp topping over the top of casserole, if you made it, then sprinkle with the almonds, if using. If you are not using the crisp topping, sprinkle the top with the extra 3 tablespoons brown sugar.
7. Bake for 40 to 45 minutes, until the oats are soft (try a small spoonful to test it) and the fruit juices are bubbling. Serve warm.

ASIAN-STYLE CHICKEN NOODLE SALAD (📷 page 287)

When I lived in Malaysia, Asian-style chicken salad was a staple on the weekends. Use whatever noodles you want, from rice noodles to thin quinoa noodles. If you have Thai chili paste, add a teaspoonful for even more flavor. For vegetarians, sautéed firm tofu strips can stand in for the chicken.

SERVES 6

Noodles

8 ounces (240 g) Asian rice or soba noodles, or other thin pasta, such as thin linguine or angel hair

1 tablespoon toasted sesame oil

2 tablespoons seasoned rice vinegar

2 tablespoons lite soy sauce

Splash of chili oil or hot sauce or a pinch of red pepper flakes, optional

Egg Pancake Strips (recipe follows)

Chicken Salad

1 tablespoon minced fresh ginger

1 small garlic clove, cut in half

2 tablespoons seasoned rice vinegar

2 tablespoons lite soy sauce

1 tablespoon fresh lime juice, or to taste

1 tablespoon canola oil

2 teaspoons toasted sesame oil

1 teaspoon brown sugar

1¼ pounds (600 g) cooked chicken, shredded or cut into small pieces (about 4½ cups/1.25 l)

2 tablespoon very finely sliced fresh kaffir lime leaves or 2 teaspoons grated lime zest

3 tablespoons thinly sliced scallions

3 tablespoons chopped fresh cilantro

Garnishes

1 cup (150 g) seedless cucumber matchsticks

1 cup (100 g) carrot matchsticks or grated

2 cups (160 g) fresh mung bean sprouts (see How to Clean Fresh Mung Bean Sprouts, page 215)

½ cup (30 g) thinly sliced scallions

3 tablespoons chopped fresh cilantro

3 tablespoons chopped roasted peanuts

1. Cook the noodles according to the package directions. Drain and place in a large bowl. Add the remaining noodle ingredients, toss to combine, and adjust the seasoning. Set aside at room temperature.

2. Make the Egg Pancake Strips (page 286).

3. To make the chicken salad, in the bowl of a mini food processor, combine the ginger, garlic, rice vinegar, soy sauce, lime juice, canola oil, sesame oil, and brown sugar and process, scraping down the sides of the bowl as needed, until smooth. Adjust the seasoning. Place the cooked chicken in a bowl, add the dressing, and toss to combine. Add the kaffir lime leaves, scallions, and cilantro and toss again. Adjust the seasoning and set aside. (The salad can be made up to 12 hours in advance; cover and refrigerate.)

4. When you are ready to serve, arrange the reserved noodles on one side of a very large platter. Arrange the chicken salad on the other side, and around it, make small piles of the cucumbers, carrots, bean sprouts, and egg strips. Garnish with the scallions, cilantro, and peanuts and serve.

(RECIPE CONTINUES)

370 CALORIES IN

Protein: 24 g; Carbohydrates: 41 g; Fat: 12 g; Fiber: 2 g; Sodium: 548 mg; Carb Choices: 2½; Diabetic Exchange: 2 Starch, 2 Vegetable, 3 Lean Meat

370 CALORIES OUT

Women: Walk: 90 minutes | Jog: 42 minutes

Men: Walk: 75 minutes | Jog: 36 minutes

CALORIE COMBOS

2 cups (40 g) salad greens (without dressing): 20 cals

Hot-and-Sweet Cucumber, Carrot, and Red Bell Pepper Salad (page 77): 61 cals

Thai-Style Hot-and-Sour Shrimp Soup (page 59): 83 cals

CALORIE CUTS

The chicken and noodles contain the most calories in this dish. The chicken has 107 calories and 3 grams of fat per serving, and the noodles have 133 calories and zero fat per serving. You might want to cut back a bit on the chicken and noodles, and omit the peanuts, which have 26 calories and 2 grams of fat per serving.

EGG PANCAKE STRIPS

1 large egg, lightly beaten
Pinch of salt
1 teaspoon vegetable oil

To make the egg pancake strips for the garnish, beat the egg with the pinch of salt in a small bowl. Grease a small skillet with the vegetable oil and heat over medium-low heat. Add the egg and swirl to thinly coat the pan, as you would a very thin pancake. Cook until firm, about 45 seconds, then flip the egg like a pancake and cook the other side until firm. Transfer to a plate and dab with paper towels to remove any grease. When the egg is cool, roll it up and slice it into thin strips; set aside.

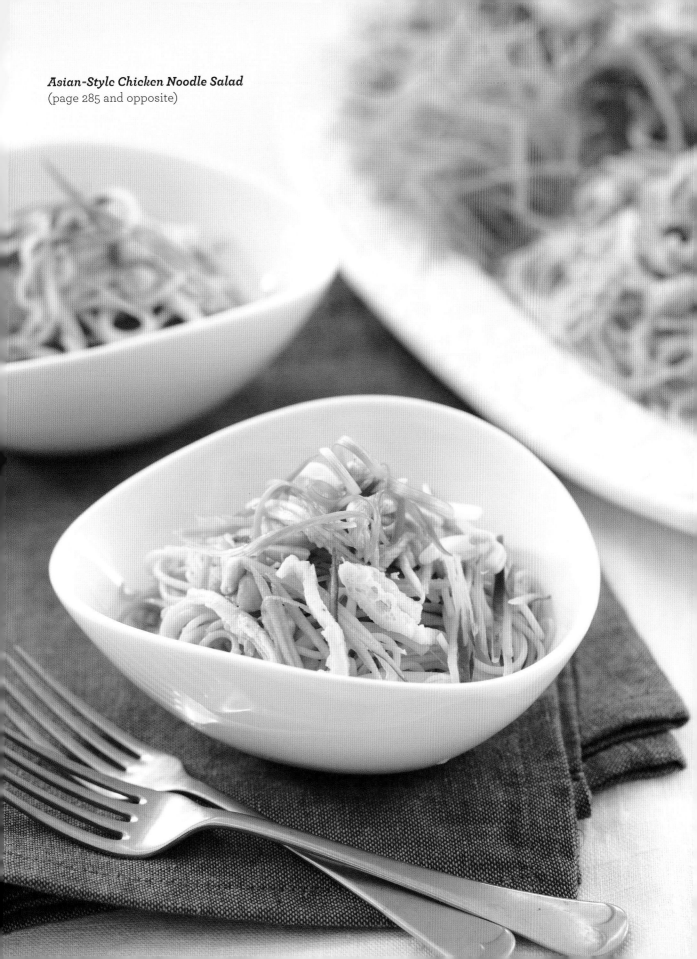

Asian-Style Chicken Noodle Salad
(page 285 and opposite)

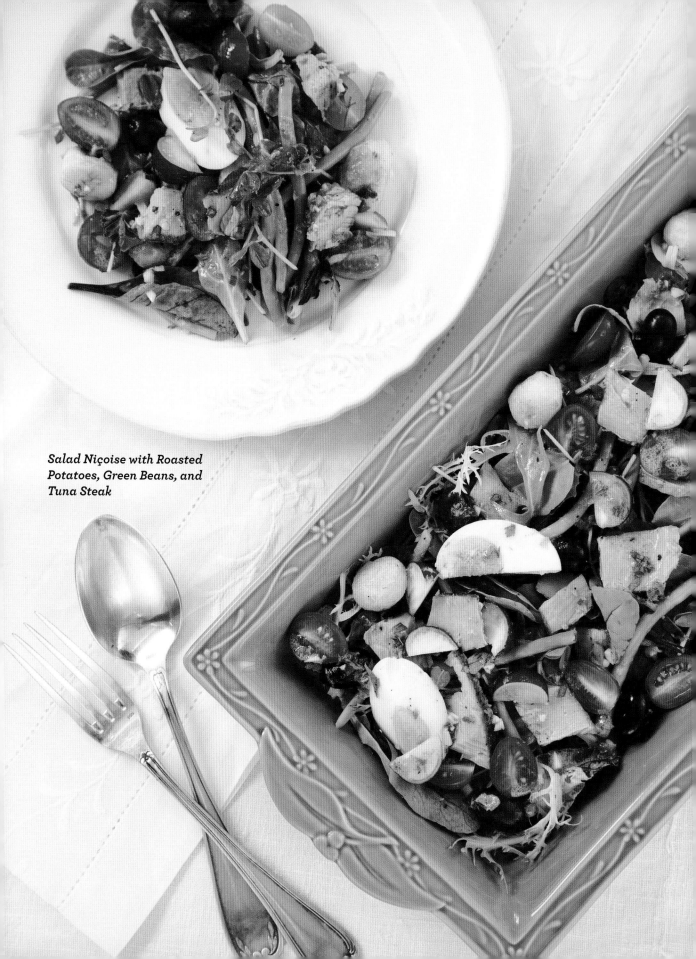

Salad Niçoise with Roasted Potatoes, Green Beans, and Tuna Steak

SALAD NIÇOISE WITH ROASTED POTATOES, GREEN BEANS, AND TUNA STEAK

Roasting the potatoes, green beans, and tuna makes for a jazzy update of a beloved classic. If you're short on time, by all means, use canned tuna, and pick up some boiled potatoes from a salad bar, along with the green beans and anything else that looks appealing. I like to garnish the salad with fresh sprouts or thinly sliced celery, cucumber, or fennel, but the dish also works well without. Whole Foods and gourmet stores often have an excellent assortment of brined and marinated olives, artichoke hearts, fava beans, and other vegetables that would be delicious in this salad. The dressing can be made up to 5 days in advance, covered, and refrigerated. Leftovers are great on any greens.

SERVES 4

Salad Niçoise Dressing

¼ cup (60 ml) fresh lemon juice, or to taste

2 teaspoons Dijon mustard

¼ cup (60 ml) extra virgin olive oil, or to taste

2 tablespoons water

2 tablespoons medium capers, drained

3 tablespoons chopped fresh flat-leaf parsley

2 tablespoons finely sliced fresh chives or scallions

Salad

2 tablespoons extra virgin olive oil

12 ounces (360 g) small new potatoes, halved, or quartered if large

Salt and freshly ground pepper, to taste

8 ounces (240 g) French-style green beans, ends trimmed

1 pound (480 g) tuna steaks, rinsed and patted dry with paper towels

1 teaspoon dried oregano

8 cups (250 to 300 g) baby greens

¼ cup (40 g) pitted Kalamata or green olives

1 cup (170 g) grape or cherry tomatoes, halved

2 hard-boiled eggs, cut into wedges

2 tablespoons chopped fresh flat-leaf parsley

2 tablespoons chopped fresh dill

Handful of fresh alfalfa sprouts, optional

1. To make the dressing, combine all of the ingredients in a small bowl and whisk until well blended. Cover and refrigerate until ready to use.

2. Preheat the oven to 450°F (230°C).

3. In a medium bowl, combine 1 tablespoon of the olive oil, the potatoes, salt, and pepper and toss until the potatoes are well coated. Transfer the potatoes and any excess oil to a baking sheet with sides and spread them out in an even layer; set the bowl aside. Roast the potatoes for 20 minutes, or until they are almost soft when pierced with the tip of a knife.

4. Add the green beans to the reserved greased bowl, along with ½ tablespoon more olive oil and a sprinkle of salt and pepper, and toss to combine, then move the potatoes on the baking sheet a bit to make room for the beans and spread the beans out on the baking sheet. Set the bowl aside again. Roast the potatoes and beans for 10 to 12 minutes longer, until the potatoes feel soft. Transfer the cooked vegetables to a

(RECIPE CONTINUES)

379 CALORIES IN

Protein: 36 g; Carbohydrates: 26 g; Fat: 15 g; Fiber: 6 g; Sodium: 517 mg; Carb Choices: 2; Diabetic Exchange: 5 Very Lean Meat, 2 Starch, 1 Fat

379 CALORIES OUT

Women: Walk: 92 minutes | Jog: 44 minutes

Men: Walk: 77 minutes | Jog: 36 minutes

CALORIE COMBOS

1 whole wheat roll: 76 cals

Gently Cooked Gazpacho (page 60): 87 cals

Quick Zucchini-Basil Soup (page 62): 99 cals

Gingery Squash Soup (page 63): 118 cals

7 whole wheat crackers: 120 cals

plate to cool. Set the baking sheet aside. Keep the oven on.

5. Add the remaining ½ tablespoon olive oil to the greased bowl, then add the tuna steaks; season with salt, pepper, and the oregano; and toss to coat the fish. Transfer the tuna to the baking sheet and drizzle any oil in the bowl over it. Roast for 5 minutes, then flip the steaks and roast for 5 to 7 minutes, until the desired doneness. (Note: Some people prefer tuna on the rare side, so adjust the timing accordingly.) Transfer the fish to a plate to cool.

6. When ready to serve, divide the baby greens evenly among 4 large plates, or use a large platter for everyone to serve themselves. Arrange one-quarter of the tuna, potatoes, and green beans artfully on top of the greens on each plate, or arrange on the platter. Add the olives, cherry tomatoes, and hard-boiled eggs. Whisk the dressing, then drizzle it over the salad. Add the herbs and sprouts, if using, and serve promptly.

HOW TO MAKE PERFECT HARD-BOILED EGGS

I'm always amazed when a hard-boiled egg comes out perfectly cooked, meaning that the yolk has set without being too hard or creamy in the middle. After many eggs, I've learned the result has less to do with boiling and more to do with letting the eggs cook off the heat. Place your large eggs in a single layer in a saucepan, cover with water, and add a generous sprinkling of salt. Bring to a boil and cook for 3 minutes (if your "large" eggs look really big, add another extra minute or 2 to the boiling time), then remove the saucepan from the heat, cover, and let stand for 15 minutes. Remove the eggs, run under cold water to cool, crack the shells on the counter, and peel.

SOBA NOODLES WITH TOFU, KALE, AND MISO DRESSING

I like to pair these soft soba noodles with robust kale for a wonderful contrast of textures and flavors. If you can find fresh Asian noodles, use them. I love this dish with sautéed baby bok choy, and when I'm looking for something fresh, not cooked, I add baby arugula instead of kale. I simply arrange it around the noodles so people can help themselves. If you prefer, use your favorite greens instead of the kale.

SERVES 4

Miso Dressing

½ cup (125 ml) hot water

½ teaspoon cornstarch

3 tablespoons yellow miso

2 teaspoons lite soy sauce

2 to 3 tablespoons seasoned rice vinegar

Pinch of sugar

Red pepper flakes, to taste

Freshly ground pepper, to taste

Noodles

6 ounces (180 g) soba noodles or any Asian noodles

1 to 2 teaspoons toasted sesame oil, to taste

Tofu and Greens

1 tablespoon vegetable oil

14 ounces (420 g) firm tofu, drained, patted dry, sliced into 2-inch (5 cm) by ½-inch (1.25 cm) rectangles, and patted dry again

Salt, to taste

8 ounces (240 g) shiitake or cremini mushrooms, rinsed, stems trimmed, and sliced

Freshly ground pepper, to taste

1 garlic clove, minced

8 ounces (240 g) kale, thinly sliced (if leaves are large, cut them in half before slicing)

½ cup (30 g) sliced scallions (1-inch/2.5 cm pieces)

1. To make the dressing, in a small bowl, combine the ingredients and mix well; set aside.

2. Cook the noodles according to the package directions. Drain well, then place the noodles in a large serving bowl or on a platter and toss with the sesame oil. Cover with foil to keep warm; set aside.

3. Line a large plate with paper towels. In a large nonstick skillet, heat ½ tablespoon of the vegetable oil over medium-high heat. Add the tofu and sauté, turning frequently, until lightly browned. Transfer the tofu to the serving bowl, arranging it over the noodles, and re-cover with the foil. (Do not rinse the skillet.)

4. Add the remaining ½ tablespoon vegetable oil to the skillet and heat over medium-high heat. Add the mushrooms, season lightly with salt and pepper, and sauté, stirring, for 3 to 4 minutes, until they release their juices. Move the mushrooms to one side of the skillet, then add the garlic to the cleared space and sauté for 30 seconds. Add the kale and scallions and cook for 3 minutes. Make a space in the middle of the greens and add the reserved dressing. Stir all of the ingredients together and cook until the sauce is slightly thickened. Adjust the seasoning, and then spoon the sauce over the noodles and tofu. Serve promptly.

349 CALORIES IN

Protein: 19 g; Carbohydrates: 45 g; Fat: 12 g; Fiber: 7 g; Sodium: 1,010 mg; Carb Choices: 2½; Diabetic Exchange: 2 Starch, 2 Vegetable, 2 Medium-Fat Meat

349 CALORIES OUT

Women: Walk:
85 minutes | Jog: 40 minutes

Men: Walk:
71 minutes | Jog: 34 minutes

CALORIE COMBOS

Broiled Portobello Mushrooms with Herbs (page 86): 23 cals

Hot-and-Sweet Cucumber, Carrot, and Red Bell Pepper Salad (page 77): 61 cals

2 cups (40 g) salad greens with 1 tablespoon Balsamic Vinaigrette (page 150): 73 cals

Gently Cooked Gazpacho (page 60): 87 cals

Broccolini with Sesame and Spice (page 96): 99 cals

Quick Zucchini-Basil Soup (page 62): 99 cals

Gingery Squash Soup (page 63): 118 cals

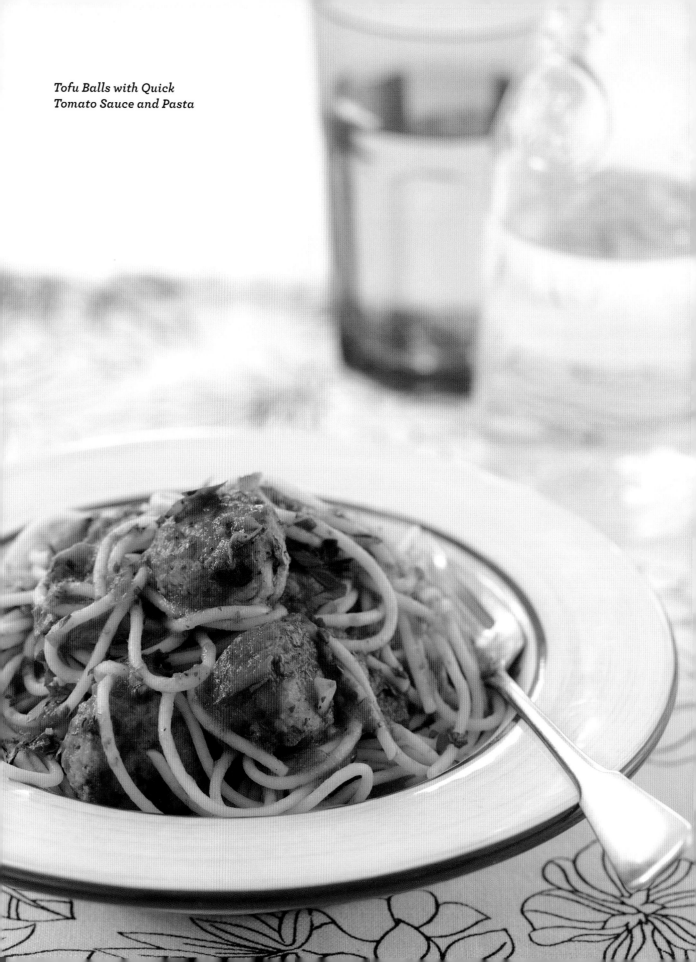

Tofu Balls with Quick Tomato Sauce and Pasta

TOFU BALLS WITH QUICK TOMATO SAUCE AND PASTA

I love these tofu balls. Here I pair them with pasta and tomato sauce, but you can serve them solo with the Creamy Cocktail Sauce (page 136) or the Fresh Mint, Cilantro, and Green Chile Chutney (page 143). To save time, you could substitute a high-quality store-bought pasta sauce and use fresh noodles that cook quickly. The tomato sauce can be refrigerated for up to 1 week or frozen for up to 1 month. The tofu balls can be refrigerated for a few days; do not freeze.

SERVES 6

Tomato Sauce

3 tablespoons vegetable oil

2 garlic cloves, minced

1 tablespoon Italian seasoning

2 pounds (1 kg) ripe tomatoes, coarsely chopped (heaping 5 cups, 1.25 ml)

1 tablespoon chopped fresh rosemary or thyme

½ cup (125 ml) canned tomato sauce

Salt and freshly ground pepper, to taste

Tofu Balls (makes about 35)

One 14-ounce (397 g) package firm tofu, drained, finely crumbled, and blotted dry with paper towels

¾ cup (60 g) panko bread crumbs

3 large eggs, lightly beaten

⅓ cup (30 g) grated Parmesan cheese

1 tablespoon Italian seasoning

1 teaspoon Old Bay seasoning, or to taste

⅓ cup (15 g) chopped fresh cilantro, basil, or dill

¼ cup (35 g) drained, diced jarred roasted red peppers

Salt and freshly ground pepper, to taste

1 tablespoon vegetable oil

Pasta

8 ounces (240 g) thin dried pasta, such as angel hair, spaghettini, or thin linguine, or fresh thin pasta

3 tablespoons chopped fresh basil or flat-leaf parsley

Grated Parmesan cheese, for serving

1. To make the tomato sauce, in a large saucepan, heat the vegetable oil over medium-high heat. Add the garlic and Italian seasoning and sauté, stirring constantly, for 1 minute. Add the tomatoes and rosemary and cook, stirring occasionally, until the tomatoes have softened, about 7 minutes. Add the tomato sauce, stir, and simmer until the desired consistency, about 7 minutes longer. Adjust the seasoning, with salt and pepper and set aside.

2. To make the tofu balls, combine all of the ingredients except the vegetable oil in a large bowl and mix until well blended. Before you shape the balls, you may want to make a test to check the seasoning: form about 1 tablespoon of the tofu mixture into a patty and cook in a little oil in a small skillet. Taste, and adjust the seasoning in the remaining mixture, if necessary.

3. Line a baking sheet with baking paper for easy cleanup. Using a rounded tablespoon

(RECIPE CONTINUES)

---

352 CALORIES IN

Protein: 18 g; Carbohydrates: 40 g; Fat: 14 g; Fiber: 6 g; Sodium: 292 mg; Carb Choices: 2½; Diabetic Exchange: 2 Starch, 2 Vegetable, 2 Medium-Fat Meat

352 CALORIES OUT

Women: Walk:
86 minutes | Jog: 40 minutes

Men: Walk:
72 minutes | Jog: 34 minutes

CALORIE COMBOS

Broiled Portobello Mushrooms with Herbs (page 86): 23 cals

2 cups (40 g) salad greens with 1 tablespoon Almost-Fat-Free Dieter's Lemony Dressing (page 140): 38 cals

Roasted Asparagus with Dill and Lemon Zest (page 88): 47 cals

Broiled Zucchini with Parmesan (page 90): 49 cals

Lemony Dill Cabbage Slaw (page 78): 63 cals

Greek-Style Broccoli (page 91): 71 cals

2 cups (40 g) salad greens with 1 tablespoon Balsamic Vinaigrette (page 150): 73 cals

Maple-Glazed Carrots (page 95): 98 cals

Brussels Sprouts with Parmesan and Pine Nuts (page 99): 118 cals

CALORIE CUTS

Instead of pasta, use a lower-calorie grain, such as ½ cup (125 ml) plain cooked couscous (88 cals), ½ cup plain cooked white rice (103 cals), ½ cup plain cooked brown rice (108 cals), or ½ cup plain cooked quinoa (111 cals).

for each one, form balls with the tofu mixture and place them on the baking sheet.

4. Heat the oil in a large nonstick skillet over medium heat. Add the tofu balls, in batches, and cook for 3 to 4 minutes, rolling them around as they cook to keep them as round as possible. The outside should be light golden brown and the inside cooked through. If they begin to brown too quickly, reduce the heat.

Transfer the cooked balls to a bowl, cover with foil, and set aside.

5. Cook the pasta according to the package directions. Drain and return the pasta to the pot. Add the desired amount of sauce and mix well. Place a portion of the sauced pasta on each plate and top with tofu balls and basil. Pass the Parmesan cheese at the table.

BEAN AND MUSHROOM ENCHILADAS

I've kept these enchiladas simple, calling only for refried beans and mushrooms (I use portobello here, but you can use any kind). Other veggies I've used with great success include sautéed sliced zucchini, yellow squash, and red bell peppers, and leftover grilled or roasted vegetables. The tomatillo sauce can be made up to 2 days in advance, covered, and refrigerated. I call for 1 cup (280 g) of refried beans, which is not a full 16-ounce (454 g) can. You can use all of the beans, which makes the enchiladas a bit heavy, or save the leftovers for quesadillas or dips. The assembled casserole can be refrigerated for up to 3 hours. Any leftovers are best heated in a microwave.

SERVES 6

Tomatillo Sauce

1 pound (about 500 g) tomatillos, husks removed, rinsed, and quartered

1 large sweet onion, coarsely chopped

2 garlic cloves, halved

2 to 3 tablespoons minced jalapeño chile, or to taste

10 ounces canned diced tomatoes or 1¼ cups (310 ml) diced ripe tomatoes

1 cup (250 ml) low-sodium fat-free vegetable stock

Bean and Mushroom Filling

1 tablespoon vegetable oil

1 pound (480 g) portobello mushrooms, rinsed, stems trimmed, and sliced into ¼-inch (6 mm) thick by 1-inch (2.5 cm) long strips

1 teaspoon roasted ground cumin

1 teaspoon dried oregano

¼ teaspoon salt, or to taste

Freshly ground pepper, to taste

1 cup (280 g) refried beans

2 tablespoons milk, or as needed

Sixteen 5- to 6-inch (13 to 15 cm) soft corn tortillas

1½ cups (6 ounces/180 g) shredded reduced-fat Monterey Jack cheese

1. To make the sauce, place the tomatillos, onion garlic, and jalapeños in a food processor and pulse just until coarsely pureed; you want the sauce to have some texture. Transfer the mixture to a large saucepan, add the tomatoes and stock, and bring to a boil. Reduce the heat and simmer for about 15 minutes, stirring occasionally. The finished sauce should be the consistency of slightly chunky pureed canned tomatoes. Set aside.

2. Center an oven rack and preheat the oven to 400°F (200°C).

3. To prepare the filling, heat the vegetable oil in a large nonstick skillet over medium-high heat. Add the mushrooms, cumin, and oregano and sauté, stirring occasionally, for about 10 minutes, or until the mushrooms are soft. Season with the salt and pepper to taste. Set aside.

4. Place the refried beans in a bowl and mix with the milk to thin them; if necessary, add a little more milk or water. Set aside.

5. To assemble, spread 1 cup of the sauce in the bottom of a 9 x 13-inch (23 x 33 cm) baking dish. Dip a tortilla into the remaining sauce to thoroughly moisten it. (Note: This is a very important step; failure to do this will result in cracked tortillas, which will make rolling them difficult.) Place it on a

(RECIPE CONTINUES)

chopping board or large plate. Spread about 3 tablespoons of the refried beans on the tortilla, then add about 2 tablespoons of the sautéed mushrooms. Roll up the tortilla and place it seam side down in the baking dish. Repeat with the remaining tortillas and filling, arranging the tortillas close together. Top the enchiladas with the remaining sauce and sprinkle with the cheese.

6. Bake until the enchiladas are heated through and the cheese is melted and golden, about 20 minutes. Serve promptly.

HOW TO SLICE PORTOBELLO MUSHROOMS

Portobellos are just about the biggest, meatiest, and tastiest mushrooms out there. Most people throw them on the grill or broil them, but they are also good sliced and added to casseroles, stir-fries, and other dishes. After trimming the stems and rinsing the mushrooms, slice each cap into 3 or 4 strips, then slice each strip into the desired size and thickness. When cooked, the mushrooms tend to give off purple-brown juices, akin to the color of balsamic vinegar.

VEGETARIAN STIR-FRIED RICE (📷 page 299)

There is something about stir-fried rice that is universally appealing to all ages and all nationalities. And with a few cooking tips in mind, stir-fried rice is easy and delicious. The first thing is the rice. Brown rice, which has a springiness and wonderful nuttiness, is great, but long-grain white rice works well, too. Ideally, the rice should be cooked a day in advance, covered, and refrigerated. Next comes the sauce. Make sure it's flavorful, which can be achieved by using garlic, ginger, scallions, and Asian sauces. The vegetables follow. They should be cooked to the crisp-tender stage. The sliced thin omelet is easy and authentic. Also, for nonvegetarians, feel free to add thin strips of chicken, ham, or shrimp. In Malaysia, I always garnished fried rice with crispy fried shallots and a drizzle of homemade garlic oil. For more tips, see How to Stir-Fry Rice, below.

SERVES 6

Sauce for Stir-Fried Rice

2½ tablespoons soy sauce, or to taste

1 tablespoon hoisin sauce

Freshly ground pepper, to taste

Fried Tofu

½ tablespoon vegetable oil

6 ounces (180 g) firm tofu, cut into ¼-inch (6 mm) cubes and blotted dry with paper towels

Salt and freshly ground pepper, to taste

Egg Pancake Strips

1 teaspoon vegetable oil

1 large egg, lightly beaten

Stir-Fry

1½ tablespoons vegetable oil

1 small onion, finely diced

1 tablespoon minced garlic

1 tablespoon minced fresh ginger

6 cups (730 g) cooked rice

2 teaspoons toasted sesame oil, or to taste

½ cup (70 g) thinly sliced green beans

½ cup (80 g) very thinly sliced or cubed carrots

½ cup (80 g) frozen corn, thawed

½ cup (30 g) thinly sliced scallions

Salt and freshly ground pepper, to taste

Pinch of red pepper flakes, optional

1. To make the sauce, in a small bowl, mix the ingredients until well combined; set aside.
2. To make the fried tofu, line a large plate with paper towels. In a very large nonstick skillet, heat the vegetable oil over medium-high heat. Season the tofu with salt and pepper, then sauté it, turning frequently, until lightly browned on all sides, 3 to 5 minutes. Transfer to the prepared plate and set aside. (Do not rinse the skillet.)
3. To make the egg pancake strips for the garnish, return the skillet to medium-low heat and add the vegetable oil. Brush it over the bottom, then add the egg and swirl to thinly coat the pan, as you would for a very thin pancake. Cook until firm, about 45 seconds, then flip the egg like a pancake and cook the other side until firm. Transfer to a large plate and dab with paper towels to remove any grease. Set the skillet aside. When the egg is cool, roll it up and slice it into thin strips; set aside.

(RECIPE CONTINUES)

367 CALORIES IN

Protein: 9 g; Carbohydrates: 61 g; Fat: 10 g; Fiber: 2 g; Sodium: 694 mg; Carb Choices: 3½; Diabetic Exchange: 3 Starch, 2 Vegetable, 1 Medium-Fat Meat

367 CALORIES OUT

Women: Walk:
89 minutes | Jog: 42 minutes

Men: Walk:
75 minutes | Jog: 35 minutes

CALORIE COMBOS

Napa Cabbage with Ginger and Oyster Sauce (page 89): 48 cals

Hot-and-Sweet Cucumber, Carrot, and Red Bell Pepper Salad (page 77): 61 cals

Japanese Eggplant in Sweet Chili Sauce (page 94): 86 cals

2 cups (40 g) salad greens with 1 tablespoon Benihana-Style Ginger-Sesame Dressing (page 155): 89 cals

Broccolini with Sesame and Spice (page 96): 99 cals

4. To make the stir-fry, return the skillet to medium-high heat and heat the vegetable oil. Add the onions and sauté for 1 minute. Add the garlic and ginger and sauté for 1 minute, then add the rice and increase the heat to high. Sauté, stirring occasionally, until the rice is heated through.

5. Push the rice to one side of the skillet and add the sesame oil to the empty space. Add the green beans, carrots, and corn and sauté, stirring, until crisp-tender, about 2 minutes. Add the scallions and sauté for 1 minute, then mix the vegetables with the rice. Make a well in the center of the rice, add the reserved sauce, and stir until it boils, then add the tofu and mix everything again. Season with salt, pepper, and pepper flakes, if using, garnish with the reserved egg pancake strips, and serve promptly.

HOW TO STIR-FRY RICE

Here are some pointers for a perfect stir-fry every time.

- Make your sauce in advance.
- Ingredients should be of a uniform small size so they cook evenly and quickly.
- Ingredients should be dry when added so they don't create steam.
- When frying the rice, the flame should be high enough that the "rice dances in the wok," a common Chinese saying. This is particularly important when cooking the rice, because you don't want it to steam. Instead, you want the part that hits the skillet to sizzle.
- No need to rinse the skillet in between the cooking steps; just wipe it out if needed. The important thing is to keep the food from sticking. If it does stick, add 1 tablespoon of vegetable oil and continue cooking.
- Instead of egg strips for garnish, in Step 5, you can add a beaten egg or two after you sauté the vegetables and add the scallions. Push the vegetables to the side, scramble the egg, then mix the egg and the vegetables into the rice. Proceed with the recipe.

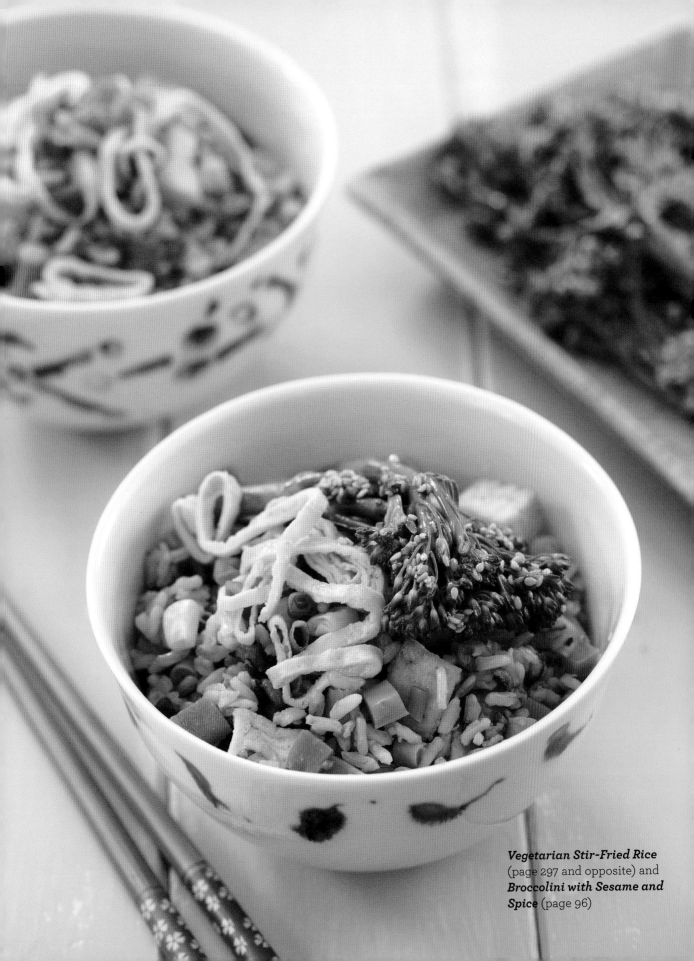

Vegetarian Stir-Fried Rice
(page 297 and opposite) and
Broccolini with Sesame and Spice (page 96)

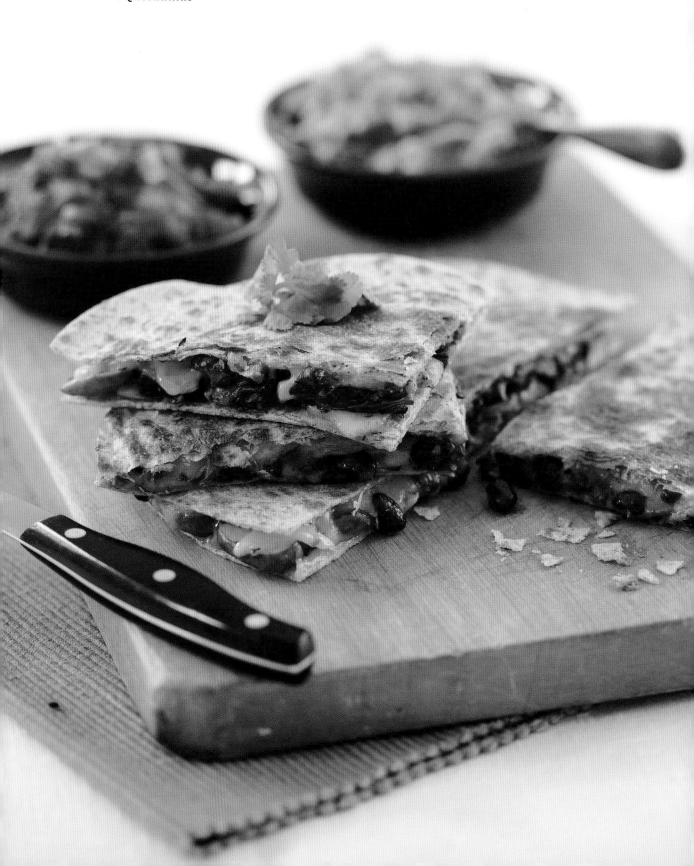

Black Bean, Spinach, and
Mushroom Quesadillas

BLACK BEAN, SPINACH, AND MUSHROOM QUESADILLAS

In my family, when we make quesadillas, we all craft our own versions and therefore everyone is happy. My daughter loves to add vegetables, while my son keeps his very basic. This recipe calls for black beans, fresh baby spinach, and mushrooms, but feel free to throw any other vegetables into the mix. Cilantro adds a fantastic kick. Homemade Pico de Gallo and Yummy Guacamole make an ordinary quesadilla extraordinary. Any extra black beans are great in a salad.

SERVES 4

½ tablespoon extra virgin olive oil

1 teaspoon minced garlic

8 ounces (240 g) cremini mushrooms, rinsed, stems trimmed, and sliced

¼ teaspoon chili powder, or to taste

4 cups (6 ounces/135 g) loosely packed baby spinach

1 cup (160 g) canned black beans, rinsed and drained

2 tablespoons minced fresh or jarred jalapeño chiles, optional

Salt and freshly ground pepper, to taste

Four 9- to 10-inch (23 to 25 cm) whole wheat tortillas or smaller corn tortillas

1 cup (120 g) shredded reduced-fat Monterey Jack cheese

Fresh cilantro leaves, for garnish

1. In a large nonstick skillet, heat the olive oil over medium-high heat. Add the garlic and cook for 20 seconds, then add the mushrooms and chili powder and sauté, stirring occasionally, for 5 minutes, or until the mushrooms are light golden and most of the juices they release have evaporated. Add the spinach and stir until wilted, then add the black beans and jalapeños and stir until well combined. Season with salt and pepper, transfer to a bowl, and set aside. Wipe out the skillet with paper towels and set aside.

2. Lay the tortillas on a flat surface. Sprinkle one half of each round with an equal amount of cheese, then divide the mushroom filling equally over the cheese. Fold each tortilla in half.

3. Reheat the skillet over medium heat. Place one of the quesadillas in the skillet (add a second one if it fits) and cook for about 3 minutes on each side, or until the cheese melts and the inside is warm. Continue to cook the remaining quesadillas. Serve promptly.

388 CALORIES IN

Protein: 26 g; Carbohydrates: 44 g; Fat: 15 g; Fiber: 5 g; Sodium: 851 mg; Carb Choices: 2½; Diabetic Exchange: 2 Starch, 2 Vegetable, 3 Lean Meat

388 CALORIES OUT

Women: Walk: 94 minutes | Jog: 45 minutes

Men: Walk: 79 minutes | Jog: 37 minutes

CALORIE COMBOS

1 tablespoon jarred salsa: 5 cals

Radish-Tomato-Cucumber Salsa (page 135): 12 cals

Pico de Gallo (page 137): 16 cals

2 cups (40 g) salad greens with 1 tablespoon Almost-Fat-Free Dieter's Lemony Dressing (page 140): 38 cals

Roasted Asparagus with Dill and Lemon Zest (page 88): 47 cals

Broiled Zucchini with Parmesan (page 90): 49 cals

Lemony Dill Cabbage Slaw (page 78): 63 cals

Greek-Style Broccoli (page 91): 71 cals

2 cups (40 g) salad greens with 1 tablespoon Balsamic Vinaigrette (page 150): 73 cals

Yummy Guacamole (page 157): 86 cals

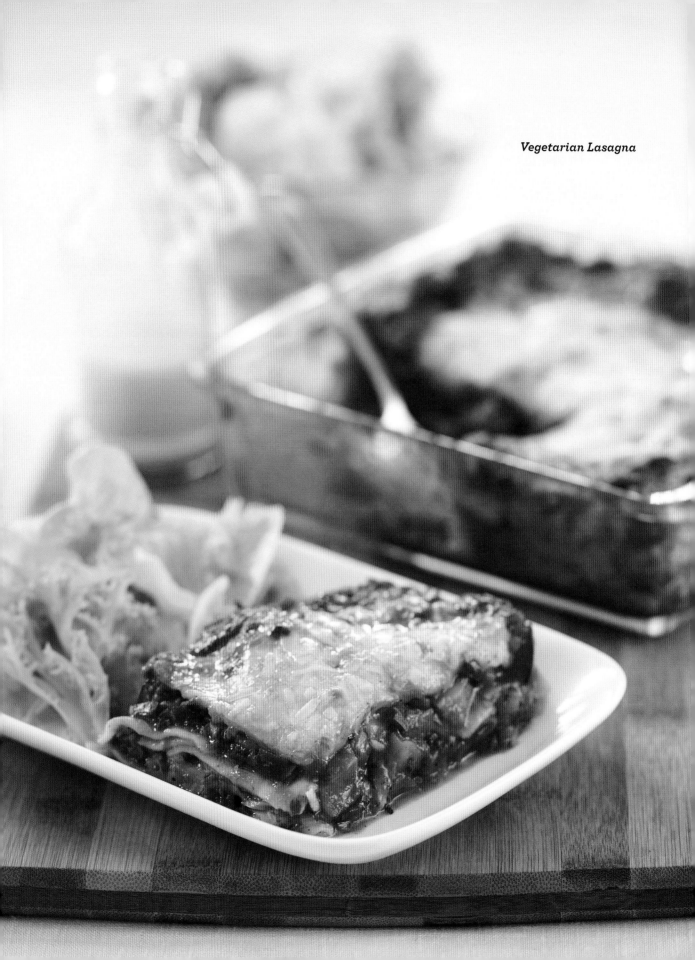

Vegetarian Lasagna

VEGETARIAN LASAGNA

Lasagna is one of those recipes that is hard to quantify perfectly on paper. There are so many variables at play, from how thick or runny your sauce is to how absorbent your no-boil noodles are, that you just have to trust your best judgment. One thing to keep in mind is that no-boil noodles require a little more liquid than cooked noodles do during the baking process, or they can become dry. Barilla oven-ready lasagna noodles work really well. Avoid the very thin no-bake noodles. In this recipe I've given a mix of vegetables. You can use all or choose your favorites. You should have about 7 cups of vegetables diced small or sliced, which will shrink down to about 4 cups after cooking. To make things really easy, I call for jarred tomato sauce, to which I add some canned tomato sauce. Your total amount of sauce plus cooked vegetables should be about 7 cups. To keep the calories at bay, the amount of mozzarella cheese is on the low side. If you're not concerned with calories, feel free to add more mozzarella or your favorite cheese. The lasagna can be assembled up to 12 hours in advance and refrigerated before baking, and the baked lasagna freezes well for weekday dinners.

SERVES 6

390 CALORIES IN

Protein: 21 g; Carbohydrates: 49 g; Fat: 13 g; Fiber: 7 g; Sodium: 1,291 mg; Carb Choices: 3; Diabetic Exchange: 3 Starch, 2 Medium-Fat Meat

390 CALORIES OUT

Women: Walk: 95 minutes | Jog: 45 minutes

Men: Walk: 80 minutes | Jog: 37 minutes

CALORIE COMBOS

2 cups (40 g) salad greens with 1 tablespoon Almost-Fat-Free Dieter's Lemony Dressing (page 140): 38 cals

Greek-Style Broccoli (page 91): 71 cals

Lemony Dill Cabbage Slaw (page 78): 63 cals

2 cups (40 g) salad greens with 1 tablespoon Balsamic Vinaigrette (page 150): 73 cals

Tomato Vegetable Sauce (makes scant 7 cups, 1.75 l)

2 tablespoons vegetable oil

1 onion, chopped

2 garlic cloves, minced

1 tablespoon Italian seasoning

1 tablespoon dried oregano

1 small zucchini (5 ounces/150 g), cut into small dice (1 cup/250 ml)

1 small red bell pepper (3 ounces/90 g), cored, seeded, and cut into small dice (1 cup/250 ml)

1 very small eggplant (6 ounces/180 g), cut into a small dice (2 cups/500 ml)

8 ounces (240 g) cremini or button mushrooms, rinsed, stems trimmed, and thinly sliced (3 cups/750 ml)

A sprinkle of salt and freshly ground pepper

One 24-ounce (680 g) high-quality jarred pasta sauce

One 15-ounce (425 g) can tomato sauce

¼ cup (10 g) chopped fresh basil, to taste

For Assembly

One 9-ounce (255 g) box no-boil or oven-ready lasagna noodles, such as Barilla

3 cups (12 ounces/360 g) shredded part-skim low-moisture mozzarella cheese

1. To make the sauce, heat the oil in a very large nonstick saucepan over medium-high heat. Add the onions and sauté for 2 minutes. Add the garlic, Italian seasoning, and oregano and sauté for 30 seconds, then add the zucchini, red bell peppers, eggplant, mushrooms, and a sprinkle of salt and pepper. Cook, stirring occasionally, until the vegetables are soft, about 7 minutes. Add the pasta sauce and tomato sauce, stir well, and remove from the heat.

2. To assemble the lasagna, spread a heaping 1 cup (250 ml) of the sauce over the bottom of a deep 9 x 9-inch (23 x 23 cm) square baking dish. Cover with some of the lasagna noodles. Break some of the noodles lengthwise to fill in any gaps on the sides of the pan.

(RECIPE CONTINUES)

3. Cover the noodles with a heaping 1 cup (250 ml) of the sauce, then sprinkle one-quarter of the mozzarella cheese evenly over the sauce. Repeat this layering process of noodles, sauce, and cheese two more times. For the final fourth layer of noodles, place the noodles on top of the cheese, then spread the remaining sauce over them and top with the remaining cheese. You will have some noodles left over. (At this point, the lasagna can be covered with plastic wrap and refrigerated for up to 12 hours.)

4. To bake, center an oven rack and preheat the oven to 375°F (190°C). Cover the lasagna with a piece of foil and bake for 45 minutes (or slightly longer, about 15 minutes, if coming straight out of the refrigerator).

5. Remove the foil and bake for 10 more minutes, or until a knife inserted into the middle of the lasagna indicates soft noodles and most of the sauce has been absorbed. Remove from the oven, cover with foil, and allow to rest for 15 minutes before slicing.

ASPARAGUS AND MUSHROOM RISOTTO

One thing I'm sure you'll like about this risotto is that I've reduced the amount of stirring that goes along with making a traditional risotto. I just don't have the time to hover over a saucepan of rice, and I doubt you do, either. I've used asparagus and mushrooms, which I precook separately to keep them al dente, but feel free to swap them with your favorite vegetables. I sometimes use sliced leeks instead of chopped onions. Also, because all rice is different, you may need to adjust the amount of liquid to reach your desired consistency. Keep in mind that risotto thickens quite a bit as it cools, so it's better to have it be a little more on the runny side than on the stiff side when serving. A heavy-bottomed saucepan with a lid is a must here.

SERVES 6

4 cups (1 liter) low-sodium fat-free vegetable stock

2 cups (500 ml) water

2 cups (8 ounces/240 g) sliced asparagus (½-inch/1.25-cm pieces)

1 tablespoon vegetable oil

1 pound (480 g) cremini or shiitake mushrooms, rinsed, stems trimmed, and thinly sliced

2 tablespoons unsalted butter

1 onion, chopped

1 garlic clove, minced

2 cups (400 g) Arborio rice

1 cup (250 ml) white wine

1 teaspoon salt, or to taste

½ cup (50 g) grated Parmesan cheese

Freshly ground pepper, to taste

3 tablespoons chopped fresh flat-leaf parsley

3 tablespoons chopped fresh chives

1. Combine the stock and water in a saucepan and bring to a simmer; set aside.

2. Meanwhile, cook the asparagus in a large saucepan of boiling salted water for 2 minutes; drain and set aside.

3. In a large saucepan or Dutch oven, heat the vegetable oil over medium-high heat. Add the mushrooms and sauté, stirring occasionally, for 5 minutes, or until most of the juices they release have evaporated. Remove the mushrooms and set aside. (Do not rinse the saucepan.)

4. Add the butter to the saucepan and melt over medium heat. Add the onions and sauté for 5 minutes. Add the garlic and sauté for 1 minute. Add the rice and cook, stirring frequently, for 3 minutes, or until the edges of the grains are translucent.

5. Add the wine and cook for 3 minutes. Add 4 cups of the warm stock mixture and the salt, stir, and bring to a boil. Reduce the heat to low, cover, and simmer for 8 minutes, then uncover and stir well. Cook for 5 more minutes, covered. Stir again, add more of the stock or water if needed (usually another ½ cup [125 ml] is required at this point; or if you've run out of stock mixture, add water intead), and continue to cook, covered, for 5 minutes. Almost all of the liquid should be absorbed and the rice should be soft.

(RECIPE CONTINUES)

---

392 CALORIES IN

Protein: 14 g; Carbohydrates: 56 g; Fat: 10 g; Fiber: 3 g; Sodium: 662 mg; Carb Choices: 3½; Diabetic Exchange: 3 Starch, 2 Medium-Fat Meat

392 CALORIES OUT

Women: Walk:
95 minutes | Jog: 45 minutes

Men: Walk:
80 minutes | Jog: 38 minutes

CALORIE COMBOS

2 cups (40 g) salad greens with 1 tablespoon Almost-Fat-Free Dieter's Lemony Dressing (page 140): 38 cals

2 cups (40 g) salad greens with 1 tablespoon Balsamic Vinaigrette (page 150): 73 cals

6. Add 1 cup of the stock mixture and stir. Add the Parmesan cheese and the cooked asparagus and mushrooms. Stir until the vegetables are well heated and the Parmesan is melted. Thin the risotto with a bit of the extra stock mixture (you'll have about ½ cup [125 ml] left at this point), if needed. Season with salt and pepper, garnish with the parsley and chives, and serve promptly.

BROILED SALMON WITH SCALLION-GINGER SAUCE

If you're looking for a homemade version of a teriyaki sauce for salmon, and you love scallions, look no further. Serve this salmon with soba noodles, brown rice, or quinoa tossed with a bit of toasted sesame oil and chopped fresh cilantro. I usually add a medley of vegetables, steamed or quickly sautéed, and top them with some of the sauce.

SERVES 4

Scallion-Ginger Sauce

¼ cup (60 ml) water

2 tablespoons lite soy sauce

1 teaspoon seasoned rice vinegar

2 tablespoons seasoned rice wine

2 tablespoons brown or granulated sugar

¼ teaspoon cornstarch

2 teaspoons vegetable oil

1 cup (60 g) sliced scallions

2 tablespoons minced peeled fresh ginger

1 tablespoon minced green chile

Salmon

Canola oil cooking spray

4 skinless center-cut salmon fillets, about 6 ounces (180 g) each, rinsed and patted dry with paper towels

¼ cup (10 g) chopped fresh cilantro, for garnish

1. To make the sauce, in a small bowl, mix the water, soy sauce, rice vinegar, rice wine, sugar, and cornstarch; set aside. In a small skillet, heat the vegetable oil over medium heat. Add the scallions, ginger, and green chiles and sauté for 2 minutes. Add the reserved sauce mixture and cook, stirring occasionally, until the sauce begins to thicken, about 3 minutes, and set aside.

2. To broil the salmon, position an oven rack one or two rungs down from the heating element and preheat the broiler to high. Line a baking sheet with sides with foil, grease it with cooking spray, and arrange the fillets on it, skinned side down. Place the fish under the broiler and cook for 10 to 12 minutes, depending on the thickness. Check every 5 minutes, to avoid burning. (There is no need to turn the fish, but you can if you want to.) The fish should be cooked through when flaked with the tip of a knife in the thickest part of the flesh.

3. Meanwhile, rewarm the sauce over low heat.

4. Transfer the salmon to a serving platter or individual plates, and pass the sauce in a bowl at the table.

307 CALORIES IN

Protein: 35 g; Carbohydrates: 11 g; Fat: 13 g; Fiber: 1 g; Sodium: 434 mg; Carb Choices: 1; Diabetic Exchange: 5 Lean Meat, 1 Vegetable

307 CALORIES OUT

Women: Walk:
75 minutes | Jog: 35 minutes

Men: Walk:
63 minutes | Jog: 30 minutes

CALORIE COMBOS

Napa Cabbage with Ginger and Oyster Sauce: (page 89): 48 cals

Japanese Eggplant in Sweet Chili Sauce (page 94): 86 cals

2 cups (40 g) salad greens with 1 tablespoon Benihana-Style Ginger-Sesame Dressing (page 155): 89 cals

Broccolini with Sesame and Spice (page 96): 99 cals

½ cup (80 g) plain white rice: 103 cals

½ cup (90 g) plain brown rice: 108 cals

½ cup (65 g) plain quinoa: 111 cals

1 cup (200 g) plain udon noodles: 210 cals

BAKED MARINATED SALMON WITH MUSTARD-DILL SAUCE

This salmon can also be pan-fried, broiled, or grilled. The mustard-dill sauce is also lovely on smoked salmon, burgers (all kinds from veggie burgers to salmon burgers), and grilled or broiled chicken. If you don't have whole-grain Dijon mustard, just add a little bit more of the regular Dijon, and feel free to adjust; some people don't like too much of a mustardy taste. Fresh dill is the only way to go here; avoid the dried stuff. The sauce can be made up to 2 days in advance, covered, and refrigerated.

SERVES 4

Dill Marinade

3 tablespoons fresh lemon juice

1½ tablespoons extra virgin olive oil

3 tablespoons chopped fresh dill

Sprinkle of salt and freshly ground pepper

4 skinless center-cut salmon fillets, about 6 ounces (180 g) each, rinsed and patted dry with paper towels

Mustard-Dill Sauce

2 tablespoons Dijon mustard, or to taste

2 teaspoons whole-grain Dijon mustard, or to taste

¼ cup (60 ml) fat-free sour cream

1 teaspoon extra virgin olive oil

3 tablespoons finely chopped fresh dill

Pinch of sugar

Salt and freshly ground pepper, to taste

1. To marinate the salmon, combine all of the marinade ingredients in a Pyrex baking dish and mix well, then add the salmon and turn to coat evenly with the marinade. Cover and refrigerate for at least 1 hour and up to 6 hours.

2. To make the sauce, combine all of the ingredients in a small bowl and mix well. Cover and refrigerate.

3. Center an oven rack and preheat the oven to 400°F (200°C).

4. Place the salmon skinned side down on a foil-lined baking sheet with sides. Bake for 10 to 15 minutes, depending on the thickness, until cooked through when flaked with the tip of a knife in the thickest part of the flesh. (There is no need to turn the fish, but you can if you want to.)

5. Transfer the salmon to individual plates or a serving platter and evenly divide the sauce over the top, or serve it on the side.

Broiling Note: To broil the salmon, line a baking sheet with foil and lightly grease the foil. Place the salmon fillets skinned side up on the baking sheet and broil under high heat until cooked through, turning once. The time will depend on the thickness of the salmon and your broiler: 8 to 10 minutes is the norm. The fish should be cooked through when flaked with the tip of a knife in the thickest part.

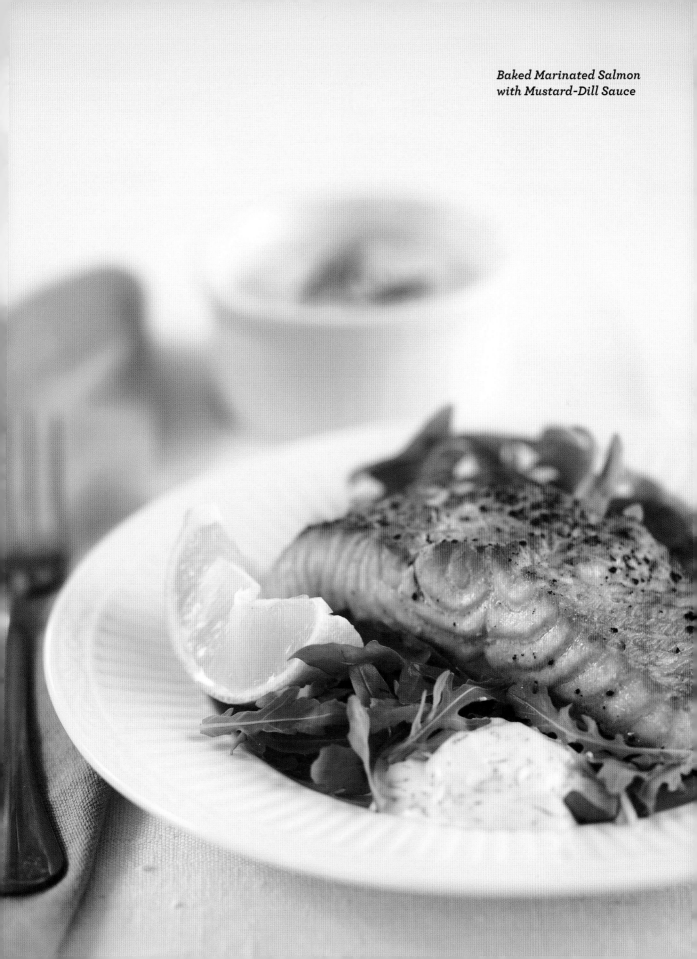

*Baked Marinated Salmon
with Mustard-Dill Sauce*

363 CALORIES IN

Protein: 36 g; Carbohydrates: 3 g; Fat: 22 g; Fiber: 1 g; Sodium: 364 mg; Carb Choices: 0; Diabetic Exchange: 5 Medium-Fat Meat

363 CALORIES OUT

Women: Walk: 88 minutes | Jog: 42 minutes

Men: Walk: 74 minutes | Jog: 35 minutes

CALORIE COMBOS

Napa Cabbage with Ginger and Oyster Sauce (page 89): 48 cals

Sautéed Baby Bok Choy and Red Bell Peppers (page 92): 79 cals

Japanese Eggplant in Sweet Chili Sauce (page 94): 86 cals

2 cups (40 g) salad greens with 1 tablespoon Benihana-Style Ginger-Sesame Dressing (page 155): 89 cals

Broccolini with Sesame and Spice (page 96): 99 cals

½ cup (80 g) plain white rice: 103 cals

½ cup (100 g) plain udon noodles: 105 cals

½ cup (90 g) plain brown rice: 108 cals

½ cup (65 g) plain quinoa: 111 cals

CALORIE CUTS

Skip the sesame seeds and save 50 calories and 4 grams of fat per serving.

SESAME-COATED SALMON WITH SOY SAUCE–LIME DRIZZLE

A super-simple, sure-to-impress salmon recipe for two. One of my recipe testers had this to say: "The skin turned out crunchy and the meat tender and juicy! I added only a little of the sauce on top. Yummy!" Now, if you want to get fancy, use a combination of white and black sesame seeds. The drizzle, which goes with anything from fried tofu to grilled steaks, can be made up to 3 days in advance, covered and refrigerated. I love this dish with udon noodles and sautéed Asian greens, such as the Sautéed Baby Bok Choy and Red Bell Peppers or the Napa Cabbage with Ginger and Soy Sauce.

SERVES 2

Soy Sauce–Lime Drizzle

1 tablespoon lite soy sauce

1 teaspoon fresh lime juice, or to taste

Pinch of sugar

1 to 2 drops toasted sesame oil

2 teaspoons minced seeded red chile, optional

Salmon

2 tablespoons white sesame seeds

1 teaspoon grated lime zest

2 skinless center-cut salmon fillets, each about 6 ounces (180 g), rinsed and patted dry with paper towels

1 tablespoon vegetable oil

1. To make the drizzle, combine all of the ingredients in a small bowl and mix until the sugar has dissolved. Adjust the seasoning and set aside.

2. To make the salmon, in a very small bowl, mix together the sesame seeds and lime zest. Place the salmon on a large plate, skinned side down. Divide the sesame topping in half and press half of it onto the top and bottom of each fillet, patting gently to adhere. Cook, or cover and refrigerate for up to 12 hours.

3. To cook the salmon, heat the vegetable oil in a medium nonstick skillet over medium-low heat. Add the fillets and cook the first side for 5 minutes. (Note: You might want to use a splatter guard or a piece of foil loosely placed over the skillet to catch any splatters.) Adjust the heat as needed, erring on the low side so as not to burn the sesame seeds before the salmon is cooked. Using a wide spatula, very carefully turn the fillets and cook for 4 to 5 minutes on the other side; the cooking time will depend on the thickness of the fillets. The fish should be cooked though when flaked with the tip of a knife in the thickest part of the flesh.

4. Transfer the salmon to individual plates, spoon a little bit of the drizzle over the top, and serve the rest on the side.

PAN-SEARED SCALLOPS WITH SPINACH PASTA

Because scallops are so expensive, I like to pair them with something special. This sauce is so flavorful that all the scallops need is a light sprinkle of salt and pepper before you cook them. Be careful not to overprocess the sauce, or it will lose its pretty bright green color. A mini processor is ideal for small jobs like this. The tomatoes add color and flavor. I call for fresh spinach pasta, but you can use any kind of fresh or dried pasta. A green salad would round out the meal.

SERVES 4

Sauce

1 tablespoon medium capers, drained

⅓ cup (40 g) green olives with pimientos

1 garlic clove, cut in half

1 teaspoon grated lemon zest

1 tablespoon fresh lemon juice, or to taste

2 tablespoons extra virgin olive oil

½ cup (20 g) loosely packed fresh cilantro leaves

⅓ cup (10 g) loosely packed fresh dill

Freshly ground pepper, to taste

Pinch of sugar

2 cups (330 g) cherry tomatoes, halved

Scallops and Pasta

12 ounces (360 g) fresh spinach pasta or other pasta

2 tablespoons extra virgin olive oil

1 pound (480 g) sea scallops (tough side muscle removed, if necessary), rinsed and blotted dry with paper towels

Light sprinkle of salt and freshly ground pepper

1. To make the sauce, combine all of the ingredients except the tomatoes in the bowl of a mini food processor and pulse to a chunky puree; do not overprocess. Set aside at room temperature. (If serving the sauce later, cover it with plastic wrap pressed flush against the surface and refrigerate. The sauce can be made up to 12 hours in advance.)

2. Bring a large pot of salted water to a boil. Cook the pasta according to the package directions, drain, cover, and set aside. (The cooked pasta will be tossed with the sauce, and the cooked scallops will be placed on top of the pasta.)

3. To cook the scallops, have a large plate ready for the seared scallops. Heat 1 tablespoon of the olive oil in a large skillet over medium-high heat. Lightly season the scallops with salt and pepper, then add them to the skillet and cook for 4 minutes on each side, or until cooked through. (Note: Cut into a scallop to check for doneness.) Transfer to the plate and cover with aluminum foil. (Do not rinse the skillet.)

4. Add the remaining 1 tablespoon olive oil to the skillet and heat over medium-high heat. Add the cherry tomatoes and sauté until they give off their juices, about 4 minutes. Add the reserved sauce and stir until heated through, then add the reserved cooked pasta and toss until well combined.

5. Divide the pasta among 4 serving plates and arrange the scallops on top. Serve promptly.

390 CALORIES IN

Protein: 21 g; Carbohydrates: 40 g; Fat: 16 g; Fiber: 4 g; Sodium: 1,053 mg; Carb Choices: 2½; Diabetic Exchange: 2 Starch, 3 Medium-Fat Meat

390 CALORIES OUT

Women: Walk:
95 minutes | Jog: 45 minutes

Men: Walk:
80 minutes | Jog: 38 minutes

CALORIE COMBOS

Broiled Portobello Mushrooms with Herbs (page 86): 23 cals

Roasted Asparagus with Dill and Lemon Zest (page 88): 47 cals

Broiled Zucchini with Parmesan (page 90): 49 cals

2 cups (40 g) salad greens with 1 tablespoon Classic Red Wine Vinaigrette (page 146): 62 cals

Lemony Dill Cabbage Slaw (page 78): 63 cals

Greek-Style Broccoli (page 91): 71 cals

CALORIE CUTS

Skip the pasta and save 166 calories and 1 gram of fat per serving.

391 CALORIES IN

Protein: 15 g; Carbohydrates: 49 g; Fat: 15 g; Fiber: 3 g; Sodium: 1,120 mg; Carb Choices: 3; Diabetic Exchange: 3 Starch, 2 Medium-Fat Meat

391 CALORIES OUT

Women: Walk:
95 minutes | Jog: 45 minutes

Men: Walk:
80 minutes | Jog: 38 minutes

CALORIE COMBOS

Hot-and-Sweet Cucumber, Carrot, and Red Bell Pepper Salad (page 77): 61 cals

2 cups (40 g) salad greens with 1 tablespoon Benihana-Style Ginger-Sesame Dressing (page 155): 89 cals

CALORIE CUTS

Skip the peanuts and save 68 calories and 6 grams of fat per serving.

SHRIMP PAD THAI

Almost everyone loves pad Thai. I've had some amazing versions in all kinds of eating establishments, from street food stalls in Bangkok to the dining rooms of swank Thai restaurants. What I discovered when attending the Baipai Thai Cooking School in Bangkok is that the secret to a good pad Thai involves two things: first, the freshness of the ingredients is essential; and second, it must be prepared at the last minute. Authentic pad Thai recipes often call for dried shrimp, palm sugar, and tamarind paste, but because most Western kitchens do not have these on hand, I've omitted them. I did keep the Chinese garlic chives, which look like chives and have a very strong garlicky flavor, because I've seen them in Whole Foods on occasion. The shrimp can be replaced with chicken, pork, or tofu. It is key to have all the ingredients ready before you start cooking. Serve with lots of fresh herbs, bean sprouts, and lime wedges.

SERVES 6

10 ounces (300 g) pad Thai rice noodles (the kind that look like linguine, not the thin rice vermicelli)

Pad Thai Sauce

3 tablespoons fish sauce

3 tablespoons fresh lime juice

1½ tablespoons lite soy sauce

1 tablespoon brown sugar

Pinch of cayenne or red pepper flakes, optional

Shrimp and Vegetables

10 ounces (300 g) large shrimp, peeled, deveined, and cut in half lengthwise (see How to Clean Shrimp, page 123)

Salt and freshly ground pepper, to taste

3 tablespoons vegetable oil

3 garlic cloves, minced

1 cup (60 g) sliced garlic chives or scallions (about 1 inch/2.5 cm long)

6 ounces (2 cups, 180 g) fresh mung bean sprouts, root ends trimmed (see How to Clean Fresh Mung Bean Sprouts, page 215)

1 tablespoon finely diced red chiles, or to taste, optional

2 large eggs, lightly beaten

Garnishes

Fresh cilantro leaves

Fresh basil leaves, preferably Thai basil

½ cup (50 g) salted roasted peanuts or cashews

Fresh mung beans sprouts

Lime wedges

1. To cook the noodles, bring a pot of water to a boil. Add the noodles, turn off the heat, and let them sit in the hot water for 4 minutes. Drain, rinse under cold running water, and drain again. Set aside.

2. To make the sauce, in a small bowl, combine the ingredients and stir until the sugar has dissolved; set aside.

3. Place the shrimp in a bowl and season with salt and pepper; set aside.

4. In a large wok or nonstick skillet, heat 1 tablespoon of the vegetable oil over medium-high heat. Add one-third of the garlic and sauté until golden, then add the garlic chives and bean sprouts and sauté, stirring constantly, for 1 minute. Transfer the vegetables to a large bowl and set aside. (Do not rinse the skillet.)

5. Add the remaining 2 tablespoons vegetable oil to the wok and heat over medium-high heat. Add the remaining garlic and the red chiles, if using, and sauté for 30 seconds, then add the shrimp and sauté for 2 minutes. Add the reserved noodles and bean sprout mixture and, using large chopsticks or tongs, toss the noodles until everything is combined.

6. Move the noodles out to the sides of the wok to form a well in the center. Add the beaten egg to the well and toss the contents of the wok until everything is well combined and the eggs coat the noodles as they cook. Add the reserved sauce, mix well, and adjust the seasoning. Transfer to a large serving platter, garnish with any of the garnishes you like, and serve promptly.

SLOW-COOKER GINGER-GARLIC CHICKEN WITH VEGETABLES

I designed this recipe specifically for a slow cooker, but you can also use a Dutch oven (I give instructions for both). Feel free to change the vegetables: green beans, snow peas, carrots, shiitake mushrooms, and broccolini are all great options. I use a whole chicken rather than parts because the meat stays moist and juicy. To save time, pulse the garlic and ginger in a mini food processor until minced. If you don't have fish sauce, increase the soy sauce by 1 tablespoon. Brown rice or a whole grain is the perfect pairing for the chicken and sauce.

SERVES 5

Chicken Stew

¼ cup (40 g) packed brown sugar

3 tablespoons minced fresh ginger

3 large garlic cloves, smashed and peeled

3 tablespoons lite soy sauce (plus 1 tablespoon if not using fish sauce)

2 tablespoons fresh lemon or lime juice

1 tablespoon fish sauce, optional

3 scallions, trimmed and cut into thirds or quarters

5 fresh cilantro sprigs

¼ teaspoon red pepper flakes, or to taste, optional

One 2½-pound (1.25 kg) whole chicken, rinsed and all visible fat trimmed

2 to 3 teaspoons cornstarch

2 tablespoons water

Vegetables

1 tablespoon vegetable oil

1 garlic clove, minced

1 red bell pepper, cored, seeded, and thinly sliced

6 ounces (180 g) green beans, ends trimmed, and cut into thirds

10 ounces (300 g) bok choy, preferably baby bok choy, heads sliced lengthwise in half or, if large, into quarters

1. Combine all of the stew ingredients except the chicken, cornstarch, and water in a slow cooker and mix well. Add the chicken and turn to coat. Turn the chicken breast side up, and make sure some of the seasonings are on top of the chicken. Cover and cook on low for 2 hours, or on high for 1½ hours. Then turn the chicken over, so the breast side is down, and cook on low for 2 hours longer, or on high for 45 minutes, until the juices run clear when the thick part of the thigh is pierced with the tip of a knife. (Note: The cooking time will depend on your slow cooker and the size of the chicken.)

2. *Alternatively*, to braise the chicken in the oven, preheat the oven to 250°F (120°C). Place the chicken stew, without the cornstarch and water, in an ovenproof casserole dish with a lid (or use foil to cover it tightly) and cook for 2 to 3 hours, until the chicken is done when tested as above.

3. While the chicken is cooking, sauté the vegetables. In a large nonstick skillet, heat ½ tablespoon of the vegetable oil over medium-high heat. Add the garlic and cook for 30 seconds. Add the red bell peppers and green beans and sauté, stirring occasionally, for 2 minutes; add 1 tablespoon water if necessary to prevent the vegetables from overbrowning. Transfer to a deep serving platter and cover with foil

to keep warm. Add the remaining ½ tablespoon vegetable oil to the skillet and heat over medium-high heat. Add the bok choy and sauté for 2 minutes. If the greens stick to the skillet, add 1 tablespoon water to the skillet. Transfer to the serving platter and cover.

4. Once the chicken is cooked, carefully transfer it to a chopping board and cover with foil. Strain the cooking liquid into a small saucepan. Skim any fat off the sauce. Dissolve 2 teaspoons of the cornstarch in the water, add it to the saucepan, and cook over medium heat, stirring, for 4 to 5 minutes, until the sauce is the thickened to the desired consistency. If you want to further thicken the sauce, dissolve 1 teaspoon more cornstarch in 1 tablespoon water, add it to the saucepan, and cook, stirring, until thickened.

5. To serve, carve the chicken, place it on the center of the serving platter with the vegetables surrounding it. Pour some of the sauce on top of the chicken, and serve the rest at the table.

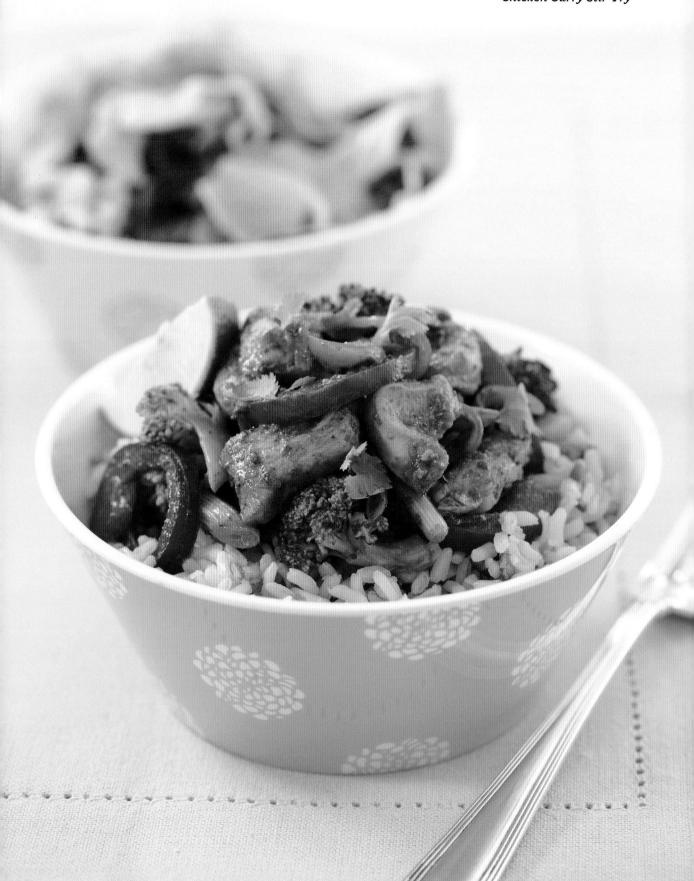

CHICKEN CURRY STIR-FRY

This dish is a staple in my repertoire because it's tasty, and it's a cinch to make. Serve with brown basmati rice, sautéed vegetables, or a green salad, and you're good to go. Another option is to serve the chicken on a bed of rice noodles, sprinkled with chopped peanuts, bean sprouts, and cilantro leaves, and garnished with lime wedges. You'll keep coming back to this one, I promise. Although this dish can be frozen, it's really best eaten on the same day it's made.

SERVES 4

1½ pounds (720 g) chicken tenderloins, cut into 1-inch (2.5 cm) slices on the diagonal

1 red bell pepper, cored, seeded, and cut into strips

1 medium sweet onion, halved lengthwise and sliced

1 tablespoon plus 1 teaspoon mild yellow curry powder

1 tablespoon plus 1 teaspoon sugar

3 tablespoons vegetable oil

2 tablespoons lite soy sauce or 1 tablespoon lite soy sauce mixed with 1 tablespoon fish sauce

3 scallions, sliced into 1-inch (2.5 cm) pieces

1½ cups (135 g) broccoli florets, blanched in boiling water for 2 minutes, or until crisp-tender

3 tablespoons whole or chopped fresh cilantro

Fresh lime juice, to taste

1. Combine the chicken, red bell peppers, onions, curry powder, sugar, 2 tablespoons of the vegetable oil, soy sauce, and the fish sauce, if using, in a bowl and mix well. Cover and refrigerate for at least 30 minutes, and up to 6 hours.

2. Heat the remaining 1 tablespoon vegetable oil in a large nonstick skillet over medium-high heat. Add half of the marinated chicken mixture and half of the scallions and sauté for 5 to 7 minutes, until the chicken is cooked. (Note: You might want to use a splatter screen.) Transfer the chicken to a serving dish and cover with foil to keep warm.

3. Reheat the skillet over medium-high heat. Add the remaining chicken, scallions, and the broccoli florets and cook in the same way. Adjust the seasoning and transfer to the serving dish. Garnish with the cilantro and sprinkle with lime juice to taste. Serve promptly.

---

352 CALORIES IN

Protein: 39 g; Carbohydrates: 14 g; Fat: 15 g; Fiber: 3 g; Sodium: 498 mg; Carb Choices: 1; Diabetic Exchange: 5 Lean Meat, 3 Vegetable

352 CALORIES OUT

Women: Walk: 86 minutes | Jog: 40 minutes

Men: Walk: 72 minutes | Jog: 34 minutes

CALORIE COMBOS

2 cups (40 g) salad greens with 1 tablespoon Almost-Fat-Free Dieter's Lemony Dressing (page 140): 38 cals

Indian-Style Cucumber Yogurt Salad (page 75): 45 cals

Tomato, Cucumber, and Radish Salad (page 76): 55 cals

Hot-and-Sweet Cucumber, Carrot, and Red Bell Pepper Salad (page 77): 61 cals

Lemony Dill Cabbage Slaw (page 78): 63 cals

2 cups (40 g) salad greens with 1 tablespoon Balsamic Vinaigrette (page 150): 73 cals

½ cup (80 g) plain white rice: 103 cals

½ cup (100 g) plain udon noodles: 105 cals

½ cup (90 g) plain brown rice: 108 cals

½ cup (65 g) plain quinoa: 111 cals

SLOW-COOKER PULLED PORK WITH WHOLE WHEAT BUNS

Pulled pork is a perennial crowd-pleaser. This recipe calls for a slow cooker, but you could use a Dutch oven or cook it in the oven on low heat. If you're short on time, use 1 cup (250 ml) of your favorite BBQ sauce mixed with 2 tablespoons water instead of the homemade sauce below. Add hot sauce if you desire, or simply jack up the heat with a pinch of cayenne. This dish is traditionally served on soft white buns, which is tasty, but I use whole wheat buns here. Leftovers can be frozen; thaw and reheat in a microwave oven.

SERVES 6

Pulled Pork Sauce

1 large onion, chopped

½ cup (125 ml) cup cider vinegar

1 teaspoon salt

½ teaspoon freshly ground pepper

¼ cup (60 ml) tomato paste

¼ cup (40 g) brown sugar

1 tablespoon Worcestershire sauce

1 tablespoon Dijon mustard

1 teaspoon garlic powder

¼ cup (60 ml) ketchup

2 tablespoons water

Pinch of cayenne, optional

Pork

2 pounds (1 kg) boneless pork shoulder, rinsed and trimmed of all visible fat

1½ teaspoons cornstarch

1 tablespoon water

6 whole wheat buns

1. To make the sauce, in a medium bowl, mix together all of the ingredients.

2. Place the pork in a slow cooker, add the sauce, and turn until the pork is well coated. Cover and cook on low for about 5 hours, or until the pork is very tender and the meat gives easily when poked with a fork. (Note: The timing will depend on your slow cooker.)

3. Transfer the cooked pork to a bowl and set aside to cool. Transfer the sauce to a medium saucepan and skim off as much fat as possible. If you have more than 1½ cups (375 ml) sauce, simmer the sauce over low heat until reduced to that amount; otherwise, just bring it to a simmer. Dissolve the cornstarch in the water and add it to the sauce, stirring until the sauce thickens; set aside.

4. As soon as the pork is cool enough to handle, shred it, using 2 forks and a small knife. Add the pulled pork to the sauce in the saucepan and reheat it over low heat. Place some of the pork in each of the buns, if using, and serve promptly.

CHICKEN AND RICE STOVE-TOP CASSEROLE (📷 page 321)

Get out your cast-iron casserole or Dutch oven for this chicken and rice dish. Brown and white rice have different cooking times and require different amounts of water, so you will need to adjust the recipe to the type of rice you use. My original recipe calls for chorizo sausage as well as chicken, but after calculating the nutritional breakdown with both, I decided to just add the chicken, which is still great.

SERVES 7

Chicken Marinade

1 teaspoon garlic powder

1 teaspoon paprika

½ teaspoon turmeric

2 teaspoons Italian seasoning or dried oregano

1 teaspoon roasted ground cumin

1 tablespoon extra virgin olive oil or vegetable oil

Freshly ground pepper, to taste

Sprinkle of salt

1¼ pounds (600 g) skinless bone-in chicken thighs and/ or drumsticks, scored (see How to Score Bone-In Chicken Parts, page 245)

1¼ pounds (600 g) chicken tenderloins

Casserole

2 tablespoons vegetable oil

1 large onion, chopped

2 large garlic cloves, minced

1 medium red bell pepper, cored, seeded, and cut into small dice

8 ounces (240 g) shiitake mushrooms, rinsed, stems removed, and thinly sliced

½ teaspoon paprika

1½ cups (300 g) white rice, rinsed

⅓ cup (80 ml) white wine

One 14-ounce (350 g) can diced tomatoes, drained, or 2 cups (500 ml) diced fresh tomatoes

2¼ cups (560 ml) low-sodium fat-free chicken stock

½ cup (70 g) frozen peas, cooked

½ cup (17 g) thinly sliced scallions

Squeeze of fresh lemon juice, to taste

¼ cup (15 g) chopped fresh cilantro or flat-leaf parsley, optional

1. To marinate the chicken, combine the marinade ingredients in a bowl or baking dish and mix well, then add all of the chicken. Prick all of the chicken with a fork and turn until well coated. Cover and refrigerate for at least 6 hours, and up to 24 hours.

2. In a large deep skillet or Dutch oven (it should be large and deep enough to cook the chicken and rice together), heat 1 tablespoon of the vegetable oil over medium-high heat. Add the chicken thighs and drumsticks and cook until golden brown on both sides, about 7 minutes per side. (Note: The chicken will not be cooked through at this point.) Transfer the chicken to a heatproof bowl. (Do not rinse the skillet.)

3. Reheat the skillet, without adding any oil, and sauté the chicken tenderloins for 3 minutes. Add them to the bowl with the chicken parts. (Do not rinse the skillet.)

4. Add the remaining 1 tablespoon vegetable oil to the pan and heat over medium

(RECIPE CONTINUES)

371 CALORIES IN

Protein: 31 g; Carbohydrates: 36 g; Fat: 11 g; Fiber: 4 g; Sodium: 486 mg; Carb Choices: 2; Diabetic Exchange: 4 Very Lean Meat, 2 Starch, 1 Vegetable, 1 Fat

371 CALORIES OUT

Women: Walk:
90 minutes | Jog: 43 minutes

Men: Walk:
76 minutes | Jog: 36 minutes

CALORIE COMBOS

2 cups (40 g) salad greens with 1 tablespoon Almost-Fat-Free Dieter's Lemony Dressing (page 140): 38 cals

Tomato, Cucumber, and Radish Salad (page 76): 55 cals

2 cups (40 g) salad greens with 1 tablespoon Classic Red Wine Vinaigrette (page 146): 62 cals

Lemony Dill Cabbage Slaw (page 78): 63 cals

Greek-Style Broccoli (page 91): 71 cals

Maple-Glazed Carrots (page 95): 98 cals

CALORIE CUTS

The best way to save calories here is to reduce the amount of oil. If you cut 1 tablespoon you will save 30 calories and 7 grams of fat per serving. Add a little bit of water if things start to stick to the pan.

heat until hot. Add the onions and garlic and sauté for 3 minutes. Add the red bell peppers, mushrooms, paprika, and rice and sauté for 2 minutes. Add the wine and cook for 2 minutes, then add the diced tomatoes and chicken stock and bring to a boil over high heat. Add the chicken thighs and drumsticks, (not the tenderloins), placing them evenly around the pan, slightly covered by the rice, cover the skillet, and simmer for 15 minutes, checking occasionally to make sure the liquid level is okay and adding more water if necessary. Add the chicken tenderloins to the pan, cover again, and cook for 15 minutes, or until the chicken and rice are completely cooked, again checking occasionally to make sure the liquid level is okay.

5. Scatter the cooked peas and scallions on top. Add the lemon juice to taste and adjust the seasoning. Garnish with the cilantro if desired, and serve promptly.

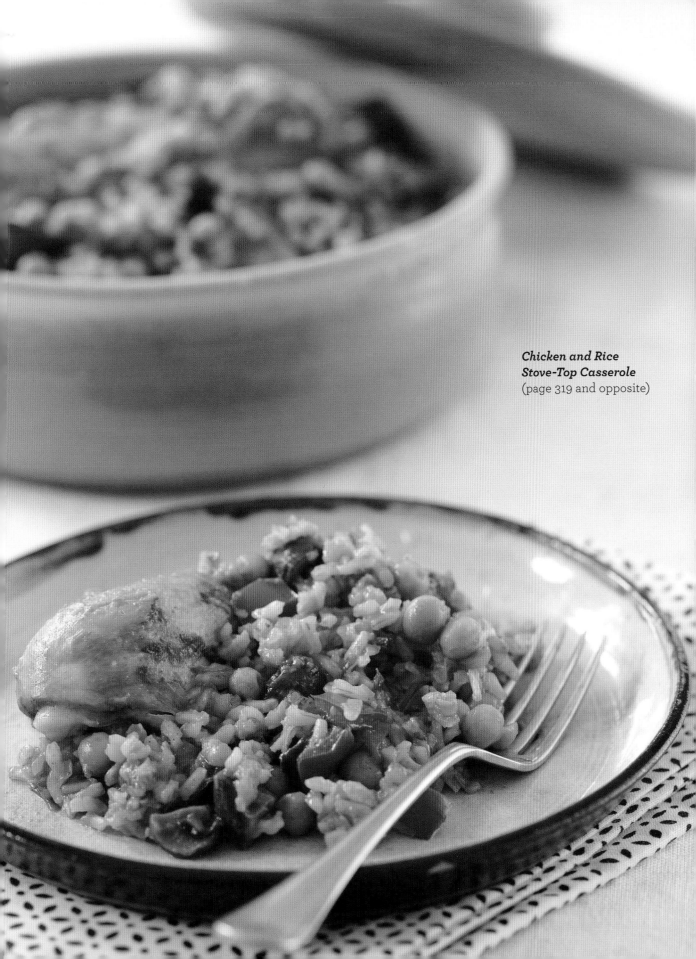

**Chicken and Rice
Stove-Top Casserole**
(page 319 and opposite)

*Vietnamese-Style Caramelized
Pork over Rice Noodles with Herbs*

VIETNAMESE-STYLE CARAMELIZED PORK OVER RICE NOODLES WITH HERBS

In authentic Vietnamese restaurants, you may recall seeing piles of fresh vegetables and herbs on many dishes (including this one) or they are sometimes arranged on a platter on the table for diners to help themselves. Despite the long list of steps, this dish is easy to prepare, especially if you stagger the steps and do some of the prep in advance. For an extra kick, add a dash of chili sauce or chili oil to the noodles. Elephant brand rice noodles are the best. To save time, pick up some of the ingredients, such as the shredded carrots, scallions, and sliced cucumbers, from a salad bar. You can marinate the pork ahead and then freeze it; thaw before cooking. Firm tofu, sliced and marinated, can be used in place of the pork: pan-fry the tofu until hot. Traditional garnishes include a mix of whole fresh herbs leaves, such as mint, Thai basil, and cilantro; lime wedges; roasted nuts; and bottled hot chili sauce, if you want more heat.

SERVES 4

1 pound (480 g) pork tenderloin

Vietnamese-Style Pork Marinade

⅓ cup (75 g) sugar

⅓ cup (60 g) chopped shallots

¼ cup (60 ml) fresh lime juice

2 tablespoons lite soy sauce

2 tablespoons water

Rice Noodles and Vegetables

8 ounces (240 g) thin rice noodles (also called rice vermicelli)

2 teaspoons toasted sesame oil

¼ cup (60 ml) seasoned rice vinegar

1 tablespoon fish sauce, or to taste

½ teaspoon sugar

2 tablespoons lite soy sauce

Pinch of red pepper flakes

1 cup (100 g) coarsely shredded carrots

1 cup (65 g) peeled, halved, and sliced seedless cucumbers

½ cup (30 g) thinly sliced scallions

¼ cup (15 g) fresh cilantro leaves

1 tablespoon vegetable oil

1½ cups (100 g) fresh mung bean sprouts, roots trimmed and rinsed (see How to Clean Fresh Mung Bean Sprouts, page 215)

3 tablespoons fresh mint leaves

¼ cup (10 g) fresh Thai basil leaves, torn or cut if large

4 tablespoons chopped salted peanuts

Lime wedges, for garnish

1. Slice the pork tenderloin on the diagonal into ½-inch (1.25 cm) slices. Place it in a Pyrex baking dish, cover, and refrigerate until ready to marinate.

2. To make the marinade, in a small skillet or heavy-bottomed saucepan, cook the sugar over medium heat, without stirring, until it becomes a light golden caramel color; do not let it get too brown or burn, or it will taste bitter. Add the shallots, lime juice, soy sauce, and water and bring to a boil. Remove from the heat and allow to cool completely, then pour the marinade over the reserved pork. Turn to make sure all sides are well coated, then cover and

(RECIPE CONTINUES)

394 CALORIES IN | I SERVING WITHOUT GARNISHES

Protein: 23 g; Carbohydrates: 61 g; Fat: 5 g; Fiber: 3 g; Sodium: 874 mg; Carb Choices: 3½; Diabetic Exchange: 3 Very Lean Meat, 3 Starch, 2 Vegetable

394 CALORIES OUT

Women: Walk:
96 minutes | Jog: 45 minutes

Men: Walk:
80 minutes | Jog: 38 minutes

CALORIE COMBOS

2 cups (40 g) salad greens with 1 tablespoon Almost-Fat-Free Dieter's Lemony Dressing (page 140): 38 cals

Tomato, Cucumber, and Radish Salad (page 76): 55 cals

Hot-and-Sweet Cucumber, Carrot, and Red Bell Pepper Salad (page 77): 61 cals

¼ cup (30 g) roasted peanuts: 214 cals

CALORIE CUTS

The rice noodles are 165 calories per serving, so you can cut back on them. Also, skip the peanuts and save 54 calories per tablespoon.

refrigerate for at least 3 hours and up to 24 hours.

3. When ready to serve, soak the noodles for 10 minutes, then drain, cook them according to the package directions, drain, rinse quickly, and drain again. Place the noodles in a bowl and mix with the sesame oil to prevent sticking; set aside.

4. In a small bowl, combine the rice vinegar, fish sauce, sugar, soy sauce, and red pepper flakes, and mix until the sugar has dissolved. Add the sauce to the cooked noodles, along with the carrots, cucumbers, scallions, and cilantro, and toss until well combined. Adjust the seasoning and set aside.

5. Remove the pork from the marinade and reserve the marinade. Heat the vegetable oil in a large nonstick skillet over medium-high heat. Cook the pork, in batches, for 3 to 4 minutes, until cooked through. Transfer the cooked pork to a large plate. (Do not rinse the skillet.)

6. Add the reserved marinade to the skillet and bring to a boil. Simmer for 5 minutes, then add it to the noodles and mix gently.

7. To serve, divide the noodles among 4 large individual bowls, or place them on a very large serving platter. Arrange the pork, bean sprouts, mint, and basil leaves on top of the noodles. Sprinkle with the peanuts and serve with lime wedges on the side.

BEEF AND VEGETABLE KEBABS WITH CILANTRO-GREEN OLIVE DRIZZLE

There is something festive about kebabs. Perhaps it's the fact that they conjure up summer days of BBQs by the beach, or just plain fun times with friends. In this recipe, sirloin steak is skewered with red bell peppers, button mushrooms, and onions. Just about any sauce or salsa in this book would be a lovely. Leftovers are scrumptious in a pita pocket with a bit of feta cheese, tomatoes, cucumbers, lettuce, and/or tahini. (See the boxes on page 129 for guidance about preparing and cooking with skewers.)

SERVES 6

Beef Kebab Marinade

2 tablespoons extra virgin olive oil

3 tablespoons fresh lemon juice

½ teaspoon salt

1 teaspoon brown sugar

3 tablespoons chopped fresh rosemary

2 teaspoons garlic powder

1 teaspoon Italian seasoning

2 teaspoons dried oregano

1 teaspoon red pepper flakes

2 pounds (1 kg) boneless sirloin or top round steak, trimmed of all visible fat and cut into 1½-inch (4 cm) pieces

Cilantro-Green Olive Drizzle

3 tablespoons extra virgin olive oil

1 to 2 tablespoons water

1 garlic clove, halved

1 cup (30 g) packed fresh cilantro leaves

¼ cup (40 g) green olives with pimientos

1 tablespoon medium capers

Salt and freshly ground pepper, to taste

Kebabs

1 large red bell pepper, cored, seeded, and cut into pieces about the same size as the meat

1 large onion, cut into pieces the same size as the meat

8 ounces (240 g) button mushrooms, rinsed, stems trimmed, and halved, or quartered if large

1. To make the marinade, in a large bowl, whisk together all of the ingredients. Add the steak, poke it with a fork to allow the marinade to seep in, and mix well. Cover and refrigerate for at least 3 hours and up to 12 hours.

2. For the cilantro drizzle, combine all of the ingredients in the bowl of a food processor and pulse until fairly smooth. Adjust the seasoning, transfer to a serving bowl, and set aside at room temperature. (If you make it more than 2 hours in advance, cover with plastic wrap pressed flush against the surface of the sauce and refrigerate.)

3. To make the kebabs, thread the beef and vegetables, alternating, onto eight 12-inch (30 cm) metal or soaked bamboo skewers. Reserve the remaining marinade for basting the skewers.

4. For a charcoal grill: Light a chimney starter filled with charcoal briquettes. When the coals are hot, spread them evenly over the bottom of the grill and set the cooking grate in place. Cover and heat until hot, about 5 minutes. For a gas grill: Turn all the

(RECIPE CONTINUES)

304 CALORIES IN

Protein: 24 g; Carbohydrates: 7 g; Fat: 21 g; Fiber: 1 g; Sodium: 290 mg; Carb Choices: ½; Diabetic Exchange: 3 High-Fat Meat

304 CALORIES OUT

Women: Walk: 74 minutes; Jog: 35 minutes

Men: Walk: 62 minutes; Jog: 29 minutes

CALORIE COMBOS

2 tablespoons crumbled reduced-fat feta: 35 cals

Indian-Style Cucumber Yogurt Salad (page 75): 45 cals

Tomato, Cucumber, and Radish Salad (page 76): 55 cals

2 cups (40 g) salad greens with 1 tablespoon Classic Red Wine Vinaigrette (page 146): 62 cals

Lemony Dill Cabbage Slaw (page 78): 63 cals

½ cup (75 g) plain couscous: 88 cals

Grilled Vegetables (page 108): 89 cals

1 tablespoon tahini: 90 cals

½ cup (80 g) plain white rice: 103 cals

½ cup (90 g) plain brown rice: 108 cals

½ cup (65 g) plain quinoa: 111 cals

Roasted New Potatoes (page 98): 118 cals

Great Green Couscous (page 105): 152 cals

1 pita bread: 165 cals

CALORIE CUTS

Skip the drizzle and save 26 calories and 3 grams of fat per serving.

burners to high, cover, and heat until hot, about 10 minutes.

5. Have a platter ready for the cooked kebabs. Oil the grill grate, then reduce the heat and grill the kebabs over medium heat, uncovered, basting at the start of cooking with the reserved marinade, and turning and moving the skewers and adjusting the heat as needed, until the vegetables and beef are nicely browned and the beef is cooked to the desired doneness, 5 to 7 minutes. Cut a piece of beef in half to check for doneness.

6. Transfer the kebabs to the serving platter and serve promptly with the cilantro drizzle.

FILET MIGNON WITH ZESTY BLACK PEPPER SAUCE

If the thought of a perfectly cooked filet mignon with a zesty black pepper sauce makes your mouth water, head to the kitchen now. This sauce can also be drizzled over grilled chicken, lamb, or almost anything else. The sauce can be made up to 3 days in advance, covered, and refrigerated.

SERVES 4

Zesty Black Pepper Sauce

1 tablespoon freshly ground black pepper

2 tablespoons ketchup

2 teaspoons Thai sweet chili sauce

1 teaspoon honey

1 tablespoon balsamic vinegar

2 teaspoons oyster sauce

2 tablespoons water

Four 4- to 5-ounce (120 to 150 g) beef tenderloin steaks, about 1 inch (2.5 cm) thick

Sprinkle of salt

1. To make the sauce, combine all of the ingredients in a small saucepan, bring to a simmer, stir, and cook for 2 minutes; set aside.
2. For a charcoal grill: Light a chimney starter filled with charcoal briquettes. When the coals are hot, spread them evenly over the bottom of the grill and set cooking grate in place. Cover and heat until hot, about 5 minutes. For a gas grill: Turn all the burners to medium-high, cover, and heat until hot, about 10 minutes.
3. Have a platter ready for the cooked steaks. Oil the grill grate. Very lightly salt the steaks, then grill them for about 4 minutes on each side, or to the desired doneness. (Note: If pan-frying, use medium-high heat, and cook for 3 to 5 minutes on each side, depending on the thickness of the steaks and desired doneness.) Transfer the steaks to the platter, cover with foil, and let rest for 5 minutes.
4. Serve the steaks with the sauce drizzled on top or in a bowl on the side.

307 CALORIES IN

Protein: 23 g; Carbohydrates: 6 g; Fat: 20 g; Fiber: 0 g; Sodium: 239 mg; Carb Choices: ½; Diabetic Exchange: 3 High-Fat Meat

307 CALORIES OUT

Women: Walk: 75 minutes; Jog: 35 minutes

Men: Walk: 63 minutes; Jog: 30 minutes

CALORIE COMBOS

Broiled Portobello Mushrooms with Herbs (page 86): 23 cals

Roasted Asparagus with Dill and Lemon Zest (page 88): 47 cals

Broiled Zucchini with Parmesan (page 90): 49 cals

2 cups (40 g) salad greens with 1 tablespoon Balsamic Vinaigrette (page 150): 73 cals

Grilled Vegetables (page 108): 89 cals

½ cup (80 g) plain white rice: 103 cals

½ cup (90 g) plain brown rice: 108 cals

Smashed Potatoes with Fresh Herbs (page 102): 144 cals

Polenta with Herbs and Cheese (page 103): 146 cals

Caesar Salad with a Light Touch (page 83): 163 cals

SPAGHETTI WITH BOLOGNESE SAUCE

A surefire crowd-pleaser. My son loves this sauce. His heart-warming comment one night was, "Why can't all spaghetti sauces taste this good?" See Calorie Cuts for the calorie values of various other starches to serve with this sauce. Freeze any leftover sauce in single-size portions for a delicious meal on busy days.

SERVES 12

Bolognese Sauce (makes about 6 cups/1.5 liters)

2 tablespoons vegetable oil or extra virgin olive oil

1 onion, finely chopped

2 garlic cloves, minced

2 teaspoons dried oregano

2 teaspoons Italian seasoning

1 pound (480 g) lean ground beef (preferably chuck) or a mix of beef and pork

½ cup (125 ml) white wine

1 cup (250 ml) whole milk

8 ounces (240 g) mushrooms (any kind), rinsed, stems trimmed, and thinly sliced

1 small red bell pepper, cored, seeded, and cut into small dice

One 15-ounce can (425 g) tomato sauce

One 14.5-ounce (411 g) can diced tomatoes, with their juices, or 1½ cups (375 ml) diced ripe tomatoes

Salt and freshly ground pepper, to taste

3 to 4 tablespoons chopped fresh basil or flat-leaf parsley, or a mix of both

10 ounces (300 g) enriched spaghetti

1. To make the sauce, in a large heavy-bottomed saucepan, heat the vegetable oil over medium-high heat. Add the onions and sauté for 3 minutes. Add the garlic, oregano, and Italian seasoning and sauté for 1 minute. Crumble the ground beef into the saucepan and sauté for 5 minutes, stirring and breaking up any large clumps with the back of a wooden spoon. Add the wine and cook, stirring, until it has evaporated. Add the milk, mushrooms, and red bell peppers and simmer gently for 30 minutes, or until most of the liquid has evaporated.

2. Add the tomato sauce and diced tomatoes and simmer for 30 minutes longer, or until the sauce has thickened to the desired consistency.

3. Meanwhile, bring a large pot of salted water to a boil. About 10 minutes before the sauce is done, add the spaghetti to the boiling water and cook according to the package directions. Drain, transfer to a serving bowl, and cover to keep warm.

4. Taste the sauce, adjust the seasoning, and add the basil. Serve promptly with the spaghetti.

SKIRT STEAK FAJITAS WITH CORN TORTILLAS

Fajitas make people happy. I give instructions for broiling the steak, but throw it on the grill if that is easier for you. If you prefer white meat, you can substitute 1¼ pounds (600 g) of boneless, skinless chicken breasts. The fixins are up to you, but Pico de Gallo, Yummy Guacamole, and a splash of hot sauce or minced jarred jalapeños are perfect accompaniments.

SERVES 6

Fajita Marinade

3 tablespoons cider vinegar

1 tablespoon chili powder

1 teaspoon dried oregano

1 tablespoon brown sugar

1 tablespoon extra virgin olive oil

2 tablespoons Worcestershire sauce

1 teaspoon garlic powder

1½ pounds (720 g) skirt steak or flank steak, trimmed of all visible fat

Tortillas and Fixins

12 corn tortillas (6-inch/15 cm diameter)

Grated reduced-fat sharp cheddar

Finely sliced romaine lettuce

Fat-free sour cream

Salsa

1. To make the marinade, in a Pyrex baking dish, combine all of the marinade ingredients and stir until blended.

2. With a sharp knife, lightly score both sides of the flank steak, only about ⅛-inch (3 mm) deep, in a crisscross pattern. Poke the steak with a fork to make holes for the marinade to seep in. Place the steak in the baking dish and turn to coat both sides. Cover with plastic wrap and refrigerate for at least 1 hour, and up to 12 hours.

3. To broil the steak, position an oven rack 4 to 5 inches (13 to 15 cm) from the heat source and preheat the broiler on high. While you broil the steak, warm the tortillas in the oven: wrap them in aluminum foil and place them on the rack underneath the rack with the steaks. They will warm from the broiler's heat as the steak cooks. (See How to Warm Tortillas Four Different Ways, page 330, for other heating options.)

4. Remove the steak from the marinade and place it on a baking sheet with sides. Broil on each side for 4 to 5 minutes, or to desired doneness. The timing will depend on the thickness of the steak and the power of your broiler. Transfer the steak to a chopping board, cover with foil, and allow it to rest for 5 minutes. Remove the tortillas from the oven when they are warmed through.

5. Slice the steak against the grain to the desired thickness. Serve promptly, with the tortillas and any fixins.

354 CALORIES IN | I SERVING WITH 2 CORN TORTILLAS

Protein: 26 g; Carbohydrates: 25 g; Fat: 17 g; Fiber: 4 g; Sodium: 172 mg; Carb Choices: 1½; Diabetic Exchange: 3 Medium-Fat Meat, 1 Starch, 2 Vegetable

354 CALORIES OUT

Women: Walk: 86 minutes; Jog: 41 minutes

Men: Walk: 72 minutes; Jog: 34 minutes

CALORIE COMBOS

½ cup (25 g) sliced romaine lettuce: 5 cals

2 tablespoons jarred salsa: 10 cals

1 tablespoon fat-free sour cream: 11 cals

Radish-Tomato-Cucumber Salsa (page 135): 12 cals

Pico de Gallo (page 137): 16 cals

Broiled Portobello Mushrooms with Herbs (page 86): 23 cals

Roasted Asparagus with Dill and Lemon Zest (page 88): 47 cals

Broiled Zucchini with Parmesan (page 90): 49 cals

1 ounce (30 g) reduced-fat cheddar cheese: 49 cals

1 corn tortilla: 52 cals

2 cups (40 g) salad greens with 1 tablespoon Balsamic Vinaigrette (page 150): 73 cals

Yummy Guacamole (page 157): 86 cals

Grilled Vegetables (page 108): 89 cals

1 whole wheat tortilla: 110 cals

CALORIE CUTS

Use only 1 tortilla, not 2, per serving and save 52 calories.

HOW TO WARM TORTILLAS FOUR DIFFERENT WAYS

1. Stove-top: In an ungreased skillet over medium heat, warm the tortillas one by one, flipping them when they begin to brown in spots and puff. Transfer to a basket or bowl lined with a cloth napkin to keep warm.

2. Microwave: Place the tortillas between 2 dampened paper towel on a microwave-safe plate. Microwave for about 1 minute, or until hot. Keep warm.

3. Grill: After grilling the meat, poultry, or other filling, wipe the grate with a cloth if necessary, then place the tortillas on the grate and cook until browned in spots and puffed. Keep warm.

4. Oven: wrap the tortillas in foil and warm them in a 350°F (180°C) oven for about 10 minutes, or until heated through. Keep warm.

YOGURT TORTE WITH PASSION FRUIT GLAZE AND BLUEBERRIES (📷 page 333)

This panna cotta–like yogurt torte, crowned with a yellow passion fruit glaze is a real stunner. If you can't find fresh passion fruit, or you're in a hurry, the glaze can be replaced with the Blueberry Sauce (page 337), Rhubarb-Raspberry Sauce (page 46), or Blueberry-Plum Sauce (page 47), spooned over or next to each slice. There are admittedly a lot of steps in this recipe, but the techniques are quite simple.

SERVES 8

Graham Cracker Crust

1 cup (100 g) graham cracker crumbs

2 tablespoons brown sugar

4 tablespoons (60 g) unsalted butter, melted

½ teaspoon ground cinnamon

Yogurt Filling

1¾ cups (450 ml) whole milk

¾ cup (180 g) sugar

1 tablespoon plus 1 teaspoon powdered gelatin

1¾ cups (420 g) nonfat plain Greek-style yogurt

1 tablespoon vanilla extract

Passion Fruit Glaze

(makes about ²/3 cup/160 ml)

1½ tablespoons cornstarch

1 tablespoon water

5 tablespoons (75 g) sugar, or to taste

6 ripe passion fruits (about 1 pound/480 g; see How to Clean Fresh Passion Fruit, page 332), to yield about 1¼ cups (310 ml) pulp

1½ cups (225 g) fresh blueberries

1. To make the graham cracker crust, center an oven rack and preheat the oven to 350°F (180°C). Line the bottom of an 8-inch (20 cm) springform pan with a circle of baking paper.

2. Combine all of the crust ingredients in a bowl and mix until well blended and the crumbs are moist. Transfer the mixture to the springform pan and press it evenly over the bottom. Bake for 8 to 10 minutes, until the crust is slightly firm to the touch. Remove from the oven and set aside to cool. (Note: The crust can be baked up to a day in advance; wrap in foil or store in an airtight container at room temperature.)

3. To make the filling, in a medium saucepan, combine the milk and sugar, stir, and heat over medium heat to just below a boil. Remove from the heat and pour 1 cup (250 ml) of the hot mixture into a Pyrex measuring cup. Add the gelatin and whisk to dissolve. Using a small strainer to catch any lumps, pour the gelatin mixture back into the saucepan. Stir and set aside to cool to room temperature.

4. Once the gelatin mixture has cooled, add the yogurt and vanilla extract and stir until well combined. (Note: Do not whisk, which would cause air bubbles.) Pour the mixture over the baked crust. Tap gently

318 CALORIES IN

Protein: 6 g; Carbohydrates: 55 g; Fat: 9 g; Fiber: 1 g; Sodium: 162 mg; Carb Choices: 3; Diabetic Exchange: 3 Starch, 2 Fat

318 CALORIES OUT

Women: Walk: 77 minutes; Jog: 36 minutes

Men: Walk: 65 minutes; Jog: 31 minutes

(RECIPE CONTINUES)

to release any air bubbles. Place a large paper towel over the top of the pan to absorb any condensation and tape down the edges, then cover with plastic wrap or aluminum foil and refrigerate for at least 3 hours, or until the filling is set.

5. To make the glaze, in a very small bowl, combine the water and cornstarch and mix until the cornstarch dissolves. In a small saucepan, combine the sugar, passion fruit juice, and cornstarch mixture and bring to a simmer over medium-low heat, stirring constantly. The glaze should be the consistency of a thick gravy. Set aside to cool.

6. When the glaze is at room temperature, pour it evenly over the top of the torte. Cover again with a paper towel and plastic wrap as in Step 4 and refrigerate until the glaze sets.

7. To unmold, have ready a deep container of hot water and a thin knife. Dip the knife in the hot water, wipe dry, and carefully run it around the sides of the pan. Release the sides of the pan and transfer the torte, still on the bottom of the pan, to a serving platter. To slice, dip the knife in the hot water, dry it, and slice, reheating and wiping the knife between slices. Garnish each slice with a scattering of blueberries. Cover and refrigerate any leftovers.

HOW TO CLEAN FRESH PASSION FRUIT

I use fresh passion fruit for the torte above. I've tried processed canned or bottled passion fruit pulp, and found it terribly disappointing. So please avoid it. Fresh passion fruits are deemed ripe when the brownish-red skin is wrinkled and shrunken. To clean them, rinse the fruit and then cut the orbs in half. Scoop out the bright yellow pulp into a bowl. Six passion fruits should yield about 1¼ cups (310 ml) pulp. Using a handheld immersion blender or a food processor, quickly pulse the pulp 3 times, or just long enough to separate the black seeds. Do *not* overprocess, or the seeds will break and impart black flecks into the sauce. Strain the pulp through a sieve into a measuring cup; you should have ⅔ to ¾ cup (160 to 180 ml) strained pulp. As an alternative to blending, add 2 tablespoons of the sugar in the recipe to the pulp and stir vigorously to separate the seeds. Strain, working the pulp through the sieve with the back of a spoon. Discard the seeds.

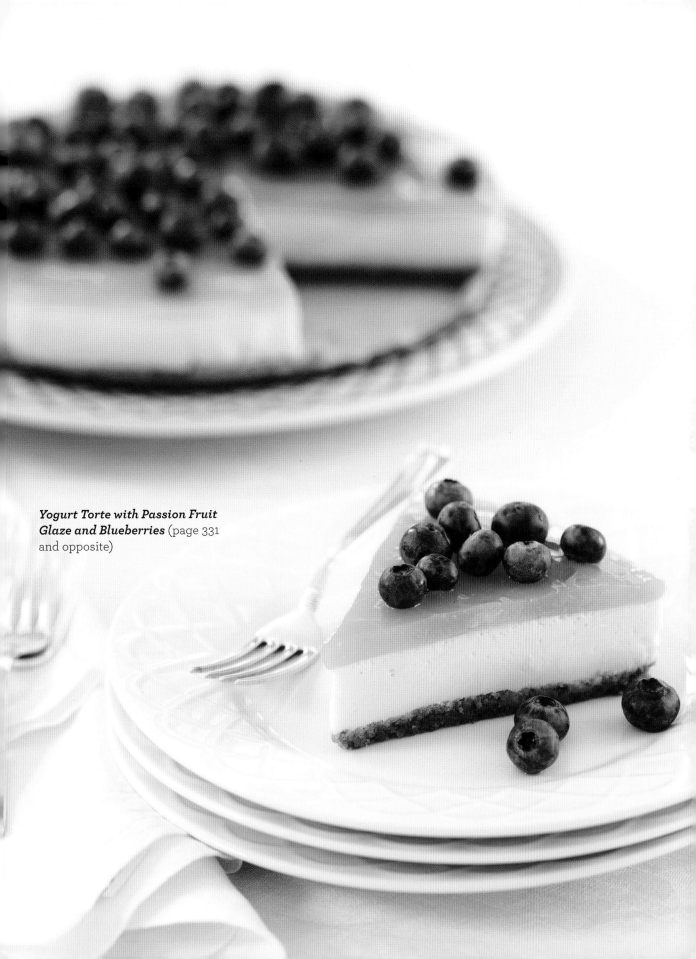

Yogurt Torte with Passion Fruit Glaze and Blueberries (page 331 and opposite)

CARROT BUNDT CAKE WITH ORANGE GLAZE

Dense and delicious, this carrot cake is perfect for dessert, coffee gatherings, or any special occasion, even birthdays. I replaced the traditional cream cheese frosting with a light orange glaze. One of my recipes testers wrote that she preferred the glaze and was happy it had fewer calories. Store any leftovers in an airtight container at room temperature for up to 3 days, or refrigerate for up to 1 week. The unglazed cake can be frozen for up to 1 month; glaze after thawing.

SERVES 15

Canola oil cooking spray

2 cups (260 g) unbleached all-purpose flour, plus flour for the Bundt pan

2 teaspoons baking soda

2 teaspoons baking powder

2 teaspoons ground cinnamon

½ teaspoon salt

1 cup (250 ml) canola oil

1 cup (160 g) packed brown sugar

3 tablespoons maple syrup

4 large eggs

2 teaspoons vanilla extract

3 cups (750 ml) finely grated carrots (about 10 ounces/300 g)

½ cup (50 g) chopped toasted walnuts or pecans

⅓ cup (60 g) dark or light raisins

Orange Glaze (makes about ¾ cup/180 ml)

1½ cups (180 g) confectioners' sugar

1 tablespoon grated orange zest

3 tablespoons orange juice

1 teaspoon hot water

1. Center an oven rack and preheat the oven to 350°F (180°F). Grease a 12-cup (3 liter) Bundt pan with cooking spray and lightly flour it; set aside.

1. Sift the flour, baking soda, baking powder, cinnamon, and salt into a large bowl.

2. In the bowl of an electric mixer, beat the canola oil, brown sugar, and maple syrup on medium speed for 2 minutes. Add the eggs and vanilla extract and continue to beat on medium speed for 2 minutes, or until the batter has slightly increased in volume. Add the reserved dry ingredients in two batches, beating on low speed for about 1 minute after each addition and scraping down the sides of the bowl as needed. Using a rubber spatula, fold in the carrots, nuts, and raisins, then transfer the batter to the prepared Bundt pan.

3. Bake for 60 minutes, or until a cake tester inserted into the middle of the cake comes out clean. Remove the cake from the oven, loosen the sides with a knife, and invert it onto a cooling rack. Let cool completely.

4. To make the glaze, mix all of the ingredients in a bowl until smooth. (The glaze can be made up to a day ahead. Cover and refrigerate.) Transfer the cake to a serving platter. Pour the glaze over the cake, allowing it to drip down the sides.

Baking Note: Instead of using a Bundt pan, grease and lightly flour a 13 x 9 x 2-inch (33 x 23 x 5 cm) baking pan or two 8- or 9-inch (20 or 23 cm) round cake pans. Bake for about 40 minutes, or until a cake tester inserted into the middle of the cake comes out clean.

APPLE BLUEBERRY CRISP (📷 page 336)

What's the difference between and crisp and a crumble? A crisp is fruit topped with a mixture of butter, sugar, flour, and, usually, nuts, then baked until the fruit is bubbly. A crumble is the same thing plus oatmeal. If you'd like to turn this crisp into a crumble, add ½ cup (50 g) old-fashioned rolled oats or 1 cup (100 g) low-fat granola without raisins or other dried fruit to the topping in Step 3. This crisp can be made in a 9-inch (23 cm) baking dish as here, but it is lovely baked in individual ovenproof molds or ramekins. You will need to adjust the baking time if you use smaller molds; bake for about 30 minutes, or until the apples are tender when pierced with the tip of a knife and the juices are bubbling. Top with low-fat or nonfat frozen yogurt, if desired. The blueberries can be replaced with an equal amount of your favorite berries. One of my testers commented that the berry and apple combination was heavenly. Her husband wanted more of the topping, which I can relate to, but it's not a such good idea if you're tracking calories. This crisp is best eaten on the same day it's made, ideally warm from the oven.

SERVES 8

Apple Blueberry Crisp Filling

About 3 pounds (1.5 kg) Granny Smith apples, peeled, cored, and sliced (7 to 8 cups/about 2 liters)

½ cup (115 g) granulated sugar

1½ teaspoons ground cinnamon

1 teaspoon vanilla extract

3 tablespoons unbleached all-purpose flour

1½ cups (225 g) fresh blueberries

Crisp Topping

½ cup (65 g) unbleached all-purpose flour

⅓ cup (60 g) packed brown sugar

5 tablespoons (75 g) chilled unsalted butter, cut into pieces

½ cup (50 g) chopped walnuts, optional

1. Center an oven rack and preheat the oven to 375°F (190°C). Have ready a 9-inch (23 cm) ungreased baking dish; any shape, square, round, or oval, will do.

2. To make the filling, combine all of the ingredients except the blueberries in a bowl and mix until well blended. Transfer half of the filling to the baking dish. Scatter evenly with the blueberries, then carefully spread the remaining filling over the blueberries. Set aside.

3. To make the topping, combine all of the ingredients except the walnuts in a bowl and quickly mix, using a pastry blender or your fingers, to the consistency of coarse cornmeal. Add the walnuts, mix again, and refrigerate if not using immediately.

4. Distribute the topping evenly over the filling. Bake for about 45 minutes, or until the apples are tender when pierced with the tip of a knife and the juices are bubbling. Remove the crisp from the oven and allow to cool slightly before serving.

329 CALORIES IN

Protein: 3 g; Carbohydrates: 56 g; Fat: 12 g; Fiber: 6 g; Sodium: 5 mg; Carb Choices: 3½; Diabetic Exchange: 3 Starch, 2 Fat

329 CALORIES OUT

Women: Walk: 80 minutes; Jog: 38 minutes

Men: Walk: 67 minutes; Jog: 32 minutes

CALORIE CUTS

Skip the walnuts in the topping and save 48 calories and almost 5 grams of fat per serving.

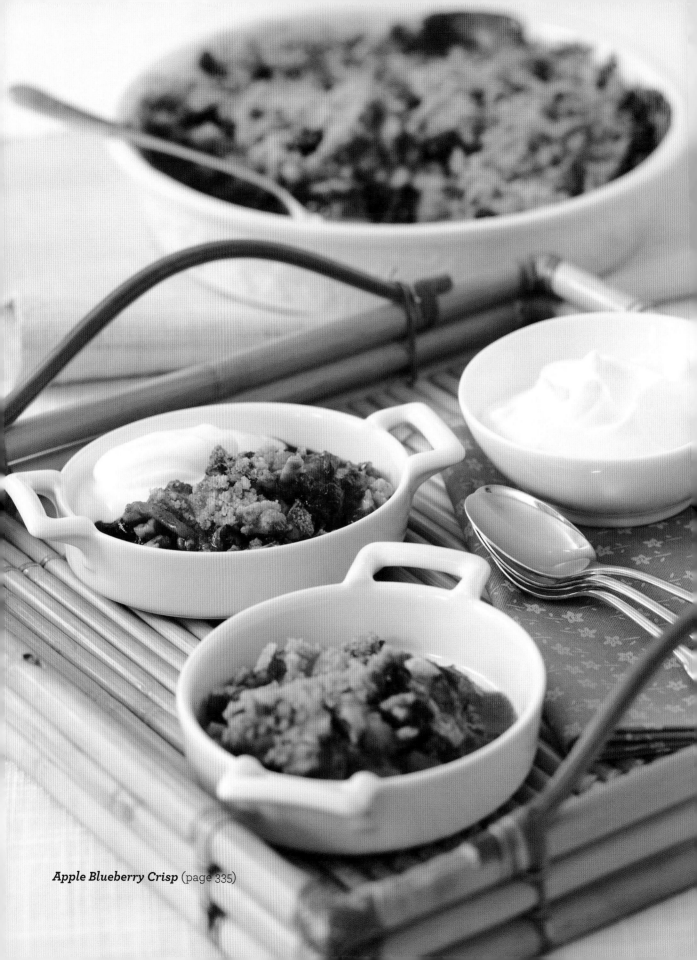

Apple Blueberry Crisp (page 335)

LEMON RICOTTA CHEESECAKE WITH BLUEBERRY SAUCE

A dessert worthy of a casual or formal dinner. The blueberry sauce can be replaced with any kind of berry puree or fruit sauce, such as the Blueberry-Plum Sauce (page 47) or Rhubarb-Raspberry Sauce (page 46). I call for reduced-fat cream cheese because it has a better consistency than nonfat. You can use a few drops of lemon extract for more intense flavor. The cheesecake is best made a day before serving. Lining the bottom of the springform pan makes it easy to lift that first slice from the pan. The sauce can be made up to 3 days ahead, covered, and refrigerated.

SERVES 8

Graham Cracker Crust

1 cup (100 g) graham cracker crumbs

4 tablespoons (60 g) unsalted butter, melted

¼ cup (40 g) finely chopped walnuts, optional

Cream Cheese Filling

One 8-ounce (240 g) package reduced-fat cream cheese

1 cup (280 g) part-skim ricotta cheese

⅓ cup plus 2 tablespoons (110 g) sugar

1 large egg

1 cup (225 g) fat-free sour cream

1 tablespoon dark or light rum, optional

2 teaspoons vanilla extract

1½ tablespoons very finely grated lemon zest

2 tablespoons fresh lemon juice

A few drop of lemon extract, optional

Blueberry Sauce (makes 1 cup/250 ml)

2 cups (300 g) fresh blueberries or frozen unsweetened blueberries

⅓ cup (75 g) sugar, or to taste

2 teaspoons cornstarch

1. To make the graham cracker crust, center an oven rack and preheat the oven to 350°F (180°C). Line the bottom of an 8-inch (20 cm) springform pan with a round of baking paper.

2. Combine all of the crust ingredients in a bowl and mix until well blended and the crumbs are moist. Transfer the mixture to the springform pan and press it evenly over the bottom. Bake for 8 to 10 minutes, until the crust is slightly firm to the touch. Remove from the oven and set aside to cool. (Note: The crust can be baked up to a day in advance; cover with foil or store in an airtight container at room temperature.)

3. To make the filling, using an electric mixer, beat the cream cheese and ricotta on medium speed until creamy, about 2 minutes. Add the sugar and beat for 30 seconds. Add the egg, sour cream, rum, if using, vanilla extract, lemon zest, lemon juice, and lemon extract, if using, and beat until well blended.

4. Pour the filling into the baked crust. Bake for 40 minutes, or until the center of the cheesecake is almost firm. The cake should still jiggle a bit in the center, but it will firm up as it cools. Remove the cheesecake from the oven and cool to room temperature, then refrigerate for at least 4 hours before serving.

(RECIPE CONTINUES)

362 CALORIES IN

Protein: 9 g; Carbohydrates: 44 g; Fat: 16 g; Fiber: 2 g; Sodium: 321 mg; Carb Choices: 2½; Diabetic Exchange: 2 Starch, 1 Fruit, 3 Fat

362 CALORIES OUT

Women: Walk: 88 minutes; Jog: 42 minutes

Men: Walk: 74 minutes; Jog: 35 minutes

CALORIE CUTS

Skip the sauce and save 56 calories per serving.

5. To make the blueberry sauce, combine all of the ingredients in a medium saucepan and bring to a boil, stirring occasionally. Reduce the heat to medium and cook until the sauce has thickened slightly, about 5 minutes. Remove from the heat.

6. To unmold the cheesecake, have ready a deep container of hot water and a thin knife. Dip the knife in the hot water, wipe dry, and carefully run it around the sides of the pan. Release the sides of the pan and transfer the cake, still on the bottom of the pan, to a serving platter. To slice, dip the knife in the hot water, dry it, and slice, reheating and wiping the knife between slices. Serve with the blueberry sauce. Cover and refrigerate any leftovers.

INGREDIENT NOTES AND RECOMMENDED BRANDS

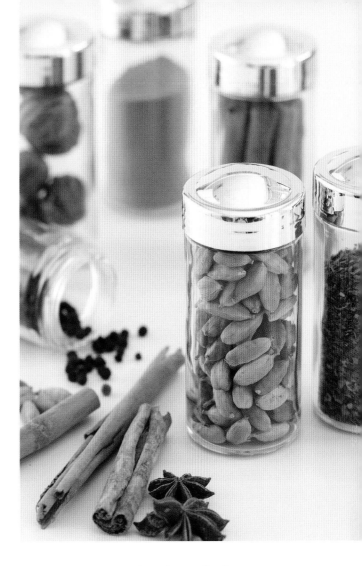

A WELL-STOCKED PANTRY is the key to easy, flavorful, and creative cooking. It will be an investment if you don't already have an array of staples and condiments on hand, or if you're new to cooking, but you'll quickly see that it is money well spent. For a list of all of the ingredients used in the recipes, see Essential Pantry (page 29). This section is designed to home in on the ingredients marked by an asterisk there. It explains what they are and how best to use and store them. Note that *The Calories In, Calories Out Cookbook* does not endorse any products, food or other, although they may be mentioned in the text or recipes. These are what I use in my cooking, and I can recommend them based on my personal experience. New products enter the market all the time, so think of these notes as a start.

Asian Ingredients

Special Note: Some of the best Asian brands have labels written in the language of their country of origin—Thai, Chinese, Japanese, or Vietnamese—which I could not transliterate.

From my experience, though, usually the pricier brands are of better quality.

Bonito Flakes: These pinkish-brown dried, fermented, and smoked fish flakes are used to flavor dashi, the base of miso soup; see How to Make Dashi (page 65). They are commonly made from skipjack tuna (also called Arctic bonito, aku, or striped tuna). *Brand:* Eden.

Coconut Milk: Nothing compares to fresh coconut milk, but if you're not in a region where coconut trees grow, you'll probably have to make do with commercial brands, which can be very good. They come in 13.5- to

14-ounce (400 ml) cans or Tetra Paks, labeled regular or lite/reduced-fat—the lite claiming a range of 25 to 75 percent less fat than the regular. I have also seen them in smaller 5.5-ounce (161 ml) containers, which are very convenient. Many people say that the lite versions are not nearly as rich and flavorful as the regular, and I agree. Thai brands are the best in my experience. Coconut milk is used extensively in Asian cuisines, in curries; satay meat, seafood, and vegetable dishes; and desserts. Once opened, any unused coconut milk should be transferred to a container, refrigerated, and used within 4 days; it can also be frozen. Be sure to use only unsweetened coconut milk in your cooking, not the sweetened coconut cream meant for cocktails. *Brands:* 365, Roland, Thai Kitchen, Aroy-D, Native Forest Organic, and Tiger Tiger.

Fish Sauce: Fish sauce is made from salted fish, usually fermented anchovies, but sometimes crab, shrimp, or squid. This thin, golden liquid has a strong, somewhat repellent scent that mellows with cooking. My advice is to purchase a good Vietnamese (*nuoc man*) or Thai (*nam pla*) fish sauce, which tend to be more refined. The cheaper sauces are often extremely salty, fishy, and smelly. For most recipes, lite soy sauce can be used as a substitute for fish sauce. Refrigerate after opening. *Brands:* Golden Boy, Aroy-D, and Thai Kitchen.

Hoisin Sauce: A thick, sweet but tangy brown sauce usually made from sugar, fermented soybean paste, garlic, dried sweet potato, salt, sesame paste, spices, and chili peppers. It is added to sauces or marinades and used as a glaze for roasted meats or as a dipping sauce for Peking duck or moo shu pork with pancakes. Refrigerate after opening. *Brands:* Lee Kum Kee and Kikkoman.

Miso: A Japanese staple used in soups, sauces, glazes, marinades, and salad dressings. Sometimes called miso paste, it is made from soybeans, salt, a yeast culture (called *koji*), and/or malted rice, barley, or wheat. The paste is left to age for at least several months, and up to 3 years. The type of malted grain determines the color, aroma, and flavor. The white and yellow are interchangeable in cooking, while the red is only used in hearty dishes that can handle its strong flavor.

- ▶ Rice miso (also called white miso) is a smooth paste that is light in flavor because of its shorter fermentation period. It is frequently used for salad dressings, sauces, soups, and marinades.

- ▶ Barley miso (also called yellow miso) is a smooth paste that is aged anywhere from 18 months to 2 years. It's the most common and most versatile in cooking and can be used like white miso.

- ▶ Hatcho miso (also called red miso) is named for the Chinese city where it originated. It is deep red, almost brown, with an earthy, meaty flavor and chunky texture. It has a longer fermentation period, from 2 to 3 years. Because the flavor is strong, it is often mixed with other types of miso or reserved for hearty dishes and sauces. Shopping online is a good way to buy miso. Store it tightly covered in your refrigerator. *Brands:* Awase, Shiro, Maruman Organic Miso, and Eden.

Oyster Sauce: A thick brown Chinese sauce usually made from oyster extract, water, sugar, and wheat flour. Many Chinese cooks believe that whenever oyster sauce (or soy sauce) is used in a recipe, a pinch of sugar should be added to the dish to counterbalance the saltiness. Choose a more expensive brand (I go by the price tag, because most are labeled only in Chinese), as the taste will be far superior to cheaper ones, which tend to contain more oyster extract. Refrigerate after opening. *Brands:* Lee Kum Kee and Kame.

Panko Bread Crumbs: These flaky Japanese bread crumbs, sometimes labeled bread flakes, are larger than their traditional fine-textured Western cousins. Most are made with wheat flour, but there are some gluten-free varieties. *Brands:* Sushi Chef and Original Organic Panko.

Seasoned Rice Vinegar: Made from fermented glutinous rice, this vinegar has a mild flavor with slightly sweet overtones. It is used in cooking and salad dressings, for pickling and brining, and in sauces. Seasoned rice vinegar is more golden and more flavorful than plain rice vinegar. Store at room temperature. *Brands:* Marukan, Nakamo, Kame, and Nishiki.

Seasoned Rice Wine: Also called *shaoxing*, rice wine should not be confused with rice vinegar. It is a product of fermented glutinous rice and is aged for at least 10 years and up to a hundred years. The price tag is usually an indicator of whether it's for cooking or for drinking. Rice wine has a rich amber color and an alcohol content similar to dry sherry. *Brands:* Marukan, Kikkoman, and Eden.

Sesame Oil: There are two types of sesame oil—a light-colored one that is pressed from untoasted seeds and a darker version that has a stronger, often almost smoky, flavor that comes from toasted seeds. The toasted version is frequently used to flavor a finished dish, hot or cold, or it can be used in salad dressings, dipping sauces, marinades, and other dishes. When cooking, the heat should not be too high, as sesame oil has a very low smoking point. Sesame oil is highly perishable; it gets bitter when past its prime. Choose dark bottles that will help preserve the flavor, and store it in the refrigerator. In my experience, the best sesame oils come from Japan. *Brands:* Kadoya, Mauhon (both Japanese brands), Lee Kum Kee, Sun Luck, and Dynasty.

Seaweed: The recipe for Miso Soup with Tofu, Shiitakes, Noodles, and Baby Spinach (page 64) includes a subrecipe for homemade dashi. This Japanese stock calls for a couple of different types of dried seaweed, which are available at Whole Foods:

- ▶ *Kombu* (also called *konbu*): A deep green, leafy dried kelp, used in salads as well as in dashi. The white powder sometimes present is simply salt residue. It should be soaked for 10 to 20 minutes before being used. *Brands:* Emerald Cove and Sea Mama.
- ▶ *Wakame:* A salty, dark-olive-green dried seaweed also used in other Japanese dishes, particularly salads. Soak *wakame* for at least 10 minutes before using. *Brands:* Eden, Emerald Cove, Shirakiku, Sea Mama, and Radiant Whole Foods.

Soy Sauce: Soy sauce is a dark, aged liquid distilled from a mixture of fermented soybeans, wheat, salt, and caramel. Read labels, and try to avoid brands with additives. Lite soy sauce is often used as a dipping sauce and in poultry and seafood dishes. Medium soy sauce has a bit more sodium and a deeper color. Dark soy sauce is heavy and salty-sweet and, in small amounts, adds a lovely depth flavor to sauces, stews, and marinades. *Brands:* King Imperial Golden Light, Pearl River Bridge, Wan Ja Shan, and Kikkoman Lite.

Sriracha Hot Sauce: A bright-red, now-trendy sauce made from chiles, sugar, salt, garlic, and distilled vinegar (shree-RA-cha is the correct pronunciation). A squirt goes well with grilled chicken or seafood, soups, marinades, salads, or anything else that begs for a bit of heat. Store in the refrigerator. *Brand:* Huy Fong Foods.

Tofu: Tofu is a high-protein, low-fat, cholesterol-free curd made from dried soybeans, which are boiled until soft, then pureed and strained. Soy milk is extracted from the boiled beans and curdled with one of two natural coagulants: nigari or calcium sulphate. Soft tofu is simply drained, not pressed, and has a silky texture. Firm and extra firm tofu is drained and pressed into bricks. Tofu can be found in regular or plain varieties, lite, seasoned, calcium-enriched, marinated, or baked. If you buy unpackaged tofu from a tub of water, make sure that the water is clear and odorless and that the store has a high turnover. Ideally, chose organic, non-GMO brands. Because of its high water content, tofu does not freeze well. Store in the refrigerator and use as soon as possible. *Brands:* Nasoya, Nature's Promise, and Morinaga.

▶ *Firm and extra-firm tofu:* A firm block of bean curd that holds its shape when cut or cooked. It is used in stir-fries and for tofu patties, and it can be grilled or broiled.

▶ *Soft or silken tofu:* A very soft white bean curd that has the consistency of lightly set Jell-O. It is slippery and tends to break apart easily. It is usually steamed and served with a sauce.

Thai-Style Sweet Red Chili Sauce: This is the sauce typically served alongside deep-fried or fresh spring rolls in Thai restaurants. The ingredients usually include cane sugar, water, pickled red chiles, garlic, rice vinegar, and salt, as well as preservatives. Refrigerate after opening. *Brand:* Thai Kitchen.

Tom Yam Red Chili Paste: This chili paste is designed specifically for *tom yam* soup. So it is only used in one recipe, but you can also add it to coconut milk–based curries. It adds heat and flavor, as well as a bit of oil, but it is well worth the few extra calories. It is quite hot, so use it in moderation. *Brands:* Thai Kitchen and Blue Elephant.

Spices and Herbs

Always check expiration dates on spice packaging before buying them. Store in an airtight container away from heat, direct sunlight, and humidity. If you open a container and the spice is no longer fragrant, toss it and buy new. You should probably invest in new spices at least once a year. Buy small jars, especially if you don't use them very often. Whenever possible, grind your spices from dry-roasted seeds (see page 237). They will be infinitely more fragrant.

Black Mustard Seeds: These tiny brown-purple seeds have a distinct peppery-mustard flavor that is unique to Indian fare. Heating releases the oils and brings out the mustard flavor. Be warned that they pop as they cook, so use a splatter screen. Yellow mustard seeds are not a suitable substitute. Black mustard seeds are used in tarkas (see How to Make a Basic Indian Tarka, page 210) for yogurt-based salads and in soups, curries, dals, pickles, chutneys, and numerous vegetable dishes. Look for them at Indian grocery stores or online. *Brands:* Swad and Kalustyan's.

Cayenne: Cayenne chiles are named for the city of Cayenne in French Guiana, South America, where the peppers are grown. The familiar pungent bright-red powder is made from dried and finely ground chiles and seeds. *Brands:* McCormick, Simply Organic, Vanns Spices, The Spice Hunter, Frontier, Swad, Indus Organic, and Kalustyan's.

Chili Powder: The chili powder used for traditional chilis, stews, and bean dishes also includes other spices and ingredients, such as dried onions, garlic, cumin, and oregano, to produce a deep, spicy flavor. Pure Asian chile powder, made only from chiles, a finely ground bright red-orange spice akin to cayenne, is a bit sweeter, with a delicate smoky finish. It is not a substitute for ordinary chili powder. *Brands:* McCormick, Simply Organic, Vanns Spices, and The Spice Hunter.

Chinese Five-Spice Powder: This light brown, spicy, slightly sweet blend of ground star anise, cloves, cinnamon, fennel seeds, and Sichuan peppercorns (sometimes other spices are added) is used in meat and poultry marinades and rubs and in other Chinese or similar dishes. *Brands:* Vanns Spices, The Spice Hunter, Frontier, Swad, and Kalustyan's.

Cinnamon, Sticks and Ground: One of the most familiar spices around the globe, used in both savory and sweet dishes. Westerners generally reserve cinnamon for sweets, including breakfast items, baked goods, and other desserts, while Indians put it in everything from garam masala, biryanis, and curries to spice-infused teas. Cinnamon sticks come from the inner bark of the tropical cassia evergreen tree. Look for unblemished sticks free of mold, dust, cracks, and other imperfections. The flavor of cinnamon can vary, depending on the country of origin; you may need to try a few different types of ground cinnamon to see what works best for you. If you want to grind cinnamon sticks into powder yourself, I strongly advise that you first use a mortar and pestle to break them up into small pieces before processing them in a spice grinder, to avoid damaging the blade. *Brands:* McCormick, Indus Organic, Simply Organic, Vanns Spices, The Spice Hunter, Swad, and Kalustyan's.

Coriander, Seeds and Ground: The seeds come from the coriander plant, perhaps better known as cilantro. After the pinkish-white flowers bloom and dry out, the seeds are harvested and dried. The whole seeds are usually cracked before using for pickling or in vegetable or other dishes. Ground coriander is most fragrant when you dry roast the seeds and then grind them yourself (see How to Roast and Grind Spices, page 237). When grinding coriander seeds, it's best to use an electric spice grinder, as the husks are difficult to crush finely by hand. I was thrilled when McCormick came out with a line of roasted ground spices, including coriander. *Brands:* Simply Organic, 365 Everyday, Whole Foods, Frontier, McCormick, Vanns Spices, The Spice Hunter, Indus Organic, Swad, and Kalustyan's.

Cumin, Seeds and Ground: Earthy and aromatic, with a slightly peppery and grassy undertone, cumin seeds turn sweet and nutty when roasted. A mainstay of savory Indian dishes, they are used in spice blends, curry bases, tarkas, rice dishes, breads, pickles, chutneys, and just about everything in between. Dry roast and grind them yourself (see How to Roast and Grind Spices, page 237), or use McCormick's roasted ground cumin. If you buy cumin seeds in bulk, check expiration dates and look for seeds that are free of stems and other debris that may be used as fillers. *Brands:* Simply Organic, 365 Everyday, Whole Foods, Frontier, McCormick, Vanns Spices, Indus Organic, The Spice Hunter, Swad, and Kalustyan's.

Curry Leaves: Curry leaves, resembling small bay leaves, come from the curry plant. The leaves release their oils when heated, lending a pleasant curry-citrus flavor to dishes. Dried leaves are not as strong as fresh, but they are still flavorful. Curry leaves, usually cooked in a tarka (see page 210), add a magical touch to yogurt-based salads, curries, rice dishes, seafoods, and soups. Unlike bay leaves, these leaves do not need to be removed from a dish before serving; they are edible.

Curry Powder: Most Westerners are familiar with the ubiquitous yellow curry powder, but, in fact, curry powders come in many flavors and colors, and often the spice combinations are custom-designed for meats, poultry, or seafood. Yellow curry powders have a base of turmeric, while the red contain dried red chile pepper and/or red pepper, which can be a bit spicy. The flavors of the two are very different. Curry powder should always be added to a dish in the early sauté phase of cooking; it should never be added directly to a liquid base as it needs direct heat to release its full flavor potential. Curry powders are a matter of personal preference, so when you find one or two you like, stick with them. *Brands:* McCormick, Frontier, Vanns Spices, Indus Organic, Swad, Sadaf, and Kalustyan's.

Fennel Seeds: These greenish-brown, small, oval seeds from a plant in the parsley family have a slightly sweet licorice-like flavor. In Indian restaurants and homes, they are sometimes served after a meal to freshen the breath and aid digestion. *Brands:* McCormick, Simply Organic, Vanns Spices, The Spice Hunter, Swad, and Kalustyan's.

Fresh Chiles: The world of chiles can be confusing, especially if you're new to cooking. The good news is that chiles are very easy to grow in a pot, so if you cannot find what you are looking for, you can grow it. Here is a lineup from hot to mild.

▶ *Habanero:* Very, very hot, slightly fruity orange, red, yellow, or green chiles. They are used in salsas, hot sauces, and marinades.
▶ *Thai bird's-eye or bird:* Tiny, very hot red, green, orange, or yellow chiles used in Southeast Asian stir-fries, curries, soups, and salads. They have a slightly nutty flavor.

- ▶ *Serrano:* Very hot bright green (when unripe) or red (ripe) peppers with a zippy, fresh flavor. They are used raw in salsas and cooked in curries, chilis, and other main courses.
- ▶ *Jalapeño:* Medium-hot to very hot, these plump green or red peppers are most commonly used to add heat to salsas, guacamole, and other Mexican dishes. They are also sold jarred or canned, whole or sliced (the jarred tend to be pickled).
- ▶ *Anaheim or California:* These mild, sweet, crisp green or red peppers are typically roasted and peeled before using in sauces and salsas. They are also sold jarred or canned, whole or diced.
- ▶ *Banana:* Mild, yellow-green, long peppers with a sweet, faintly fruity flavor, also known as Hungarian wax or *guero.* They are used in salsas, tacos, salads, pickles, and other dishes where a bit of mellow heat is desired.

Garam Masala: *Garam masala,* literally translated as "spice mix," is the cornerstone of savory Indian cooking, and just about every serious Indian cook has his or her own secret recipe. For those who lack a prized recipe, there are some good store-bought versions. *Brands:* Frontier, McCormick, Simply Organic, Vanns Spices, The Spice Hunter, Swad, and Kalustyan's.

Garlic Powder: Not to be confused with garlic salt, this is ground dried garlic cloves and nothing else. I call for garlic powder, not garlic salt, in my recipes. *Brands:* Simply Organic, 365 Everyday, Whole Foods, Frontier, McCormick, Vanns Spices, and The Spice Hunter.

Green Cardamom, Pods and Ground: These pungent camphor-and-eucalyptus-scented, pale green oval seed pods hail from the ginger family. When gently cracked open, they reveal three sections, each housing a tiny lobe of three or four brown, oily seeds. Used in many cuisines, cardamom is added to both savory and sweet dishes, teas, and coffee. The smoky brown cardamom pods are less common and much more expensive than the green, while the bleached white pods are seldom used. Ground cardamom is pungent but not as flavorful as the pods. *Brands:* Simply Organic, 365 Everyday, Whole Foods, Frontier, McCormick, Vanns Spices, The Spice Hunter, Indus Organic, Swad, and Kalustyan's.

Kaffir Lime Leaves: Fresh is the only way to go here; don't even think about using dried leaves. If necessary, hold off on making a dish that requires lime leaves until you find the fresh. The aromatic, zesty figure eight–shaped double leaves are commonly used in Southeast Asian curries, curry pastes, soups, salads, and other dishes to add a fresh lime flavor. I have found the fresh leaves in Asian specialty stores and some Whole Food stores.

Lemongrass: Fresh stalks are by far the best. The dried ones are almost flavorless, and lemongrass pastes usually taste of citric acid more than lovely lemongrass. Lemongrass is commonly added to curries, soups, salads, and stir-fries and used as a base for tisanes. Fresh lemongrass is sold in Asian specialty stores, gourmet markets, some Whole Foods stores, and certain grocery store chains, such as Giant Food, in the fresh herb section. See How to Clean and Cook with Fresh Lemongrass, page 74.

Paprika and Smoked Paprika: A delicate spice from dried sweet peppers that adds color and flavor, and some heat if it's hot paprika, to numerous cuisines around the globe. It is milder than chili powder, cayenne, or pure Asian chile powder. The smoked version adds a wonderful depth of flavor to potatoes, chicken, polenta, and other dishes. *Brands:* Simply Organic, 365 Everyday, Whole Foods, Frontier, McCormick, Vanns Spices, The Spice Hunter, and Szeged (sweet and hot).

Salt: Buying salt used to be a simple task, but now, too many options can lead to confusion. Boutique salts are in fashion, and many of these designer brands come with matching price tags. The salt sampler packages available from Amazon are a great way to experiment with different types of salt. Generally, unrefined sea salts and naturally pink Himalayan salt offer an appealingly complex salty flavor. Refined table salt, iodized or not, comes from rock deposits and is more one-dimensional on the tongue. A salt grinder is not essential, but it is fun. *Brands:* Your favorites.

Sesame Seeds: These white or black seeds are sold raw or toasted, and they are used differently, depending on the dish. If the seeds are going to be roasted or cooked in a dish, I call for raw sesame seeds. If they are used to garnish salads, soups, or noodles, I call for toasted. Both raw and toasted are readily available, but if you have the time, you can dry roast raw seeds and freeze for later use (see How to Toast and Freeze Nuts and Seeds, page 93). I don't specifically call for black sesame seeds in any of my recipes, but you may use them in almost any recipe that calls for sesame seeds for a stunning contrast of color. Because of their high oil content,

sesame seeds can go rancid quickly, so pay attention to expiration dates. Store them in the freezer if you use them infrequently. *Brands:* Sushi Chef, Sun Luck, Bob's Red Mill, and McCormick.

Star Anise, Pods and Ground: These dark brown, eight-pointed, star-shaped pods, which taste of licorice, come from the flowers of an evergreen tree grown in China and Japan. Each branch of the pods holds a shiny dark brown seed. Whole pods are added to savory and sweet dishes; be sure to remove them before serving. Ground star anise is readily available, but to grind your own, crush the pods in a mortar and pestle and then use a spice grinder (crushing them first will protect the food processor's blade). *Brands:* Vanns Spices, The Spice Hunter, Swad, and Kalustyan's.

Tandoori Spice Mix: The best tandoori spice mixes are homemade, but there are a couple of good ones on the market. Just be sure to avoid those with artificial red food coloring. *Brands:* Whole Foods Organic, Vanns Spices, Swad, and Kalustyan's.

Turmeric: Turmeric comes from a rhizome in the ginger family. Fresh, or dried and powdered, it has a mellow, warm, musky aroma and flavor, but it can become bitter if too much is used. Turmeric powder is an essential spice in Indian cooking, used in spice mixes, and to season rice, vegetables, sauces, curries, dals, and a whole range of other dishes. It does stain, so be careful when you use it. *Brands:* Simply Organic, 365 Everyday, Whole Foods, Frontier, McCormick, Vanns Spices, Indus Organic, The Spice Hunter, Swad, and Kalustyan's.

Whole Grains and Pastas

Brown Rice: Brown rice is bulkier and chewier than polished white rice and takes longer to cook, because its outer layer of bran and inner germ are still intact. If you don't cook brown rice often, store it in the refrigerator or freezer to prevent the oils in the outer husks from getting rancid. If the rice develops a musty smell, toss it. *Brands:* 365 Organic, Rice Select, and Lundberg.

Basmati Rice: A long, slender rice grain available in white and brown varieties, primarily grown in India, Pakistan, and Thailand. It is usually aged for at least a year to develop its full flavor. Basmati rice expands lengthwise when cooked, and true success is measured by how long and intact the grains are after cooking. It is advisable to soak the grains for 10 to 15 minutes before cooking (unless a recipe instructs you otherwise); keep in mind that the longer you soak the grains, the less time they need to cook. Basmati rice should be stored in a cool, dry place. Brown and white basmati are interchangeable, though the cooking time might be slightly longer for brown. *Brands:* Texmati, Royal Basmati, Rice Select, Tilda, and Village Harvest.

Cornmeal (sometimes called polenta): Cornmeal, which contains the germ and fibrous bran of corn, comes in coarse, medium, and fine grinds. White cornmeal is slightly sweeter and more delicate than the more common yellow. Instant polenta is the finest and takes only about 3 minutes to cook; coarse can take up to 20 to 30 minutes. Cornmeal is used in baking and for savory dishes such as spoon bread. *Polenta* is the Italian word for cornmeal, as well as the name of the traditional dish made from it. Fine-textured corn flour differs from cornmeal. It is sometimes interchangeable with cornmeal in baked goods, but it should not be used for polenta. *Brands:* Roland, Dellalo, Bob's Red Mill, Arrowhead Mills, and Quaker.

Couscous: Everyone loves this pasta granule because it's quick, easy, and almost foolproof. The packaged instant couscous sold in the West is presteamed and dried, which accounts for the short cooking time. Traditional couscous is steamed in a special two-tiered contraption called a *couscoussière*. A meat or vegetable stew cooks in the bottom part of the vessel, while the top is a steamer insert for cooking the couscous, which allows the grains to absorb the flavors of the stew below. Pearl-like Israeli couscous resembles springy, tiny balls of pasta more than regular couscous. *Brands:* Lundberg, Near East, Bob's Red Mill, and Rice Select.

Oats: The world of oats can be confusing; here's the skinny.

- ▶ *Quick-cooking oats:* These thin, small flakes, which cook in a matter of minutes, are commonly eaten for breakfast. They are not suitable for granola.
- ▶ *Rolled oats (also called old-fashioned rolled oats):* These thicker, rounder flakes are also eaten as porridge, but they have a longer cooking time, usually about 10 minutes over a low flame. They are used in granola, crisp toppings, and other baked goods.
- ▶ *Steel-cut oats:* Shaped like tiny pellets, these oats take the longest to cook, 30 to 40 minutes on a low simmer. Even

when cooked, they are chewy, which some people love and others don't. The good news is that a batch can be cooked in advance and then reheated for breakfast, thinned with a little bit of water or milk.

Pad Thai Noodles: These rice noodles, which are naturally gluten-free, are made from rice powder and water. They come in different shapes and sizes, most of which are intended for specific Asian dishes. Follow the package directions, as cooking times will differ according to thickness. *Brands:* A Taste of Thai, Annie Chun's, and Thai Kitchen.

Soba Noodles: Light brown in color, with a nutty flavor and chewy texture, Japanese soba noodles are commonly made from a mix of buckwheat and wheat flour. They are used in soups or salads. Soba noodles may include green tea, lemon zest, or black sesame seeds, but these flavor varieties are less popular and hard to find. Boiling time is usually about 5 minutes. *Brands:* Eden and Hakubaku.

Somen Noodles: Made from wheat flour, these very thin Japanese noodles are traditionally eaten cold with soy sauce and rice vinegar or added to soups. Udon noodles are a fine substitute. Cooking time is about 3 minutes. *Brands:* JFC, Hime, Tomoshiraga, and Hakubaku.

Udon Noodles: White Japanese udon noodles are eaten in soups and served cold with a dipping sauce. They are made from wheat flour (sometimes mixed with rice flour) and are sold fresh or dried. They can be used interchangeably with thinner somen noodles or fresh Chinese egg noodles. Boiling time

is 7 to 10 minutes; try not to overcook them. *Brands:* Eden and Hakubaku.

Dairy Products

Paneer: Paneer is a fresh white Indian cheese that can be either soft and slightly creamy or hard and dry. It is commonly made at home, especially in northern India, where it is widely consumed by vegetarians almost daily. The recipes in this book were tested using Lemos brand, which tends to be very firm and slightly dry. Other brands I've tried, such as Gopi, are moister and a bit creamier. Brands: Lemos and Gopi.

Other Staples

Extra Virgin Olive Oil: Extra virgin comes from the first pressing of green olives and has a lower acidity than regular olive oil. Oil simply labeled "olive oil" is from a second pressing or from chemical extraction of the olive debris after the first pressing. It is usually lighter and milder than extra virgin and virgin. Light and extra light olive oils are a mix of refined oils; they contain the same amount of calories as other olive oils. You may want to keep two types of olive oil on hand: a more expensive extra virgin for drizzling on salads or flavoring special dishes, and a less robust oil for everyday cooking needs. Price tags usually indicate quality, but this is not always the case; go with the flavor and acidity level you like. *Brands:* Spectrum, Filippo Berio, Bertolli, Colavita, and Pompeian.

Oat Flour: Oat flour is a slightly sweet flour that can be used like whole wheat flour. It is excellent in waffles, pancakes, muffins, cookies, and other baked goods. *Brands:* Arrowhead Mills, Bob's Red Mill, Gold Medal, Pillsbury, and King Arthur.

Onions: Yellow, white, and red onions are all interchangeable. Sweet onions usually have a higher water content and lower sulfur content (i.e., fewer tears). Some popular varieties are Maui, Vidalia, Walla Walla, Sweet Imperial, and Spring Sweet. In general, 1 superlarge onion = 1¼ to 1½ cups (310 to 375 ml) chopped onion; 1 large = 1 cup (250 ml) chopped; 1 medium = ¾ cup (180 ml) chopped; and 1 small = ½ cup (125 ml) chopped.

Stocks: Homemade stock is best, but there are a number of very good prepared low-sodium fat-free stocks on the grocery shelves. You may have to try a few to find your favorite. Even though they are low-sodium, they are sometimes quite salty, so I usually water them down a little. Avoid brands with MSG. *Brands:* 365 Organic, Kitchen Basics, Emeril's All-Natural Vegetable Stock, and Pacific.

Vegetable Oils: The range of vegetable oils can be confusing: corn, peanut, sunflower, soybean, safflower, cottonseed, and rapeseed (canola). Which is best? Healthwise and caloriewise, they are all about equal; table-spoon contains about 120 calories and 14 grams of fat. It is really a matter of taste preference, and whether you want a flavorful or neutral oil. For baking, I tend to use canola oil or safflower oil, which are completely flavorless.

Vinegars: A good supply of vinegars is the key to fantastic homemade salad dressings.

You can get as fancy as you like. *Brands:* Progresso, Heinz, Pompeian, Trader Joe's, Monari, and Federzoni.

▶ *Balsamic vinegar:* Made in Modena, northern Italy, balsamic vinegar comes from grapes fermented in wooden barrels for a minimum of 4 years and up to 40 years or more. Prices correspond to the duration of aging. White or regular brown balsamic vinegar is a welcome addition to any salad, roasted vegetables, or other dish that begs for a hint of sweetness.

▶ *Wine vinegars:* Red and white wine vinegar are the most popular, and the taste is not that different once they are mixed into a dressing. You can get fancy by using Chianti, Pinot Noir, or Champagne vinegar.

▶ *Cider vinegar:* Made from apples, cider vinegar is sweeter than wine vinegar, with a slight apple flavor. It is used in vinaigrettes, pickling, and sauces. A good substitute is cane vinegar.

FREQUENTLY ASKED QUESTIONS

By Elaine Trujillo, MS, RDN

1. *If I count my calories, am I guaranteed to lose weight?*

Counting calories is a tool that can definitely help you lose weight, but try to look beyond that. Increasing awareness of what and how much you eat, which is one of the main goals of this book, will have positive effects on your overall health. Counting calories may help you recognize eating patterns that you were unaware of, or it may help you differentiate between when you are snacking from boredom and when you are really hungry. On the flip side, you might discover that you are already following a healthy diet and staying within your ideal calorie range, and if that's the case, kudos to you! Counting calories can be both an educational and a weight-loss tool.

2. *Is it true that if I drink lots of water I'll lose weight faster?*

No, sorry, but please do keep drinking water. There are lots of benefits to drinking more water, although faster weight loss is not one of them. Generally, when you lose weight, the first few pounds lost are water weight, and it is important to replace it. Drinking lots of water may make you feel fuller, at least temporarily, so in that sense, it may aid weight loss, but it does not improve or speed up your metabolism. On the other hand, not getting enough water can lead to mild dehydration, can make you feel drained and fatigued, and may lead to overeating. Whether you are losing weight or not, it is important to stay well hydrated, and how much water you need depends on your gender, where you live, and how active you are. The Food and Nutrition Board of the Institute of Medicine set general recommendations for women at approximately 91 ounces (about 11 cups, or 2.7 liters) and men at 125 ounces (about 4 quarts, or 3.7 liters) of water, from both beverages and foods, daily.

3. *Why am I gaining weight when I'm exercising every day?*

You're not alone here, but please (please!) don't get discouraged. Some people gain weight with exercise for a variety of reasons. One is that exercise can increase appetite, so they end up consuming more calories than they otherwise would. Although exercise does cause you to burn more calories, if you eat more calories than you burn, you will not lose weight. But also keep in mind that the physiological changes associated with exercise, such as reduced blood pressure, reduced heart rate, improved insulin regulation, and cardiovascular fitness, are all extremely important health benefits. Even if you don't lose weight, you are probably changing your body's makeup by increasing muscle and decreasing body fat, which is a great thing. Regardless of what the scale might indicate, a tape measure or your looser-fitting clothes can show real progress. Bottom line? Keep moving.

4. *Are weight-loss drugs safe?*

If you have not been successful with weight loss and your BMI is greater than 30, or you have a serious medical problem, such as diabetes or high blood pressure, and your BMI is greater than 27, you may be a candidate for prescription weight-loss medications. When medication is combined with a low-calorie diet and exercise, you can lose 5 to 10 percent of your body weight over a one-year period. Many medications work by reducing your appetite and increasing the feeling of fullness, but because of the potential side effects, many are only for short-term use, usually less than twelve weeks. One of these prescription drugs, Orlistat, works by blocking fat absorption; a reduced-strength version of this medication, Alli, is available over the counter. Weight-loss drugs are not an easy answer, but under proper medical supervision, when combined with a low-calorie diet and an exercise plan, they can be a useful tool.

5. *Are sugar substitutes safe?*

The short answer is yes. Before reaching store shelves, sugar substitutes go through an approval process overseen by the U.S. Food and Drug Administration (FDA), which includes toxicology studies in animals. Seven sugar substitutes have been determined to be safe and approved for use in the United States: acesulfame K (Sunett and Sweet One), aspartame (Equal, NutraSweet), luo han guo fruit extract (Fruit-Sweetness), neotame, saccharin (Sweet'n Low), stevia (Truvia and RureVia), and sucralose (Splenda). Although these sugar substitutes have been deemed safe, however, more needs to be understood about how they affect our energy intake and metabolic functioning. For many, however, sugar substitutes can be helpful in weight management.

6. *What are sugar alcohols?*

Not to be confused with sugary alcoholic drinks, sugar alcohols, such as sorbitol and xylitol, are sugar substitutes. They add sweetness (generally they are less sweet than table sugar), with fewer calories. Because some are not completely absorbed, people may experience a laxative effect when consuming too much of them.

7. *Is there such a thing as good food and bad food?*

I prefer the words "healthy" and "unhealthy" to "good" and "bad." Some foods are healthier than others, or more *nutrient dense*, which means that they are loaded with nutrients, such as vitamins, minerals, phytonutrients, and, often, fiber, and don't have added fats and sugars. Fruits, vegetables, whole grains, eggs, beans, legumes, seafood, lean meats, nuts, and seeds are all nutrient-dense foods. Other foods fall into the category of *calorie dense*, without much nutritional benefit—these include such items as french fries, cookies, and candy bars. It helps to think of food as providing fuel and nutrients for your body. Ideally, to keep your body working at optimal performance, you want to consume more nutrient-dense foods and fewer calorie-dense foods.

8. *Does eating fat make you fat?*

This is a really tough question, so I'll start with the Atwater values: 4, 4, 9 discussed by Malden in Understanding the World of Calories (see page 4). Fat has more calories per gram than carbohydrates and protein. It clocks in at 9 calories per gram, compared to 4 calories per gram. But weight gain is a complicated and highly individualized process that involves numerous variables and cannot be blamed solely on fat intake. Even if you removed all the fat from your diet (and I don't recommend doing so), you can still gain weight. Please continue reading Questions 9 and 10 for more on healthy fats and how much dietary fat you require.

9. *What are good and bad fats?*

Fats get a bad rap, as they are often associated with overweight, obesity, and heart disease. The so-called "bad fats" include saturated fats from animal foods, which may not be as bad as once thought, and artificial trans fats that used to be added to food, but, thankfully, the FDA is banning them from the food supply. These trans fats are not to be confused with the naturally occurring trans fats in animal meats, which are healthy. Then there are the "good fats," the monos (monounsaturated) and polys (polyunsaturated) that are naturally present in olives, nuts, avocados, seafood, among other foods, and many common oils, such as canola, corn, olive, peanut, safflower, soybean, and sunflower oil. The polys provide essential fatty acids, and some sources, such as fatty fish, shellfish, walnuts, and flaxseeds, provide healthy omega-3 fatty acids. All fats have the same calories, whether they come from, say, meat or olives: 9 calories per gram.

10. *How much fat can I eat each day?*

The amount varies from person to person. However, in general, adults should aim for 20 to 35 percent of total calories from fat every day. This is the amount recommended to reduce the risk of chronic diseases, such as cardiovascular disease. It is also a good ballpark range for weight control. You can get an idea of how much fat is in the foods you are eating by checking the nutrient facts on the food label: from the "Calories from Fat," you can calculate the percentage of calories in one serving. You can do the same for each of the recipes in this book. Multiply the grams of fat by 9 to determine the calories from fat, divide the calories from fat by the total calories of that food item, and then multiply by 100. If the food has less than 20 to 35 percent of calories from fat, you are good to go.

11. *Are all calories created equal?*

No, all calories are *not* created equal. For the reasons mentioned in the answer to Question 7 above, some calories pack in tons of nutrients, while others have little or no nutritional benefits. But even beyond nutrients, calories from some foods may act differently from others metabolically. Take fat and protein, for example. They both increase satiety, so we feel fuller after eating them than when we eat carbohydrate-based foods. Eating protein while losing weight may have the added advantage of protecting your lean body mass (muscle mass) while increasing loss of body fat.

12. *If a store-bought product's calorie count differs from the calorie value listed in the Appendix, which should I use?*

Although it may be tempting to use the count with the lower calorie value, the value that is likely to be more reliable is the one on the product label. The values given in the Appendix, while extremely reliable, may differ slightly among different brand-name products of the same item.

13. *Can I drink alcohol if I am trying to lose weight?*

The calories from alcohol can add up quickly, so be sure to remember to include calories from all beverages in your daily count. Alcohol itself has 7 calories per gram, plus any additional calories from whatever you may be mixing it with. FYI, a 5-ounce glass of wine has about 125 calories, a 12-ounce bottle of beer has about 150 calories, and a 5-ounce margarita has a whopping 338 calories.

14. *What are the rules about displaying charts of calorie counts in restaurants and other eating establishments?*

Beginning with New York City in 2008, several states and municipalities have implemented regulations requiring posted nutrition information in chain restaurants. Recently the FDA proposed national regulation that would ensure calorie labeling on menus and menu boards in all chain restaurants, retail food establishments, and vending machines having twenty or more locations. This is all moving in the right direction. Stay posted.

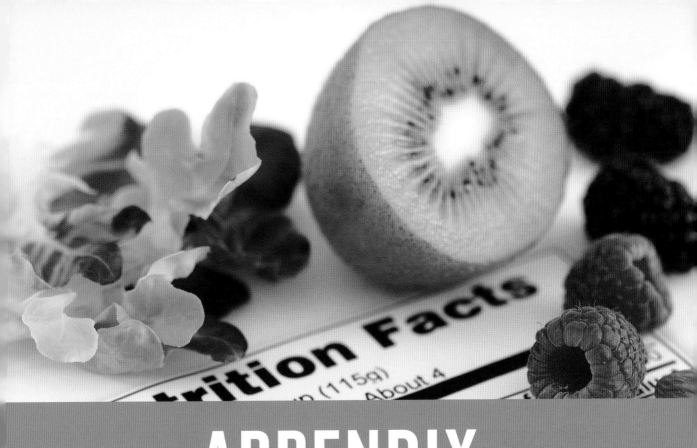

APPENDIX

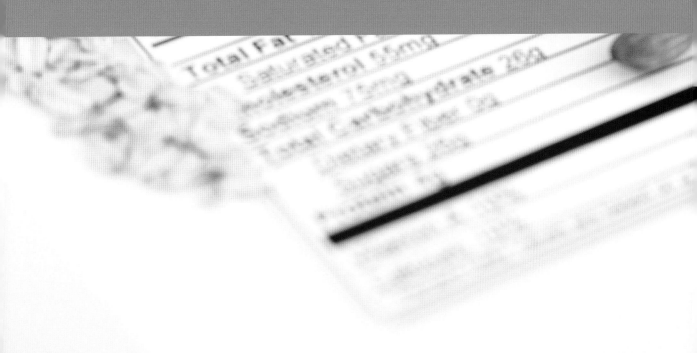

UNDERSTANDING NUTRITION TERMS AND LABELS

DEFINITIONS OF NUTRIENT CLAIMS ON LABELS*

NUTRIENT	FREE	LOW	REDUCED/LESS
Calories	<5 cal	≤40 cal	At least 25% fewer calories than an appropriate reference food
Total Fat	<0.5 g	≤3 g	At least 25% less fat than an appropriate reference food
Saturated Fat	<0.5 g saturated fat	≤1 g and ≤15% of calories from saturated fat	At least 25% less saturated fat than an appropriate reference food
Cholesterol	<2 mg	≤20 mg	At least 25% less cholesterol than an appropriate reference food
Sodium	<5 mg	≤140 mg	At least 25% less sodium than an appropriate reference food
Sugars	"Sugar Free": <0.5 g sugars	Not defined and may not be used	At least 25% less sugar than an appropriate reference food

Source: U.S. Food and Drug Administration. "Guidance for Industry: A Food Labeling Guide (9. Appendix A: Definitions of Nutrient Content Claims)." October 2009; updated 06/24/2013. http://www.fda.gov/Food/GuidanceRegulation/GuidanceDocumentsRegulatoryInformation /LabelingNutrition/ucm064911.htm.

UNDERSTANDING BODY MASS INDEX

The Body Mass Index (BMI) is a helpful tool for determining if you are at a healthy weight. It is a single number based on the ratio of your weight to your height. An ideal BMI is less than 25. Because muscle and bone are denser than fat, an athletic or muscular person may have a high BMI, but not be overweight or obese.

THERE ARE FOUR CATEGORIES OF BMI:

Underweight = less than 18.5

Normal weight = 18.5 to 24.9

Overweight = 25 to 29.9

Obese = 30 or greater

You can use the chart below to find out your BMI (note that the chart does not apply to children, athletes, and pregnant and lactating women).

Height in	Height cm	Weight lbs 100 / kgs 45.5	105 / 47.7	110 / 50	115 / 52.3	120 / 54.5	125 / 56.8	130 / 59.1	135 / 61.4	140 / 63.6	145 / 65.9	150 / 68.2	155 / 70.5	160 / 72.7	165 / 75	170 / 77.3	175 / 79.5	180 / 81.8	185 / 84.1	190 / 86.4	195 / 88.6	200 / 90.9	205 / 93.2	210 / 95.5	215 / 97.7
5'0"	152.4	19	20	21	22	23	24	25	26	27	28	29	30	31	32	33	34	35	36	37	38	39	40	41	42
5'1"	154.9	18	19	20	21	22	23	24	25	26	27	28	29	30	31	32	33	34	35	36	36	37	38	39	40
5'2"	157.4	18	19	20	21	22	22	23	24	25	26	27	28	29	30	31	32	33	33	34	35	36	37	38	39
5'3"	160	17	18	19	20	21	22	23	24	24	25	26	27	28	29	30	31	32	32	33	34	35	36	37	38
5'4"	162.5	17	18	18	19	20	21	22	23	24	24	25	26	27	28	29	30	31	31	32	33	34	35	36	37
5'5"	165.1	16	17	18	19	20	20	21	22	23	24	25	25	26	27	28	29	30	30	31	32	33	34	35	35
5'6"	167.6	16	17	17	18	19	20	21	21	22	23	24	25	25	26	27	28	29	29	30	31	32	33	34	34
5'7"	170.1	15	16	17	18	18	19	20	21	22	22	23	24	25	25	26	27	28	29	29	30	31	32	33	33
5'8"	172.7	15	16	16	17	18	19	20	21	22	22	23	24	24	25	25	26	27	28	28	29	30	31	32	32
5'9"	175.2	14	15	16	17	17	18	19	20	20	21	22	22	23	24	24	25	25	26	27	28	28	29	30	31
5'10"	177.8	14	15	15	16	17	18	18	19	20	20	21	22	23	23	24	25	25	26	27	28	28	29	30	30
5'11"	180.3	14	14	15	16	16	17	18	18	19	20	21	21	22	23	23	24	25	25	26	27	28	28	29	30
6'0"	182.8	13	14	14	15	16	17	18	18	19	19	20	21	21	22	23	24	24	25	25	26	27	27	28	29
6'1"	185.4	13	13	14	15	15	16	17	17	18	19	19	20	21	21	22	23	23	24	25	25	26	27	27	28
6'2"	187.9	12	13	14	14	15	16	16	17	18	18	19	19	20	21	21	22	23	23	24	25	25	26	27	27
6'3"	190.5	12	13	13	14	15	15	16	16	17	18	18	19	20	20	21	21	22	23	23	24	25	25	26	26
6'4"	193	12	12	13	13	14	15	15	16	17	17	18	18	19	20	20	21	22	22	23	23	24	25	25	26

To calculate your exact BMI value, multiply your weight in pounds by 703, divide by your height in inches, and then divide again by your height in inches; or divide your weight in kilograms by your height in meters, squared (kg/m^2).

Source: Obesity Education Initiative: Clinical Guidelines on the Identification, Evaluation, and Treatment of Overweight and Obesity in Adults. National Instevtes of Health, National Heart, Lung, and Blood Institute, Obesity Research 1998, 6 Supplement 2:51S-209S.

CALORIE VALUES

Calorie Value Tables

KEY TO CALORIE VALUE TABLES

Pro = Protein; Carb = Carbohydrate; g = gram; c = cup; oz = ounce; in = inch; T = tablespoon; t = teaspoon.

Carb Choice = Carbohydrate Choice (1 carbohydrate choice is approximately 15 g).

Diabetic Exchange: FR = Fruit; V = Vegetable (nonstarchy); F = Fat; S = Starch; VLM = Very Lean Meat; LM = Lean Meat; MFM = Medium-Fat Meat; HFM = High-Fat Meat; SM = Skim Milk; LFM = Low-Fat Milk; WM = Whole Milk

Free refers to foods with calorie values <20 calories.

Elaine and I are solely responsible for the selection of the foods included in this table; inclusion of brand-name and chain restaurant foods does not imply any endorsement of this book from the companies and restaurants whose foods appear here.

FRESH, COOKED & PREPARED FOODS

INGREDIENT	SERVING	CALORIES	PRO G	CARB G	FAT G	CARB CHOICE	DIABETIC EXCHANGE
FRESH FRUITS							
Apple	1 medium (182 g)	95	1	25	0	1½	1½ FR
Apricots	4 (140 g)	67	2	16	1	1	1 FR
Banana	1 medium (118 g)	105	1	27	0	2	2 FR
Blackberries	1 c (144 g)	62	2	14	1	1	1 FR
Blueberries	1 c (145 g)	83	1	21	1	1½	1½ FR
Boysenberries, frozen	1 c (132 g)	66	2	16	0	1	1 FR
Cantaloupe	1 c cubed (160 g)	54	1	13	0	1	1 FR
Cherimoya	1 (312 g)	234	5	55	2	3½	3½ FR
Cherries, sweet	1 c (154 g)	97	2	25	0	1½	1½ FR
Clementine	1 (74 g)	35	1	9	0	½	½ FR
Coconut meat	1 oz shredded (28 g)	100	1	4	9	0	2 F
Currant, red or white	1 c (112 g)	63	2	16	0	1	1 FR
Fig	1 medium (50 g)	37	0	10	0	½	½ FR
Gooseberries	1 c (150 g)	66	1	15	1	1	1 FR
Grapefruit, pink or red	1 c pulp (229 g)	96	2	24	0	1½	1½ FR
Grapes, red or green	1 c (151 g)	104	1	27	0	2	2 FR
Guava	1 (55 g)	38	1	8	0	½	½ FR
Honeydew melon	1 c melon balls (177 g)	64	1	16	0	1	1 FR
Kiwi fruit	1 (86 g)	52	1	12	1	1	1 FR
Kumquats	5 (95 g)	68	2	15	1	1	1 FR

INGREDIENT	SERVING	CALORIES	PRO G	CARB G	FAT G	CARB CHOICE	DIABETIC EXCHANGE
Lemon	1 (108 g)	22	1	12	0	1	1 FR
Lime	1 (67 g)	20	1	7	0	½	½ FR
Lychee	1 c pulp (190 g)	125	2	31	1	2	2 FR
Mandarin orange or tangerine	1 medium (88 g)	47	1	12	0	1	1 FR
Mango	1 (207 g)	124	2	31	1	2	2 FR
Mulberries	1 c (140 g)	60	2	14	1	1	1 FR
Orange	1 medium (131 g)	62	1	15	0	1	1 FR
Papaya	1 c diced (140 g)	60	1	15	0	1	1 FR
Passion Fruit	1 c pulp (23 g)	229	5	55	2	3½	3½ FR
Peach	1 medium (150 g)	59	1	14	0	1	1 FR
Pear	1 medium (166 g)	96	1	26	0	2	2 FR
Pineapple	1 c diced (155 g)	78	1	20	0	1	1½ FR
Plum	1 medium (66 g)	30	1	8	0	½	½ FR
Pomegranate	1 (282 g)	234	5	53	3	3½	3½ FR
Raspberries	1 c (123 g)	64	2	15	1	1	1 FR
Rhubarb	1 c diced (121 g)	25	1	6	0	½	1 V
Strawberries	1 c (144 g)	46	1	11	0	1	1 FR
Tamarind	1 c pulp (120 g)	287	3	75	1	5	5 FR
Tangelo	1 medium (95 g)	45	1	11	0	1	1 FR
Watermelon	1 c diced (152 g)	46	1	12	0	1	1 FR
CANNED FRUITS							
Applesauce, sweetened	½ c (123 g)	84	0	22	1	1½	1½ FR
Applesauce, unsweetened	½ c (122 g)	51	0	14	0	1	1 FR
Apricot halves in juice	½ c (122 g)	59	1	15	0	1	1 FR
Blackberries in heavy syrup	½ c (128 g)	118	2	30	0	2	2 FR
Blueberries in heavy syrup	½ c (128 g)	113	1	28	0	2	2 FR
Blueberries in light syrup	½ c (122 g)	107	1	28	1	2	2 FR
Grapefruit segments in juice	½ c (125 g)	46	1	12	0	1	1 FR
Grapefruit segments in light syrup	½ c (127 g)	76	1	20	0	1	1½ FR
Grapefruit segments in water	½ c (122 g)	44	1	11	0	1	1 FR
Mandarin orange segments in juice	½ c (125 g)	46	1	12	0	1	1 FR
Mandarin orange segments in light syrup	½ c (126 g)	77	1	20	0	1	1½ FR
Mixed fruit in heavy syrup	½ c (128 g)	92	1	24	0	1½	1½ FR
Peach halves in heavy syrup	½ c (131 g)	97	1	26	0	2	2 FR
Peach halves in juice	½ c (124 g)	55	1	14	0	1	1 FR
Pear halves in juice	½ c (124 g)	62	0	16	0	1	1 FR
Pear halves in heavy syrup	½ c (133 g)	98	0	25	0	1½	1½ FR
Pear halves in water	½ c (122 g)	35	0	10	0	½	½ FR

INGREDIENT	SERVING	CALORIES	PRO G	CARB G	FAT G	CARB CHOICE	DIABETIC EXCHANGE
Pineapple in juice	½ c crushed, sliced, or chunks (125 g)	75	1	20	0	1	1½ FR
Plums in heavy syrup	½ c (92 g)	81	0	21	0	1½	1½ FR
Plums in juice	½ c (126 g)	73	1	19	0	1	1 FR
Plums in water	½ c (125 g)	51	1	14	0	1	1 FR
Prunes in heavy syrup	½ c (117 g)	123	1	33	0	2	2 FR
Raspberries in heavy syrup	½ c (128 g)	116	1	30	0	2	2 FR
Strawberries in heavy syrup	½ c (127 g)	117	1	30	0	2	2 FR
Tropical fruit salad in heavy syrup	½ c (129 g)	111	1	29	0	2	2 FR
DRIED FRUITS							
Apples	½ c (43 g)	105	0	28	0	2	2 FR
Apricots	½ c (66 g)	158	2	41	0	3	3 FR
Banana chips	½ c (113 g)	221	1	25	14	1½	1½ FR, 2 F
Coconut, unsweetened	½ oz (14 g)	94	1	3	9	0	2 F
Cranberries, sweetened	½ c (61 g)	187	0	50	1	3	3 FR
Currants	½ c (72 g)	204	3	53	0	3½	3½ FR
Dates	½ c chopped (89 g)	251	2	67	0	4½	4½ FR
Figs	½ c (75 g)	186	3	48	1	3	3 FR
Mango	½ c (51 g)	160	1	42	0	3	3 FR
Mixed fruit	½ c (80 g)	200	2	52	0	3½	3½ FR
Persimmons	1 (34 g)	93	1	25	0	1½	1½ FR
Pineapple	½ c (61 g)	197	2	50	0	3	3½ FR
Prunes, pitted	½ c (85 g)	204	2	54	0	3½	3½ FR
Raisins	½ c (83 g)	244	2	65	0	4	4 FR
JUICES							
Açai	8 oz (236 g)	122	1	24	3	1½	1½ FR
Apple, unsweetened	8 oz (248 g)	114	0	28	0	2	2 FR
Cranberry apple	8 oz (245 g)	155	0	39	0	2½	2½ FR
Cranberry grape	8 oz (245 g)	137	1	34	0	2	2 FR
Cranberry juice cocktail	8 oz (253 g)	136	0	34	0	2	2 FR
Cranberry, light	8 oz (236 g)	40	0	10	0	½	½ FR
Cranberry raspberry	8 oz (236 g)	130	0	32	0	2	2 FR
Grape	8 oz (253 g)	152	1	37	0	2½	2½ FR
Grapefruit	8 oz (247 g)	96	1	23	0	1½	1½ FR
Mixed berry	8 oz (240 g)	120	0	30	0	2	2 FR
Orange	8 oz (248 g)	112	2	26	1	2	2 FR
Pineapple, unsweetened	8 oz (250 g)	133	1	32	0	2	2 FR
Pomegranate	8 oz (251 g)	136	0	33	1	2	2 FR

INGREDIENT	SERVING	CALORIES	PRO G	CARB G	FAT G	CARB CHOICE	DIABETIC EXCHANGE
Prune	8 oz (256 g)	**182**	2	45	0	3	3 FR
Tomato	8 oz (243 g)	**41**	2	10	0	½	2 V
Vegetable juice cocktail	8 oz (242 g)	**46**	2	11	0	1	2 V
VEGETABLES, RAW							
Alfalfa sprouts	⅓ c (15 g)	**4**	1	0	0	0	Free
Arugula or baby arugula	½ c (20 g)	**5**	1	1	0	0	Free
Avocado	¼ avocado (33 g)	**56**	1	3	5	0	1 F
Bell pepper	¼ c chopped (38 g)	**12**	0	2	0	0	Free
Carrot	¼ c grated (28 g)	**11**	0	3	0	0	Free
Carrots, baby	8 (3 in, 80 g)	**28**	1	7	0	½	1 V
Celery stalks	2 medium (80 g)	**13**	1	2	0	0	Free
Cherry tomatoes	5 (85 g)	**15**	1	3	0	0	Free
Cucumber	1 medium (201 g)	**24**	1	4	0	0	1 V
Cucumber	½ c sliced (52 g)	**8**	0	2	0	0	Free
Endive or escarole	½ c chopped (25 g)	**4**	0	1	0	0	Free
Fennel	½ bulb (117 g)	**36**	1	9	0	½	1 V
Leeks	½ c (45 g)	**27**	1	6	0	½	1 V
Lettuce, iceberg, romaine, Boston, or Bibb	½ c (36 g)	**5**	0	1	0	0	Free
Mushrooms, enoki	15 medium (45 g)	**17**	1	4	0	0	Free
Mushrooms, portobello	1 oz (28 g)	**6**	1	1	0	0	Free
Mushrooms, white	½ c (48 g)	**11**	1	2	0	0	Free
Onion	½ c chopped (80 g)	**32**	1	7	0	½	1 V
Pepper, chile, green or red	1 (45 g)	**18**	1	4	0	0	Free
Radicchio	½ c (20 g)	**5**	0	1	0	0	Free
Radishes	6 medium (27 g)	**4**	0	1	0	0	Free
Scallions or spring (green) onions	1 medium (15 g)	**5**	0	1	0	0	Free
Shallots	1 T chopped (10 g)	**7**	0	2	0	0	Free
Spinach	½ c chopped (15 g)	**3**	0	1	0	0	Free
Spinach, baby	½ c (14 g)	**3**	0	1	0	0	Free
Tomatillos	½ c chopped (66 g)	**21**	1	4	1	0	1 V
Tomato	1 medium (3 in diameter, 123 g)	**22**	1	5	0	0	1 V
Tomato	½ c diced (90 g)	**16**	1	4	0	0	Free
Turnip	1 medium (122 g)	**34**	1	8	0	½	1 V

INGREDIENT	SERVING	CALORIES	PRO G	CARB G	FAT G	CARB CHOICE	DIABETIC EXCHANGE
Watercress	½ c (17 g)	2	0	0	0	0	Free
Zucchini	½ c (57 g)	10	1	2	0	0	Free
VEGETABLES, COOKED							
Artichoke, boiled	1 medium (120 g)	64	4	14	0	1	3 V
Artichoke hearts, boiled	½ c (84 g)	45	2	10	0	½	2 V
Asparagus, boiled	½ c chopped (90 g)	20	2	4	0	0	1 V
Beans, green, boiled	½ c (63 g)	22	1	5	0	0	1 V
Beans, snap, yellow, wax, or string, boiled	½ c (63 g)	22	1	5	0	0	1 V
Beets, boiled	½ c sliced (85 g)	38	1	9	0	½	2 V
Bok choy, boiled	½ c (85 g)	10	1	2	0	0	Free
Broccoli, boiled	½ c chopped (78 g)	27	2	6	0	½	1 V
Brussels sprouts, boiled	½ c (78 g)	28	2	6	0	½	1 V
Butternut squash, baked	½ c flesh (103 g)	41	1	11	0	1	2 V
Cabbage, boiled	½ c shredded (75 g)	17	1	4	0	0	Free
Carrot, boiled	½ c sliced (78 g)	27	1	6	0	½	1 V
Cauliflower, boiled	½ c chopped (62 g)	14	1	3	0	0	Free
Collard greens, boiled	½ c chopped (95 g)	25	2	5	0	0	1 V
Dandelion greens, boiled	½ c chopped (53 g)	18	1	3	0	0	Free
Eggplant, boiled	½ c cubed (50 g)	18	0	0	1	0	Free
Jicama, boiled	½ c flesh (53 g)	19	0	4	0	0	Free
Kohlrabi, boiled	½ c flesh (83 g)	24	1	6	0	½	1 V
Leek, boiled	½ c chopped (65 g)	18	1	4	0	0	Free
Mushrooms, boiled	½ c pieces (78 g)	22	2	4	0	0	1 V
Mustard greens, boiled	½ c chopped (70 g)	11	2	1	0	0	Free
Nopale (cactus leaves), cooked	½ c (75 g)	11	1	3	0	0	Free
Okra, boiled	½ c (80 g)	18	2	4	0	0	Free
Parsnip, boiled	½ c sliced (78 g)	55	1	13	0	1	2 V
Pumpkin, boiled	½ c mashed (123g)	25	1	6	0	½	1 V
Rutabaga, boiled	½ c cubed (120 g)	47	2	10	0	½	2 V
Sauerkraut, canned	½ c (118 g)	22	1	5	0	0	1 V
Snow peas	½ c (32 g)	34	3	6	0	½	1 V

INGREDIENT	SERVING	CALORIES	PRO G	CARB G	FAT G	CARB CHOICE	DIABETIC EXCHANGE
Spinach, boiled	½ c chopped (90 g)	21	3	3	0	0	1 V
Squash, all varieties, sliced, boiled	½ c sliced (90 g)	18	1	4	0	0	Free
Swiss chard, boiled	½ c chopped (88 g)	18	2	4	0	0	Free
Water chestnuts, canned, with liquid	½ c (70 g)	35	1	9	0	½	1 V
Zucchini, boiled	½ c (90 g)	14	1	2	0	0	Free

STARCHY VEGETABLES, BEANS, AND PEAS							
Beans, black, boiled	½ c (86 g)	114	8	20	0	1	1 S, 1 VLM
Beans, fava or broad, boiled	½ c (85 g)	94	6	17	0	1	1 S, 1 VLM
Beans, great Northern, boiled	½ c (89 g)	104	7	18	0	1	1 S, 1 VLM
Beans, kidney, boiled	½ c (89 g)	112	8	20	0	1	1 S, 1 VLM
Beans, lima, boiled	½ c (85 g)	105	6	20	0	1	1 S, 1 VLM
Beans, mung, boiled	½ c (101 g)	106	7	19	0	1	1 S, 1 VLM
Beans, navy, boiled	½ c (91 g)	127	7	24	1	1½	1 S, 1 LM
Beans, pinto, boiled	½ c (86 g)	122	8	22	1	1½	1 S, 1 LM
Beans, refried, canned	½ c (119 g)	108	6	18	1	1	1 S, 1 V
Black-eyed peas, boiled	½ c (86 g)	100	7	18	1	1	1 S, 1 VLM
Corn on the cob, yellow, sweet	1 medium ear (90 g)	77	3	17	1	1	1 S
Corn, kernels, sweet, boiled	½ c (82 g)	77	3	18	1	1	1 S
Edamame, boiled	½ c (90 g)	127	11	10	6	½	2 V, 1 LM
Chickpeas (garbanzo beans)	½ c (76 g)	105	5	17	2	1	1 S, 1 VLM
Lentils, boiled	½ c (99 g)	115	9	20	0	1	1 S, 1 VLM
Peas, boiled	½ c (80 g)	67	4	13	0	1	2 V
Plantains	½ c sliced (77 g)	89	1	24	0	1½	2 S
Potato, baked	1 medium (173 g)	161	4	37	0	2½	2 S
Potato, boiled (with skin)	½ c (78 g)	67	1	16	0	1	1 S
Potato, french fries	14 (70 g)	114	2	19	4	1	1 S, 1 F
Potato, mashed, with whole milk and butter	½ c (104 g)	118	2	17	4	1	1 S, 1 F
Soybeans, dry-roasted	½ c (86 g)	388	34	28	19	2	2 S, 4 MFM
Split peas, boiled	½ c (98 g)	116	8	21	0	1½	1 S, 1 VLM
Succotash (corn and lima beans), boiled	½ c (96 g)	110	5	23	1	1½	1 S, 1 V
Sweet potato, baked, peeled	1 medium (100 g)	90	2	21	0	1½	1 S
Taro root, cooked	½ c sliced (66 g)	94	1	23	0	1½	1 S
Yam, baked or boiled	½ c (68 g)	78	1	18	0	1	1 S

BREADS AND STARCHES (WHOLE GRAIN)							
Barley, pearled, cooked	½ c (79 g)	97	2	22	0	1½	1½ S

INGREDIENT	SERVING	CALORIES	PRO G	CARB G	FAT G	CARB CHOICE	DIABETIC EXCHANGE
Bread, pumpernickel	1 slice (32 g)	80	3	15	1	1	1 S
Bread, rye	1 slice (32 g)	83	3	15	1	1	1 S
Bread, whole wheat	1 slice (44 g)	120	4	22	3	1½	1½ S
Brown rice, long-grain cooked	½ c (98 g)	108	3	22	1	1½	1½ S
Buckwheat groats, roasted	½ c (84 g)	77	3	17	1	1	1 S
Bulgur (cracked wheat), cooked	½ c (91 g)	75	3	17	0	1	1 S
Chapati (Indian flatbread)	1 (40 g)	137	4	22	5	1½	1 S, 1 F
Cornmeal, yellow, whole grain	¼ c (31 g)	110	2	23	1	1½	1½ S
Crackers, whole wheat	7 (28 g)	120	3	20	4	1	1 S, 1 F
Hot dog bun, whole wheat	1 (43 g)	100	5	19	2	1	1 S
Kamut, cooked	½ c (86 g)	126	6	26	1	2	1½ S
Millet, cooked	½ c (120 g)	143	4	28	1	2	2 S
Oat bran	½ c (47g)	116	8	31	3	2	2 S
Oatmeal, cooked	½ c (117 g)	83	3	14	2	1	1 S
Spaghetti, whole wheat, cooked	1 c (140 g)	174	7	37	1	2½	2½ S
Popcorn, air-popped	2 c (16 g)	62	2	12	1	1	1 S
Quinoa, cooked	½ c (93 g)	111	4	20	2	1	1½ S
Sandwich bun, whole wheat	1 (53 g)	110	6	23	2	1½	1½ S
Sorghum	2 T (24 g)	81	3	18	1	1	1 S
Tortilla, corn	1 (24 g)	52	1	11	1	1	1 S
Tortilla, whole wheat	1 (47 g)	110	4	22	1	1½	1½ S
Triticale	¼ c (48 g)	161	6	35	1	2	2 S
Wheat germ	2 T (14 g)	52	3	7	1	½	½ S
Rolls, whole wheat	1 (28g)	76	2	15	1	1	1 S
BREADS AND STARCHES (REFINED GRAINS)							
Bagel, plain	1 (3.5 in diameter, 71 g)	182	7	36	1	2½	2½ S
Baguette	2 oz (57 g)	150	5	30	1	2	2 S
Bread, low carb	1 slice (42 g)	100	6	12	3	1	1 S, ½ F
Bread, sourdough	1 slice (2 g)	72	3	14	0	1	1 S
Bread, white	1 slice (25 g)	66	2	12	1	1	1 S
Bread, white, reduced-calorie	1 slice (23 g)	48	2	10	1	½	½ S
Cornbread, prepared with 2% milk	1 piece (65 g)	173	4	28	5	2	2 S, 1 F
Couscous	½ c (79 g)	88	3	18	0	1	1 S
Crackers, crispbread, rye	1 (10 g)	37	1	8	0	½	½ S
Crackers, matzo (plain)	1 (28 g)	112	3	24	0	1½	1½ S
Croissant, with butter	1 (57 g)	231	5	26	12	2	2 S, 2½ F
Croutons (plain)	¼ c (8 g)	31	1	6	1	½	½ S
Focaccia	2 oz (57 g)	180	5	28	5	2	2 S, 1 F
Hamburger bun	1 (43 g)	120	4	22	2	1½	1½ S

INGREDIENT	SERVING	CALORIES	PRO g	CARB g	FAT g	CARB CHOICE	DIABETIC EXCHANGE
Hot dog bun	1 (43 g)	**120**	4	22	2	1½	1½ S
Naan (Indian bread)	1 (85 g)	**234**	7	39	6	2½	2 S, 2 F
Noodles, egg, cooked	1 c (160 g)	**221**	7	40	3	2½	2½ S
Noodles, Japanese-style	1 c (78 g)	**210**	8	43	1	3	2 S, 1 LM
Noodles, rice, cooked	1 c (78 g)	**210**	8	43	1	3	2 S, 1 LM
Noodles, soba	1 c (190 g)	**188**	10	41	0	3	2 S, 1 VLM
Orzo	1 c (155 g)	**210**	7	42	1	3	2 S, 1 VLM
Polenta	¼ c (35 g)	**130**	3	27	1	2	2 S
Spaghetti, cooked	1 c (140 g)	**221**	8	43	1	3	3 S
Spaghetti, spinach, cooked	1 c (140 g)	**182**	6	37	1	2½	2½ S
Pita	1 (6½ in diameter, 60 g)	**165**	5	33	1	2	2 S
Ravioli, cheese, cooked	1 c (242 g)	**191**	6	33	4	2	2 S, 1 F
Rice, long-grain white, boiled	½ c (79 g)	**103**	2	22	0	1½	1½ S
Roll, hard, white	1 (57 g)	**167**	6	30	2	2	2 S
Roll, ciabatta	1 (43 g)	**100**	3	19	2	1	1S
Taco shells, hard	2 (26 g)	**124**	2	17	6	1	1 S, 1 F
Tortilla, flour	1 (30 g)	**90**	2	15	2	1	1 S
MILK AND MILK PRODUCTS (DAIRY AND NONDAIRY)							
Almond milk	8 oz (240 ml, 243 g)	**60**	1	8	3	½	½ S
Buttermilk, 1%	8 oz (240 ml, 245 g)	**98**	8	12	2	1	1 SM
Buttermilk, 2%	8 oz) (240 ml, 245 g)	**137**	10	13	5	1	1 LFM
Buttermilk, whole	8 oz (240 ml, 245 g)	**152**	8	12	8	1	1 WM
Chocolate milk, 1% fat	8 oz (240 ml, 250 g)	**158**	8	26	3	2	1 SM, 1 S
Chocolate milk, 2%	8 oz (240 ml, 250 g)	**190**	7	30	5	2	1 LFM, 1 S
Chocolate milk, whole	8 oz (240 ml, 250 g)	**208**	8	26	8	2	1 WM, ½ S
Condensed milk, sweetened	4 oz (120 ml, 153 g)	**491**	12	83	13	5½	1 WM, 3 S, 2 F
Cream, half-and-half, fat-free	2 oz (60 ml, 60 g)	**36**	2	5	1	0	½ SM
Cream, heavy whipping	2 oz (60 ml, 30 g)	**104**	1	1	11	0	2 F
Creamer, nondairy, liquid	2 oz (60 ml, 60 g)	**80**	0	8	4	½	½ S, 1 F
Creamer, nondairy, powder	1 oz (2 T, 30 ml, 12 g)	**60**	0	6	3	½	½ S, ½ F

INGREDIENT	SERVING	CALORIES	PRO G	CARB G	FAT G	CARB CHOICE	DIABETIC EXCHANGE
Evaporated milk, fat-free	8 oz (240 ml, 255 g)	**199**	19	28	1	2	2 SM
Evaporated milk, 2%	8 oz (240 ml, 240 g)	**200**	16	24	4	1½	1 LFM, 1 S
Evaporated milk, whole	8 oz (240 ml, 252 g)	**338**	17	25	19	1½	2 WM, 1 F
Half-and-half	2 oz (60 ml, 60 g)	**79**	2	3	7	0	2 F
Kefir	8 oz, (240 ml, 226 g)	**142**	8	10	8	½	1 WM
Milk, cow's, fat-free	8 oz (240 ml, 245 g)	**83**	8	12	0	1	1 SM
Milk, cow's, 1%	8 oz (240 ml, 244 g)	**102**	8	12	2	1	1 SM
Milk, cow's, 2%	8 oz (240 ml, 244 g)	**122**	8	12	5	1	1 LFM
Milk, cow's, whole	8 oz (240 ml, 244 g)	**149**	8	12	8	1	1 WM
Milk, goat, whole	8 oz (240 ml, 244 g)	**168**	9	11	10	1	1 WM
Rice milk	8 oz (240 ml, 245 g)	**120**	0	25	2	1½	1½ S
Soy milk, plain	8 oz (240 ml, 240 g)	**80**	8	7	3	½	1 SM
Soy milk, all flavors, low-fat	8 oz (240 ml, 243 g)	**104**	4	17	2	1	1 SM
Sour cream, fat-free	4 oz (120 ml, 128 g)	**95**	4	20	0	1	1 SM
Sour cream, light	4 oz (120 ml, 96 g)	**132**	3	7	10	½	½ SM, 1 F
Sour cream	4 oz (120 ml, 96 g)	**185**	2	3	19	0	4 F
YOGURT (DAIRY AND NONDAIRY)							
Frozen yogurt, soft, low-fat or fat-free, chocolate or vanilla	8 oz (240 ml, 190 g)	**220**	8	46	0–4	3	1 SM, 2 FR
Greek yogurt, fruit varieties, fat-free	8 oz (240 ml, 226 g)	**187**	19	27	0	2	2 SM
Greek yogurt, plain	8 oz (240 ml, 226 g)	**150**	22	11	5	1	1 LFM, 1 VLM
Greek yogurt, plain, fat-free	8 oz (240 ml, 226 g)	**133**	24	9	0	½	1 SM, 1 VLM
Frozen yogurt, hard, low-fat, vanilla	8 oz (240 ml, 187 g)	**260**	8	50	3	3	1 LFM, 2 FR
Soy yogurt, fruit varieties	8 oz (240 ml, 226 g)	**200**	10	30	4	2	1 LFM, 2 FR

INGREDIENT	SERVING	CALORIES	PRO G	CARB G	FAT G	CARB CHOICE	DIABETIC EXCHANGE
Yogurt, fruit varieties, fat-free	8 oz (240 ml, 245 g)	**233**	11	47	0	3	1 SM, 2 FR
Yogurt, fruit varieties, fat-free, low-calorie, sweetened	8 oz (240 ml, 241 g)	**123**	11	19	0	1	1 LFM
Yogurt, fruit varieties, low-fat	8 oz (240 ml, 245 g)	**243**	10	46	3	3	1 LFM, 2 FR
Yogurt, plain, fat-free	8 oz (240 ml, 245 g)	**144**	26	10	0	½	1 LFM
Yogurt, plain, low-fat	8 oz (240 ml, 245 g)	**154**	13	17	4	1	1 WM
Yogurt, plain, whole	8 oz (240 ml, 245 g)	**150**	9	11	8	1	1 WM
CHEESES							
Alpine Lace, Swiss, reduced-fat	1 oz (28 g)	**90**	8	1	6	0	1 HFM
American	1 oz (28 g)	**105**	5	1	9	0	1 HFM
Blue	1 oz (28 g)	**100**	6	1	8	0	1 HFM
Brie	1 oz (28 g)	**95**	6	0	8	0	1 HFM
Camembert	1 oz (28 g)	**85**	6	0	7	0	1 HFM
Cheddar	1 oz (28 g)	**114**	7	0	9	0	1 HFM
Cheddar or American, fat-free	1 oz (21 g)	**31**	5	3	0	0	1 VLM
Cheddar, 50% reduced-fat	1 oz (28 g)	**70**	8	1	5	0	1 MFM
Colby	1 oz (28 g)	**112**	7	1	9	0	1 HFM
Colby, low-fat	1 oz (28 g)	**49**	7	1	2	0	1 LM
Cottage, 1% fat	½ c (113 g)	**81**	14	3	1	0	2 VLM
Cottage, 2% fat	½ c (113 g)	**97**	13	4	3	0	2 LM
Cottage, 4% fat	½ c (105 g)	**103**	12	4	5	0	1 HFM
Cream cheese	1 oz (2 T, 28 g)	**99**	2	1	10	0	2 F
Cream cheese, fat-free	1 oz (2 T, 30 g)	**32**	5	2	0	0	1 F
Cream cheese, low-fat	1 oz (2 T, 30 g)	**69**	3	2	5	0	1½ F
Feta	1 oz (28 g)	**75**	4	1	6	0	1 MFM
Feta, reduced-fat	1 oz (28 g)	**58**	6	1	4	0	1 LM
Fontina	1 oz (28 g)	**110**	7	0	9	0	1 HFM
Goat, hard	1 oz (28 g)	**128**	9	1	10	0	1 MFM, 1 F
Goat, soft	1 oz (28 g)	**76**	5	0	6	0	1 MFM
Gouda	1 oz (28 g)	**101**	7	1	8	0	1 HFM
Gruyère	1 oz (28 g)	**117**	8	0	9	0	1 HFM
Mexican blend	1 oz (28 g)	**101**	7	0	8	0	1 HFM
Mexican blend, low-fat	1 oz (28 g)	**80**	7	1	6	0	1 MFM
Monterey Jack	1 oz (28 g)	**106**	7	0	9	0	1 HFM
Monterey Jack, low-fat	1 oz (28 g)	**88**	8	0	6	0	1 MFM
Muenster	1 oz (28 g)	**104**	7	0	8	0	1 HFM

INGREDIENT	SERVING	CALORIES	PRO G	CARB G	FAT G	CARB CHOICE	DIABETIC EXCHANGE
Muenster, low-fat	1 oz (28 g)	77	7	1	5	0	1 MFM
Mozzarella, whole-milk	1 oz (28 g)	85	6	1	6	0	1 MFM
Mozzarella, part-skim-milk	1 oz (28 g)	72	7	1	5	0	1 MFM
Paneer, 1% fat	1 oz (28 g)	90	8	12	2	1	1 SM
Parmesan	1 oz (28 g)	111	10	1	7	0	1 HFM
Parmesan or Romano, grated	1 T (5 g)	22	2	0	1	0	1 VLM
Provolone	1 oz (28 g)	100	7	1	8	0	1 HFM
Provolone, reduced-fat	1 oz (28 g)	77	7	1	5	0	1 MFM
Ricotta, part-skim-milk	¼ c (62 g)	85	7	3	5	0	1 MFM
Ricotta, whole-milk	¼ c (62 g)	107	7	2	8	0	1 HFM
Swiss	1 oz (28 g)	108	7	2	8	0	1 HFM
Swiss, low-fat	1 oz (28 g)	49	8	1	1	0	1 LM
FISH AND SEAFOOD							
Catfish, breaded and fried	4 oz (113 g)	260	21	9	15	½	1 S, 1 HFM, 2 F
Catfish, farmed, cooked	4 oz (113 g)	163	21	0	8	0	3 LM
Catfish, wild, cooked	4 oz (113 g)	119	21	0	3	0	3 VLM
Clams, cooked	4 oz (113 g)	168	29	6	2	½	3 LM
Cod, Atlantic, cooked	4 oz (113 g)	119	26	0	1	0	3 VLM
Crabmeat, lump	4 oz (113 g)	81	16	0	2	0	2 VLM
Crayfish or crawfish, assorted species, cooked	4 oz (113 g)	99	20	0	1	0	3 VLM
Flounder or sole, baked or broiled	4 oz (113 g)	132	27	0	2	0	4 VLM
Mahi mahi, cooked	4 oz (113 g)	124	27	0	1	0	4 VLM
Monkfish, cooked	4 oz (113 g)	110	21	0	2	0	3 VLM
Mussels, blue, cooked	4 oz (113 g)	195	27	8	5	½	4 VLM, 1 F
Pollock, Atlantic, cooked	4 oz (113 g)	134	28	0	1	0	4 VLM
Rockfish, Pacific, cooked	4 oz (113 g)	124	25	0	2	0	4 VLM
Salmon, Atlantic, farmed, cooked	4 oz (113 g)	234	25	0	14	0	3 MFM
Salmon, Atlantic, wild, cooked	4 oz (113 g)	206	29	0	9	0	4 LM
Salmon, Chinook or King, cooked	4 oz (113 g)	243	26	0	15	0	4 LM
Salmon, Coho, farmed, cooked	4 oz (113 g)	201	28	0	9	0	4 LM
Salmon, pink, canned, drained solids, without skin and bones	4 oz (113 g)	154	28	0	5	0	4 VLM
Scallops, bay or sea, cooked	4 oz (113 g)	126	23	6	1	½	3 VLM
Shrimp, cooked	4 oz (113 g)	135	26	2	2	0	4 VLM

INGREDIENT	SERVING	CALORIES	PRO G	CARB G	FAT G	CARB CHOICE	DIABETIC EXCHANGE
Snapper, assorted species, cooked	4 oz (113 g)	145	30	0	2	0	4 VLM
Squid (calamari), steamed or boiled	4 oz (113 g)	119	20	4	2	0	3 VLM
Swordfish, cooked	4 oz (113 g)	195	27	0	9	0	4 LM
Tilapia, cooked	4 oz (113 g)	145	30	0	3	0	4 VLM
Tilefish, cooked	4 oz (113 g)	167	28	0	5	0	3 LM
Tuna, white, canned in oil	4 oz (113 g)	211	30	0	9	0	4 LM
Tuna, white, canned in water	4 oz (113 g)	145	27	0	3	0	4 VLM
Tuna, light, canned in oil	4 oz (113 g)	225	33	0	9	0	4 LM
Tuna, light, canned in water	4 oz (113 g)	132	29	0	1	0	4 VLM
Tuna steak	4 oz (113 g)	212	21	2	12	0	3 MFM

RED MEATS							
Beef							
Bottom round, braised	4 oz (113 g)	261	37	0	11	0	5 LM
Chuck, blade roast, braised	4 oz (113 g)	347	30	0	24	0	4 MFM, 1 F
Chuck eye steak, grilled	4 oz (113 g)	314	28	0	22	0	4 MFM
Chuck for stew, braised	4 oz (113 g)	217	37	0	8	0	4 LM
Corned (brisket), cooked	4 oz (113 g)	285	21	1	22	0	3 HFM
Eye of round, roasted	4 oz (113 g)	191	33	0	5	0	5 VLM
Flank steak, broiled	4 oz (113 g)	260	35	0	12	0	5 LM
Ground, 95% lean /5% fat, baked	4 oz (113 g)	197	31	0	7	0	4 LM
Ground, 90% lean /10% fat, baked	4 oz (113 g)	243	30	0	13	0	4 LM
Ground, 85% lean /15% fat, baked	4 oz (113 g)	272	29	0	16	0	5 LM
Ground, 75% lean /25% fat, baked	4 oz (113 g)	288	28	0	19	0	4 MFM
Ground, 70% lean /30% fat, baked	4 oz (113 g)	273	27	0	17	0	4 MFM
Jerky	2 oz (57 g)	232	19	6	15	½	3 MFM
Sausage, cooked	4 oz (113 g)	376	21	0	32	0	3 HFM, 2 F
Short loin, T-bone, porterhouse steak, broiled	4 oz (113 g)	365	26	0	28	0	3 HFM, 1 F
Short ribs, braised	4 oz (113 g)	335	35	0	21	0	5 LM, 1 F
Skirt steak, grilled	4 oz (113 g)	278	33	0	16	0	5 LM
Strip loin or New York steak, broiled	4 oz boneless (113 g)	243	36	0	9	0	5 VLM, 1 F
Tenderloin, filet mignon, broiled	4 oz (113 g)	219	32	0	9	0	4 LM
Lamb							
Australian, chop, broiled	4 oz (113 g)	266	29	0	16	0	4 LM, 1 F
Australian, leg, shank, roasted	4 oz (113 g)	196	21	0	12	0	3 MFM
Australian, loin, broiled	4 oz (113 g)	186	22	0	10	0	3 LM
Australian, shoulder, braised	4 oz (113 g)	353	34	0	23	0	5 MFM

INGREDIENT	SERVING	CALORIES	PRO G	CARB G	FAT G	CARB CHOICE	DIABETIC EXCHANGE
Leg and shoulder, cubed, braised	4 oz (113 g)	253	38	0	10	0	5 LM
Pork							
Ham, cured, 11% fat, roasted	4 oz (113 g)	202	26	0	10	0	4 LM
Ham, extra lean, 5% fat	4 oz (113 g)	119	19	1	4	0	3 VLM
Hot dog, beef, cooked	1 (45 g)	141	5	2	13	0	1 HFM, 1 F
WHITE MEATS							
Chicken, boneless, skinless breast, roasted	4 oz (113 g)	187	35	0	4	0	5 VLM
Chicken, boneless, skin-on breast, roasted	4 oz (113 g)	223	34	0	9	0	5 VLM, 1 F
Chicken, ground, cooked	4 oz (113 g)	214	26	0	12	0	4 LM
Chicken, leg, roasted, meat and skin	4 oz (113 g)	209	27	0	10	0	4 LM
Chicken, leg, roasted, meat only,	4 oz (113 g)	197	27	0	9	0	4 VLM, 1 F
Chicken, boneless, skinless thigh, roasted	4 oz (113 g)	201	27	0	9	0	5 VLM, 1 F
Chicken, thigh, roasted	4 oz (113 g)	260	26	0	17	0	4 LM, 1 F
Duck, roasted, meat and skin	4 oz (113 g)	382	22	0	32	0	3 HFM, 2 F
Duck, roasted, meat only	4 oz (113 g)	228	27	0	13	0	4 LM
Pork, ground, 96% lean/4% fat, cooked	4 oz (113 g)	209	36	1	7	0	4 LM
Pork, ground, 84% lean/16% fat, pan-broiled	4 oz (113 g)	340	31	0	24	0	3 HFM, 1 VLM
Pork, ground, 72% lean/28% fat, pan-broiled	4 oz (113 g)	426	26	1	36	0	4 MFM, 3 F
Pork, bone-in country-style ribs, broiled	4 oz (113 g)	245	32	0	13	0	4 LM, 1 F
Pork, boneless country-style ribs, broiled	4 oz (113 g)	210	22	0	13	0	3 MFM
Pork, boneless sirloin chops, braised	4 oz (113 g)	194	32	0	6	0	4 VLM, 1 F
Pork shoulder, braised	4 oz (113 g)	266	28	0	16	0	4 LM, 1 F
Pork, Polish sausage, cooked	4 oz (113 g)	370	16	2	33	0	2 HFM, 4 F
SOY PRODUCTS							
Miso	2 T (34 g)	68	4	9	2	½	1 MFM
Tofu, firm	4 oz (113 g)	79	9	2	5	0	1 MFM
Tofu, soft	4 oz (113 g)	69	7	2	4	0	1 MFM
NUTS AND SEEDS							
Almonds, dry-roasted	¼ c (35 g)	205	7	7	18	½	3 F, 1 LM
Brazil nuts	¼ c (33 g)	218	5	4	22	0	4 F, 1 VLM
Cashew, dry-roasted	¼ c (34 g)	197	5	11	16	1	3 F, 1 S
Filberts (hazelnuts)	¼ c (34 g)	212	5	6	21	½	4 F, 1 VLM

INGREDIENT	SERVING	CALORIES	PRO G	CARB G	FAT G	CARB CHOICE	DIABETIC EXCHANGE
Flaxseeds, ground	¼ c (28 g)	150	5	8	12	½	3 F
Macadamia nuts, dry-roasted	¼ c (34 g)	241	3	4	25	0	4 F, 1 LM
Mixed nuts, dry-roasted	¼ c (34 g)	203	6	9	18	½	3 F, 1 LM
Peanuts, dry-roasted	¼ c (37 g)	214	9	8	18	½	3 F, ½ S, 1 VLM
Pecans, dry-roasted	¼ c (59 g)	201	3	4	21	0	3 F, 1 LM
Pine nuts	¼ c (34 g)	232	5	5	24	0	4 F, 1 LM
Pistachios, dry-roasted	¼ c (31g)	174	6	9	14	½	3 F, ½ S
Pumpkin seeds, dry-roasted	¼ c (57 g)	326	17	8	28	½	4 F, 2 MFM
Soy nuts	¼ c (28 g)	120	11	10	5	½	1 F, 1 S
Sunflower seeds, dry-roasted	¼ c (32 g)	186	6	8	16	½	3 F, ½ S
Walnut halves	¼ c (25 g)	164	4	3	16	0	4 F
NUT BUTTERS							
Almond	1 T (16 g)	98	3	3	9	0	2 F
Cashew	1 T (16 g)	94	3	4	8	0	2 F
Peanut, smooth or crunchy	1 T (16 g)	94	4	4	8	0	2 F
Sesame	1 T (15 g)	89	3	3	8	0	2 F
FATS, CONDIMENTS, AND MISCELLANEOUS COMPONENTS							
Agave syrup, lite	1 T (21 g)	60	0	16	0	1	1 FR
Anchovies, canned in oil, drained	4 (16 g)	34	5	0	2	0	1 VLM
Bonito flakes	1 T (1 g)	3	1	0	0	0	Free
Bread crumbs, plain	¼ c (27 g)	107	4	19	1	1	1½ S
Bread crumbs, panko	¼ c (14 g)	50	2	10	0	½	½ S
Butter, salted or unsalted	1 T (14 g)	102	0	0	12	0	2 F
Butter, whipped	1 T (9 g)	67	0	0	7	0	1 F
Capers, canned, drained	1 t (3 g)	1	0	0	0	0	Free
Chocolate chips, semisweet	1 oz (60 pieces; 28 g)	136	1	18	9	1	1 S, 1 F
Cocoa powder, unsweetened	1 T (5 g)	11	1	3	1	0	Free
Jelly or jam	1 T (21 g)	56	0	15	0	1	1 FR
Fish sauce	1 T (18 g)	6	1	1	0	0	Free
Hoisin sauce	1 T (16 g)	35	1	7	1	½	½ S
Honey	1 T (21 g)	64	0	17	0	1	1 F
Horseradish, prepared	1 T (15g)	7	0	2	0	0	Free
Hot sauce	1 t (5 g)	1	0	0	0	0	Free
Ketchup	1 T (15 g)	15	0	4	0	0	Free
Margarine, tub, fat-free	1 T (15 g)	6	0	1	0	0	Free
Margarine, tub, 20% fat	1 T (15 g)	26	0	0	3	0	1 F
Margarine, tub, 60% fat	1 T (14 g)	77	0	0	9	0	2 F
Margarine, hard or tub (80% fat)	1 T (14 g)	101	0	0	11	0	2 F
Mayonnaise, fat-free	1 T (16 g)	10	0	2	0	0	Free

INGREDIENT	SERVING	CALORIES	PRO g	CARB g	FAT g	CARB CHOICE	DIABETIC EXCHANGE
Mayonnaise, light	1 T (15 g)	49	0	1	5	0	1 F
Mayonnaise	1 T (13 g)	90	0	0	10	0	2 F
Molasses	1 T (20 g)	58	0	15	0	1	1 FR
Mustard, Dijon	1 T (15 g)	15	0	0	0	0	Free
Mustard, yellow	1 T (15 g)	10	1	1	1	0	Free
Nutella	1 T (19 g)	100	2	11	6	1	1 S
Oil, canola, corn, olive, peanut, sesame, or soybean	1 T (14 g)	120	0	0	14	0	3 F
Olives, black, canned	3 (13 g)	15	0	1	1	0	Free
Olives, green, canned	3 (14 g)	20	0	1	2	0	½ F
Olives, green, with pimientos	2 (15 g)	15	0	1	1	0	Free
Oyster sauce	1 T (16 g)	8	0	2	0	0	Free
Peppers, banana or peperoncini, jarred	3 (1 oz, 28 g)	10	0	2	0	0	Free
Peppers, jalapeño	1 (14 g)	4	0	1	0	0	Free
Peppers, jalapeño, sliced canned	21 slices (1 oz, 28 g)	5	1	1	0	0	Free
Pepper, red bell, canned	¼ c halves (30 g)	5	0	1	0	0	Free
Pickles, dill	1 medium (65 g)	8	0	2	0	0	Free
Pickle relish	1 T (15 g)	19	0	5	0	0	Free
Rice wine, seasoned	1 T (15 g)	40	0	10	0	½	½ S
Salad dressing, blue-cheese, low-calorie	1 T (15 g)	15	1	0	1	0	Free
Salad dressing, blue-cheese	1 T (15 g)	71	0	1	8	0	2 F
Salad dressing, Caesar, fat-free	1 T (17 g)	22	0	5	0	0	1 V
Salad dressing, Caesar, low-calorie	1 T (15 g)	17	0	3	1	0	Free
Salad dressing, Caesar	1 T (15 g)	80	0	0	9	0	2 F
Salad dressing, French, fat-free	1 T (15 g)	21	0	5	0	0	1 V
Salad dressing, French, low-fat	1 T (15 g)	36	0	5	2	0	½ S
Salad dressing, French	1 T (15 g)	73	0	2	7	0	2 F
Salad dressing, honey mustard, fat-free	1 T (15 g)	25	0	6	0	½	1 F
Salad dressing, honey mustard, reduced-calorie	1 T (15 g)	31	0	4	2	0	1 F
Salad dressing, honey mustard	1 T (15 g)	70	0	4	6	0	1½ F
Salad dressing, Italian, fat-free	1 T (14 g)	7	0	1	0	0	Free
Salad dressing, Italian, reduced-calorie	1 T (14 g)	28	0	1	3	0	1 F
Salad dressing, Italian	1 T (15 g)	43	0	2	4	0	1 F
Salad dressing, ranch, fat-free	1 T (14 g)	17	0	4	0	0	Free

INGREDIENT	SERVING	CALORIES	PRO g	CARB g	FAT g	CARB CHOICE	DIABETIC EXCHANGE
Salad dressing, ranch, reduced-calorie	1 T (15 g)	31	0	1	3	0	1 F
Salad dressing, ranch	1 T (14 g)	68	0	1	7	0	2 F
Salad dressing, Russian, low-calorie	1 T (16 g)	23	0	4	1	0	1 V
Salad dressing, Russian	1 T (15 g)	53	0	5	4	0	1 F
Salad dressing, Thousand Island, low-calorie	1 T (15 g)	29	0	4	2	0	½ S
Salad dressing, Thousand Island	1 T (16 g)	59	0	2	6	0	1 F
Salsa, jarred	1 T (16 g)	4	0	1	0	0	Free
Salt, table	1 t (6 g)	0	0	0	0	0	Free
Seaweed, wakame	¼ c (20 g)	9	1	2	0	0	Free
Seaweed, wakame, dried	¼ c (5 g)	13	1	2	0	0	Free
Soy sauce, lite	1 T (15 g)	10	1	1	0	0	
Soy sauce, regular	1 T (18 g)	10	1	1	0		Free
Sugar, brown	1 t (3 g)	11	0	3	0	0	Free
Sugar, brown	¼ c (36 g)	137	0	35	0	2	2 FR
Sugar, granulated	1 t (4 g)	16	0	4	0	0	Free
Sugar, granulated	¼ c (50 g)	195	0	50	0	3	3 FR
Syrup, maple	1 T (20 g)	51	0	13	0	1	1 FR
Syrup, pancake, lite	1 T (15 g)	25	0	7	0	½	½ FR
Tomatoes, sun-dried, in oil, drained	¼ c (28 g)	59	1	6	4	½	1 V, 1 F
Vinegar, balsamic	1 T (16 g)	14	0	3	0	0	Free
Vinegar, red, white, or cider	1 T (15 g)	3	0	0	0	0	Free
Vinegar, rice, seasoned	1 T (15 g)	18	0	4	0	0	Free
Worcestershire sauce	1 T (17 g)	13	0	3	0	0	Free
BREAKFAST FOODS							
Bacon, pork, cured	2 cooked slices (16 g)	87	6	0	7	0	1 LM, 1 F
Cereal, All-Bran	1 c (62 g)	160	8	46	2	3	2 S
Cereal, bran flakes	1 c (40 g)	128	4	32	1	2	1½ S
Cereal, Cheerios	1 c (30 g)	110	3	22	2	1½	1½ S
Cereal, Chex, corn	1 c (31 g)	120	2	26	1	2	1½ S
Cereal, Chex, wheat	1 c (62 g)	213	7	51	1	3½	2½ S
Cereal, corn flakes	1 c (28 g)	100	2	24	0	1½	1½ S
Cereal, Froot Loops	1 c (29 g)	110	1	25	1	1½	1½ S
Cereal, Frosted Flakes	1 c (40 g)	147	1	36	0	2½	2 S
Cereal, granola	1 c (122 g)	597	18	65	29	4	4 S, 6 F
Cereal, granola, low-fat	1 c (110 g)	426	9	90	6	6	5 S, 1 F
Cereal, Kashi GoLean	1 c (52 g)	140	13	30	1	2	2 S
Cereal, Kashi GoLean Crisp	1 c (68 g)	240	12	47	5	3	3 S

INGREDIENT	SERVING	CALORIES	PRO g	CARB g	FAT g	CARB CHOICE	DIABETIC EXCHANGE
Cereal, muesli, dried fruit and nut	1 c (85 g)	289	8	66	4	4½	3 S, 1 F
Cereal, Product 19	1 c (30 g)	100	2	25	0	1½	1 S
Cereal, Raisin Bran	1 c (59 g)	190	5	45	2	3	2½ S
Cereal, Rice Krispies	1 c (26 g)	104	2	23	0	1½	1½ S
Cereal, shredded wheat, large biscuit	2 (47 g)	159	5	37	1	2½	2 S
Cereal, shredded wheat, small biscuit	1 c (30 g)	105	4	24	1	1½	1½ S
Cereal, Special K	1 c (31 g)	120	6	23	1	1½	1½ S
Cream of Wheat, cooked with water	1 c (237 g)	130	5	25	1	1½	1½ S
Donut, glazed	1 (42 g)	180	3	25	8	1½	1½ S, 1½ F
Egg, fried	1 large (46 g)	90	6	0	7	0	1 HFM
Egg, hard-boiled	1 large (50 g)	78	6	1	5	0	1 MFM
Eggs, scrambled, with milk and butter	2 large (122 g)	182	12	2	13	0	2 HFM
French toast	2 slices (130 g)	298	10	33	14	2	2 S, 1 MFM, 1 F
Grits, white corn, cooked with water	1 c (242 g)	172	4	36	1	2½	2 S
Jam, Concord grape, sugar-free,	1 T (17 g)	10	0	5	0	0	Free
Jam or preserves	1 T (20 g)	56	0	14	0	1	1 FR
Jam, preserves or marmalade, all-flavors, low sugar	1 T (18 g)	26	0	7	0	½	½ FR
Muffin, blueberry	1 (3 in diameter by 2 in high; 57 g)	224	3	28	11	2	1½ S, 2 F
Muffin, corn	1 muffin (2½ in diameter by 2 in high; 57 g)	174	3	29	5	2	1½ S, 1 F
Muffin, oat bran	1 muffin (2½ in diameter by 2 in high; 57 g)	154	4	28	4	2	1½ S, 1 F
Oatmeal, instant, prepared with water	1 c (234 g)	166	6	28	4	2	2 S
Omelet, cheese	1 large egg (75 g)	140	9	2	10	0	1 HFM, 1 F
Omelet, vegetable with onions, peppers, tomatoes, mushrooms	1 large egg (145 g)	173	8	6	13	½	1 HFM, 1 F, 1 V
Pancake, plain	3 (4 in diameter; 114 g)	259	7	32	11	2	2 S, 2 F
Sausage links, pork breakfast	2 (43 g)	187	5	2	17	0	2 HFM
Sausage links, meatless breakfast	2 (45 g)	70	8	5	3	0	2 MFM
Syrup, maple	1 T (20 g)	51	0	13	0	1	1 FR
Syrup, pancake, lite	1 T (15g)	25	0	7	0	½	½ FR
Waffle, plain, frozen	1 (72 g)	197	5	30	6	2	2 S, 1 F

INGREDIENT	SERVING	CALORIES	PRO G	CARB G	FAT G	CARB CHOICE	DIABETIC EXCHANGE
CANDY, COOKIES, AND ICE CREAM							
Candy and Candy Bars							
Almond Joy	1.7 oz bar (50 g)	239	2	30	13	2	2 S, 2 F
Butterfinger	2 oz bar (60 g)	270	4	43	11	3	2 S, 2 F
Caramels	2 (20 g)	77	1	16	2	1	1 S
Charms Blow Pop Lollipop	1 (18 g)	60	0	16	0	1	1 S
Chocolate, dark	1 oz (28 g)	156	1	17	9	1	1 S, 2 F
Chocolate, milk	1.5 oz (44 g)	235	3	26	13	2	2 S, 2 F
Fruit Roll-Ups	1 (14 g)	50	0	12	1	1	½ S
Fudge, chocolate	2 pieces (34 g)	140	1	26	4	2	1 S, 1 F
Gummi Bears	22 (42 g)	150	3	34	0	2	2 S
Jelly beans	15 (43 g)	159	0	40	0	2½	2 S
Kit Kat	1.9 oz bar (55 g)	286	3	35	15	2	2 S, 3 F
M&Ms, milk chocolate	1.6 oz bag (48 g)	240	2	34	10	2	2 S, 2 F
Milky Way	2 oz bar (58 g)	260	2	41	10	2	2 S, 2 F
Peanut brittle	1.5 oz (43 g)	207	3	30	8	2	2 S, 1 F
Raisinets	¼ c (45 g)	190	2	32	8	2	2 S, 1 F
Reese's Peanut Butter Cups	1 (35 g)	190	0	17	11	1	1 S, 2 F
Skittles	10 (11 g)	43	0	10	0	½	½ S
Snickers	2 oz bar (59 g)	280	4	35	14	2	2 S, 3 F
Tootsie Roll, chocolate flavor	2 pieces (13 g)	51	0	12	0	1	½ S
Twizzlers licorice twists	4 (45 g)	150	1	34	1	2	2 S
Cookies							
Almond biscotti	1 (32 g)	110	3	20	3	1	1 S, 1 F
Chocolate Chip	2 (2 in diameter, 32 g)	156	2	19	9	1	1 S, 2 F
Fig Newtons	2 (31 g)	110	1	22	2	1½	1 S, 1 F
Oatmeal raisin	2 (3 in diameter, 30 g)	131	2	21	5	1½	1 S, 1 F
Peanut butter	2 (3 in diameter, 40 g)	190	4	24	10	1½	1 S, 2 F
Rice Krispies Treats	1 bar (22 g)	90	1	17	3	1	1 S
Ice Cream and Frozen Desserts							
Chocolate ice cream	½ c (66 g)	143	3	19	7	1	1 S, 1½ F
Frozen custard, vanilla	½ c (98 g)	216	4	21	13	1½	1½ S, 2 F
Milk shake, chocolate	1 c (166 g)	211	6	34	6	2	1 LFM, 1 S
Milk shake, vanilla or strawberry	1 c (166 g)	245	6	33	11	2	1 WM, 1 S
Sherbet, all flavors	½ c (97 g)	134	1	29	2	2	1½ S
Sorbet	½ c (113 g)	240	0	60	0	4	3 S
Vanilla ice cream	½ c (74 g)	160	4	19	8	1	1 S, 2 F

CHIPS, CRACKERS, AND PRETZELS

INGREDIENT	SERVING	CALORIES	PRO G	CARB G	FAT G	CARB CHOICE	DIABETIC EXCHANGE
Breadsticks, plain	2 (7 g)	25	1	5	0	0	½ S
Cheetos	1 oz (28 g)	160	2	15	10	1	1 S, 2 F
Chex Mix	1 oz (28 g)	120	3	21	3	1½	1 S, 1 F
Chips, corn, plain	1 oz (28 g)	147	2	18	8	1	1 S, 2 F
Chips, Doritos, nacho cheese	1 oz (28 g)	150	2	17	8	1	1 S, 2 F
Chips, potato	1 oz (28 g)	150	2	15	10	1	1 S, 2 F
Chips, tortilla	1 oz (28 g)	139	2	19	7	1	1 S, 1 F
Cheese puffs or Curls	1 oz (28 g)	170	1	13	13	1	1 S, 2 F
Crackers, crispbread, rye	1 (10 g)	37	1	8	0	½	½ S
Crackers, graham, plain	Four 2½ in squares (28 g)	118	2	22	3	1½	1 S, 1 F
Crackers, matzo, egg	1 (28 g)	111	3	22	1	1½	1 S, 1 F
Crackers, Melba toast	3 (15 g)	59	2	11	0	1	1 S
Crackers, saltine	5 (15 g)	63	1	11	1	1	1 S
Crackers, wheat	5 (15 g)	68	1	10	3	½	1 S
Funyuns	1 oz (28 g)	140	2	18	7	1	1 S, 1 F
Goldfish	55 (30 g)	140	4	20	5	1	1 S, 1 F
Pita chips	1 oz (28 g)	120	3	19	4	1	1 S, 1 F
Pretzels, soft	1 (62 g)	210	5	43	2	3	2½ S
Pretzels, hard, thin	1 oz (28 g)	110	3	23	0	1½	1 S, 1 F
Rice cakes, plain	1 (9 g)	35	1	7	0	½	½ S
Vegetable chips	1 oz (28 g)	150	1	16	9	1	1 S, 2 F

BEVERAGES

INGREDIENT	SERVING	CALORIES	PRO G	CARB G	FAT G	CARB CHOICE	DIABETIC EXCHANGE
Arizona Iced Tea, lemon flavor	8 oz (227 g)	89	0	22	0	1½	1 S
Boost nutritional drink, all flavors	8 oz (256 g)	240	10	41	4	3	1 WM, 1 S
Carnation Instant Breakfast drink mix, all flavors, made with skim milk, no sugar added	9 oz (255 g)	150	13	24	1	1½	1 SM, 1 S
Carnation Instant Breakfast drink mix, all flavors, made with skim milk	9 oz (270 g)	220	13	39	1	2½	2 SM, 1 S
Coconut juice	8 oz (240 g)	44	0	10	0	½	2 V
Coconut milk	8 oz (240 g)	552	5	13	57	1	1 S, 10 F
Crystal Light Lemonade, sugar-free	8 oz (229 g)	5	0	0	0	0	Free
Ensure drink, non-chocolate flavors	8 oz (252 g)	250	9	40	6	2½	1 WM, 1 S
Gatorade, fruit flavor	8 oz (244 g)	63	0	16	0	1	1 FR
Hawaiian Punch	8 oz (240 g)	120	0	30	0	2	2 FR
Hot cocoa mix	3 T (28 g)	112	1	21	4	1½	1 S, 1 F
Hot cocoa mix, no sugar added	1 envelope (15 g)	50	2	10	0	½	1 FR

INGREDIENT	SERVING	CALORIES	PRO g	CARB g	FAT g	CARB CHOICE	DIABETIC EXCHANGE
Kool Aid, lemonade/punch/fruit drink	8 oz (248 g)	108	0	28	0	2	2 FR
Limeade, frozen	8 oz (247 g)	128	0	34	0	2	2 FR
Monster energy drink	8 oz (240 g)	100	0	27	0	2	2 FR
Red Bull	8 oz (255 g)	115	1	28	0	2	2 FR
Slim Fast, original shake, French vanilla	11 oz (325 g)	220	10	40	3	2½	1 WM, 1 S
Smoothie, Jamba Juice, Caribbean Passion	12 oz (355 g)	210	2	49	1	3	1 S, 2 FR
Smoothie, Jamba Juice, Orange Dream Machine	12 oz (355 g)	245	5	54	1	3½	4 FR
Smoothie, Jamba Juice, Strawberry Whirl	12 oz (355 g)	155	1	38	0	2½	1 S, 1 FR
Snapple, kiwi strawberry	8 oz (240 g)	110	0	27	0	2	2 FR
Snapple, tea, diet, lemon	8 oz (240 g)	10	0	0	0	0	Free
Snapple, tea, peach, lemonade	8 oz (240 g)	90	0	23	0	1½	1½ FR
Soda, 7Up	12 oz (360 g)	150	0	39	0	2½	2 S
Soda, club	12 oz (355 g)	0	0	0	0	0	Free
Soda, cola	12 oz (368 g)	136	0	35	0	2	2 FR
Soda, diet, all varieties	12 oz (360 g)	1	0	0	0	0	Free
Soda, ginger ale	12 oz (366 g)	124	0	32	0	2	2 FR
Soda, grape	12 oz (372 g)	160	0	41	0	3	2 S
Soda, orange	12 oz (372 g)	179	0	46	0	3	3 FR
Soda, root beer	12 oz (370 g)	152	0	39	0	2½	2 S
Soda, Sprite	12 oz (360 g)	144	0	39	0	2½	2 FR
Tea, prepared, unsweetened	8 oz (237 g)	2	0	1	0	0	Free
Tonic water	8 oz (244 g)	83	0	21	0	1½	1 S
COFFEE AND COFFEE DRINKS							
Coffee, brewed	8 oz (237 g)	2	0	0	0	0	Free
Coffee, with skim milk (2 T)	9 oz (268 g)	10	1	2	0	0	Free
Coffee, with whole milk (2 T)	9 oz (268 g)	19	1	1	1	0	Free
Coffee, with half-and-half (2 T)	9 oz (267 g)	39	1	1	3	0	1 F
Coffee, with 1 heaping teaspoon sugar (single packet)	8 oz (237 g)	25	0	6	0	½	½ FR
Starbucks Frappuccino	9.5 oz (281 g)	200	6	37	3	2½	2 S, 1 F
Starbucks, whipped cream, sweetened	1 serving (22 g)	70	0	2	7	0	2 F
Starbucks, espresso macchiato, doppio	2 oz (59 g)	15	1	2	0	0	Free
Starbucks caffe latte, grande, 2% milk,	16 oz (473 g)	190	12	18	7	1	1 WM, ½ S
Starbucks caffe mocha, grande, 2% milk (no whip)	16 oz (473 g)	260	13	41	8	3	1 LFM, 2 S

INGREDIENT	SERVING	CALORIES	PRO G	CARB G	FAT G	CARB CHOICE	DIABETIC EXCHANGE
Starbucks cappuccino, grande, 2%	16 oz (473 g)	120	8	12	4	1	1 LFM
Starbucks caramel macchiato, grande, 2% milk	16 oz (473 g)	240	10	34	7	2	1 WM, 1 S
Starbucks flavored latte, grande, 2% milk	16 oz (473 g)	250	12	36	6	2½	1 WM, 1 S
Starbucks iced coffee with 2% milk, grande	16 oz (473 g)	120	3	24	2	1½	1½ S
Starbucks skinny flavored latte, grande, 2% milk	16 oz (473 g)	180	12	18	6	1	1 SM, 1 S
Starbucks white chocolate mocha, grande, 2% milk, no whip	16 oz (473 g)	400	15	61	11	4	2 WM, 2 FR
ALCOHOL AND MIXERS							
Alcohol, 80 proof (gin, rum, vodka, or whiskey)	1 oz (28 g)	64	0	0	0	0	1 F
Beer	12 oz (356 g)	153	2	13	0	1	1 S, 2 F
Beer, light	12 oz (354 g)	103	1	6	0	½	2 F
Beer, nonalcoholic	12 oz (360 g)	133	1	29	0	2	1½ S
Bourbon with soda	4 oz (116 g)	106	0	0	0	0	2 F
Brandy	4 oz (120 g)	292	0	0	0	0	6 F
Cordials, 54 proof	4 oz (120 g)	425	0	53	0	3½	3 FR, 5 F
Daiquiri	5 oz (150 g)	279	0	10	0	½	½ S, 5 F
Dry sherry	5 oz (150 g)	210	1	12	0	1	1 S, 3 F
Liqueur, coffee (26.5% alcohol by volume)	4 oz (141 g)	460	0	66	0	4½	4 FR, 5 F
Long Island iced tea	5 oz (150 g)	144	0	11	0	1	1 FR, 2 F
Margarita	5 oz (155 g)	338	0	21	0	1½	1 S, 6 F
Martini	5 oz (141 g)	343	0	3	0	0	8 F
Piña colada	5 oz (157 g)	273	1	35	3	2	2 S, 2 F
Sake (rice wine)	1 oz (29 g)	39	0	1	0	0	1 F
Wine, red	5 oz (147 g)	125	0	4	0	0	3 F
Wine, white	5 oz (147 g)	124	0	3	0	0	3 F
Wine	5 oz (150 g)	80	0	10	0	½	½ S, 1 F
Wine, sweet dessert	5 oz (147 g)	235	0	20	0	1	1 S, 3 F

INGREDIENT	SERVING	CALORIES	PRO G	CARB G	FAT G	CARB CHOICE	DIABETIC EXCHANGE
PIZZA							
Domino's Pizza							
America's Favorite Feast, Thin Crust, 12 in	1 slice (104 g)	**261**	11	26	13	2	2 S, 1 HFM
America's Favorite Feast, Thin Crust, 14 in	1 slice (75 g)	**194**	7	19	10	1	1 S, 1 HFM
America's Favorite Feast, Ultimate Deep Dish, 14 in	1 slice (190 g)	**442**	17	44	22	1½	3 S, 2 HFM
Bacon Cheeseburger Feast, Hand Tossed, 14 in	1 slice (144 g)	**362**	17	34	18	2	2 S, 2 HFM
Barbecue Feast, Hand Tossed, 14 in	1 slice (137 g)	**342**	14	41	14	3	3 S, 1 HFM
Beef, Thin Crust, 14 in	1 slice (93 g)	**247**	10	19	15	1	1 S, 1 HFM, 1 F
Cheese, Thin Crust, 14 in	1 slice (75 g)	**180**	7	19	10	½	1 S, 1 HFM
Cheese, Ultimate Deep Dish, 14 in	1 slice (137 g)	**330**	12	40	14	2½	2 S, 2 MFM
Ham and Pineapple, Thin Crust, 14 in	1 slice (98 g)	**215**	9	21	11	1½	1½ S, 1 HFM
Pepperoni, Thin Crust, 14 in	1 slice (86 g)	**243**	9	19	15	1	1 S, 1 HFM, 1 F
Pepperoni and Sausage, Thin Crust, 14 in	1 slice (98 g)	**286**	11	20	18	1	1 S, 1 HFM, 2 F
Sausage, Thin Crust, 14 in	1 slice (93 g)	**255**	9	21	15	1½	1½ S, 1 HFM, 1 F
Veggie Feast, Ultimate Deep Dish, 14 in	1 slice (162 g)	**359**	13	43	15	3	3 S, 1 HFM
Papa John's							
Barbeque Chicken and Bacon, Original Crust, 14 in	1 slice (150 g)	**350**	15	44	12	3	3 S, 1 HFM
Cheese, Original Crust, 14 in	1 slice (125 g)	**290**	11	37	10	2½	2½ S, 1 HFM
Cheese, Thin Crust, 14 in	1 slice (89 g)	**220**	9	20	12	1	1½ S, 1 HFM
Pepperoni, Original Crust, 14 in	1 slice (130 g)	**330**	13	37	14	2½	3 S, 1 HFM
The Works, Original Crust, 14 in	1 slice (157 g)	**330**	13	39	14	2½	3 S, 1 HFM
Pizza Hut							
Cheese, Hand Tossed, Large, 14 in	1 slice (123 g)	**320**	15	38	12	2½	2 S, 2 MFM
Cheese Garlic Parmesan, Hand Tossed Style, Large, 14 in	1 slice (124 g)	**320**	15	39	12	2½	2 S, 2 MFM
Chicken, Mushrooms, and Jalapeño, Fit 'N Delicious, 12 in	1 slice (93 g)	**170**	11	22	5	1½	1 S, 1 MFM
Green Pepper, Red Onion, and Diced Red Tomato, Fit 'N Delicious, 12 in	1 slice (89 g)	**150**	6	24	4	1½	1 S, 1 MFM
Meat Lover's, Pan, large, 14 in	1 slice (160 g)	**480**	20	37	28	2½	2 S, 3 HFM

INGREDIENT	SERVING	CALORIES	PRO g	CARB g	FAT g	CARB CHOICE	DIABETIC EXCHANGE
Pepperoni and Mushroom, Pan, large, 14 in	1 slice (136 g)	350	14	37	17	2½	2 S, 2 HFM
Spicy Sicilian, Pan, large, 14 in	1 slice (148 g)	400	16	38	21	2½	2½ S, 2 HFM
Veggie Lover's, Pan, large, 14 in	1 slice (148 g)	330	13	38	15	2½	2 S, 2 MFM
RESTAURANT CHAINS							
Boston Market							
Apples, Hot Cinnamon, sweetened	¾ c (145 g)	210	0	47	3	3	3 F, 1 F
Brownie, Chocolate Chip, Fudge	3 oz (85 g)	320	5	49	13	3	3 S, 2 F
Coleslaw, Garden Fresh	¾ c (189 g)	300	2	27	20	2	5 V, 4 F
Macaroni and Cheese	¾ c (221 g)	200	11	35	11	2	2 S, 1 VLM, 2 F
Meat Loaf	7.6 oz (218 g)	520	29	21	36	1½	1 S, 1 V, 4 HFM
New Potatoes, Garlic Dill	¾ c (156 g)	140	3	24	3	1½	2 S
Pie, Apple	1 slice (6 oz, 163 g)	580	43	74	30	5	2 FR, 4 LFM
Potpie, Chicken, Pastry Top	1 (425 g)	800	32	59	48	4	4 S, 5 HFM
Potatoes, Mashed, Home-Style	¾ c (221 g)	270	5	36	11	2½	2 S, 2 F
Salad, Market, Chopped	14 oz (397 g)	480	9	24	40	1½	1½ S, 1 HFM, 6 F
Sandwich, Boston Meat Loaf Carver	1 (448 g)	980	47	92	46	6	6 S, 6 MFM, 1F
Sandwich, Boston Turkey Carver	12 oz (344 g)	700	50	65	26	4	4 S, 7 LM
Soup, Chicken Noodle	¾ c (414 g)	250	22	23	8	1½	1 S, 3 LM
Stuffing, Fresh Vegetable	1 c (136 g)	190	3	25	8	1½	2 S, 1 F
Sweet Potato, Casserole	¾ c (198 g)	460	4	77	16	5	5 S, 1 F
Turkey Breast, Roasted	4 oz (113 g)	150	31	0	3	0	4 VLM
Vegetables, Steamed Fresh	1 c (136 g)	60	2	8	2	½	2 V
Burger King							
Biscuit with Sausage, Egg, and Cheese	1 (191 g)	550	20	34	37	2	2 S, 3 HFM, 2 F
BK Big Fish Sandwich with Tartar Sauce	1 (640 g)	640	23	67	31	4½	4 S, 3 HFM
BK Burger Double Stacker	1 (173 g)	570	31	29	37	2	2 S, 4 HFM
BK Burger Quad Stacker	1 (283 g)	930	58	31	65	2	2 S, 7 HFM, 2 F
BK Chicken Fries	6 (85 g)	250	14	16	15	1	1 S, 2 MFM
BK Veggie Burger with mayonnaise and without cheese	1 (209 g)	400	22	43	16	3	3 S, 3 LM
Cheeseburger	1 (121 g)	310	16	28	15	2	2 S, 2 MFM
Cheeseburger, Bacon	1 (126 g)	330	18	28	17	2	2 S, 2 MFM
Cheeseburger, Double	1 (171 g)	460	27	28	27	2	2 S, 4 MFM
Cheeseburger, Double, Bacon	1 (181 g)	510	31	29	30	2	2 S, 4 MFM, 1 F
Chicken Tenders	4 (62 g)	179	11	11	10	1	1 S, 1 HFM
Cinnamon Rolls, Cini Minis	4 (108 g)	400	7	52	18	3½	3 S, 1 HFM, 1 F

INGREDIENT	SERVING	CALORIES	PRO g	CARB g	FAT g	CARB CHOICE	DIABETIC EXCHANGE
Croissan'wich with Bacon, Egg, and Cheese	1 (122 g)	340	14	26	19	2	2 S, 2 HFM
Croissan'wich with Ham, Egg, and Cheese	1(149 g)	330	18	27	17	2	2 S, 2 MFM
Croissan'wich with Sausage and Cheese	1 (106 g)	380	14	26	24	2	2 S, 2 HFM
Double Croissan'wich with Bacon, Egg, and Cheese	1 (142 g)	420	20	27	25	2	2 S, 3 MFM, 1 F
Double Croissan'wich with Ham, Egg, and Cheese	1 (196 g)	410	26	28	22	2	2 S, 3 MFM, 1 F
Double Croissan'wich with Sausage, Egg, Cheese	1 (215 g)	680	29	29	49	2	2 S, 4 HFM, 3 F
French fries, medium	1 (148 g)	440	5	56	22	4	4 S, 3 F
Hamburger	1 (110 g)	260	14	27	11	2	2 S, 2 LM
Hamburger, double	1 (147 g)	370	23	27	19	2	2 S, 3 MFM
Milk shake, chocolate	12 oz (340 g)	340	7	60	9	4	4 S, 1 F
Milk shake, vanilla	12 oz (340 g)	290	7	46	9	3	3 S, 1 F
Onion Rings, medium	1 (117 g)	400	6	47	21	3	3 S, 4 F
Pie, Dutch apple	1 (107 g)	320	2	46	14	3	3 S, 2 F
Potatoes, hash brown, large	1 (128 g)	390	3	38	25	2½	2 S, 5 S
Sandwich, Chicken, Original, with mayonnaise	1 (218 g)	630	24	46	39	3	3 S, 3 HFM, 2 F
Sandwich, Sourdough Breakfast, with Ham, Egg, and Cheese	1 (179 g)	420	21	40	19	2½	3 S, 3 LM
Sandwich, Tendercrisp Chicken with mayonnaise	1 (284 g)	800	32	68	46	4½	4 S, 4 HFM, 2 F
Sandwich, Tendergrill Chicken, without mayonnaise	1 (259 g)	410	38	49	7	3	3 S, 3 LM
Salad, Garden Tendercrisp Chicken, plain	1 (284 g)	410	27	27	23	2	2 S, 3 MFM, 1 F
Salad, Garden Tendergrill Chicken, plain	1 (286 g)	230	34	9	8	½	2 V, 3 LM
Whopper Jr, with cheese and mayonnaise	1 (159 g)	390	16	29	23	2	2 S, 2 HFM, 1 F
Chipotle							
Barbacoa Shredded Beef	4 oz (113 g)	170	24	2	7	0	3 LM
Beans, black or pinto	4 oz (113 g)	120	7	23	1	1½	1½ S
Burrito, Carnitas, chicken, or steak, on a flour tortilla with white rice, black beans, fresh tomato salsa, cheese, and sour cream	1	1010	55	105	41	7	7 S, 6 MFM
Burrito, Barbacoa, on a flour tortilla with brown rice, pinto beans, fajita vegetables, tomatillo-red chili salsa, and romaine lettuce	1	805	44	112	23	7½	7 S, 3 MFM, 1 F

INGREDIENT	SERVING	CALORIES	PRO g	CARB g	FAT g	CARB CHOICE	DIABETIC EXCHANGE
Burrito Bowl, with chicken, white rice, black beans, roasted chili-corn salsa, cheese, and romaine lettuce	1	665	53	71	23	5	5 S, 5 LM
Carnitas (pork)	4 oz (113 g)	190	27	1	8	0	4 LM
Cheese, shredded jack and white cheddar	1 oz (28 g)	100	8	0	9	0	1 HFM
Chicken	4 oz (113 g)	190	32	1	7	0	4 LM
Chips, tortilla	4 oz (113 g)	570	8	73	27	5	5 S, 1 HFM, 2 F
Cilantro-Lime Rice	3 oz (85 g)	130	2	23	3	1½	1½ S
Fajita Vegetables	2.5 oz (71 g)	20	1	4	1	0	1 V
Guacamole	3.5 oz (113 g)	170	2	8	15	½	1 V, 3 F
Steak	4 oz (113 g)	190	30	2	7	0	5 VLM
Tacos, Barbacoa, on 3 soft corn tortillas with brown rice, pinto beans, tomatillo-green chili salsa, and guacamole	3	825	40	108	28	7	7 S, 4 LM, 1 F
KFC							
Beans, barbecue baked	5.5 oz (130 g)	200	8	39	2	2½	2 S, 1 VLM
Biscuit	1 (57 g)	220	4	24	11	1½	1½ S, 2 F
Chicken Breast, Extra-Crispy	1 (176 g)	510	39	16	33	1	1 S, 5 MFM, 1 F
Chicken Breast, Original Recipe	1 (161 g)	340	38	9	17	½	½ S, 4 MFM
Chicken Drumstick, Extra-Crispy	1 (60 g)	150	12	4	10	0	2 MFM
Chicken Drumstick, Original Recipe	1 (59 g)	140	13	3	8	0	2 MFM
Chicken Filet, Grilled	1 (102 g)	140	26	1	3	0	4 VLM
Chicken Filet, Original Recipe	1 (200 g)	200	22	8	9	½	½ S, 2 MFM
Chicken Sandwich, Double Down, Grilled Filet	1 (253)	480	60	4	25	0	8 LM, 1 V
Chicken Sandwich, Double Down, Original Recipe	1 (248 g)	610	52	18	37	1	1 S, 7 MFM
Chicken Sandwich, Doublicious, Grilled Filet	1 (197 g)	380	35	35	11	2	2 S, 4 LM
Chicken Sandwich, Doublicious, Original Recipe	1 (188 g)	520	32	40	25	2½	2 S, 4 MFM, 1 F
Chicken Sandwich, Honey BBQ	1 (162 g)	310	23	42	4	3	2 S, 3 LM
Chicken Thigh, Extra-Crispy	1 (114 g)	290	17	16	18	1	1 S, 2 HFM
Chicken Thigh, Original Recipe	1 (126 g)	350	19	7	27	½	½ S, 3 HFM
Chicken Wing, Extra-Crispy	1 (52 g)	150	11	11	7	1	1 S, 1 MFM
Chicken Wing, Original Recipe	1 (47 g)	140	10	4	9	0	1 HFM, 1 F
Coleslaw	5 oz (130 g)	180	1	22	10	1½	4 V, 2 F
Corn bread muffin	1 (52 g)	210	3	28	9	2	2 S, 1 F
Green beans	1 (86 g)	20	1	3	0	0	1 V

INGREDIENT	SERVING	CALORIES	PRO g	CARB g	FAT g	CARB CHOICE	DIABETIC EXCHANGE
Hot Wings	1 (22 g)	70	4	4	4	0	1 V, 1 F
Macaroni and cheese	1 (135 g)	160	5	19	7	1	1 S, 1 MFM
Mashed potatoes with gravy	4.8 oz (145 g)	120	2	19	4	1	1 S, 1 F
Popcorn chicken, small or Individual	3.5 oz (114 g)	370	19	21	24	1½	1½ S, 2 HFM, 1 F
Potpie, chicken	1 (369 g)	690	27	57	40	4	4 S, 4 MFM, 2 F
Potato salad	5.6 oz (128 g)	200	2	24	10	1½	1½ S, 2 F
McDonald's							
Big Breakfast	1 (9.5 oz, 269 g)	767	27	47	52	3	3 S, 4 HFM, 3 F
Big Mac hamburger	1 (7.5 oz, 214 g)	540	25	45	29	3	3 S, 3 HFM
Big N' Tasty hamburger	1 (7.2 oz, 206 g)	460	24	37	24	2½	2 S, 3 HFM
Big N' Tasty hamburger, with cheese	1 (7.2 oz, 220 g)	510	27	38	29	2½	2 S, 4 MFM, 1 F
Biscuit, with Bacon, Egg, and Cheese	1 (4.9 oz, 140 g)	420	15	37	23	2½	2 S, 2 HFM, 1 F
Breakfast Burrito, Sausage	1 (3.9 oz, 111 g)	300	12	26	16	2	2 S, 1 HFM, 1 F
Cheeseburger	1 (4 oz, 114 g)	300	15	33	12	2	2 S, 1 HFM, 1 F
Chicken McGrill Sandwich, without mayonnaise	1 (199 g)	299	28	36	5	2½	2 S, 2 MFM
Chicken McNuggets	6 (3.4 oz, 95 g)	280	14	16	17	1	1 S, 2 HFM
Chicken Selects Premium Breast Strips	5 (7.7 oz, 219 g)	660	38	39	40	2½	2 S, 5 HFM
Double Cheeseburger	1 (5.8 oz, 165 g)	440	25	34	23	2	2 S, 3 HFM
Double Quarter Pounder hamburger, with cheese	1 (9.8 oz, 279 g)	740	48	40	42	2½	2 S, 7 MFM, 1 F
Egg McMuffin	1 (7.1 oz, 137 g)	300	18	30	12	2	2 S, 2 MFM
Filet-O-Fish sandwich	1 (5 oz, 142 g)	380	15	38	18	2½	2 S, 2 HFM
French fries, large	1 serving (5.4 oz, 154 g)	500	6	63	25	4	4 S, 4 F
French fries, medium	1 serving (4.1 oz, 117 g)	380	4	48	19	3	3 S, 3 F
French fries, small	1 serving (2.5 oz, 71 g)	230	3	29	11	2	2 S, 2 F
McChicken Sandwich	1 (5 oz, 143 g)	360	14	40	16	2½	2 S, 2 HFM
Premium Salad, bacon ranch with grilled chicken, no dressing	1 (11.3 oz, 321 g)	260	33	12	9	1	4 VLM, 1 S, 1 F
Quarter Pounder hamburger	1 (6 oz, 169 g)	410	24	37	19	2½	2 S, 3 LM, 2 F
Quarter Pounder hamburger, with cheese	1 (7 oz, 198 g)	510	29	40	26	2½	3 S, 3 MFM, 1 F
Panera							
Artisan Pastry, cheese	1 (106 g)	400	8	41	23	3	3 S, 1 HFM, 1 F
Artisan Pastry, fresh apple	1 (128 g)	380	7	44	19	3	3 S, 1 HFM, 1 F
Bagel, Asiago cheese	1 (4 oz, 113 g)	330	13	55	6	3½	3½ S, 1 MFM

INGREDIENT	SERVING	CALORIES	PRO G	CARB G	FAT G	CARB CHOICE	DIABETIC EXCHANGE
Bagel, blueberry	1 (4.25 oz, 120 g)	330	10	67	2	4½	4 S
Bagel, chocolate chip	1 (4.25 oz, 120 g)	370	10	69	6	4½	4 S, 1 F
Bagel, cinnamon crunch	1 (4.5 oz, 128 g)	430	9	81	8	5½	5 S, 1 F
Bagel, cranberry walnut	1 (4 oz, 113 g)	330	10	63	5	4	4 S
Bagel, Dutch apple and raisin	1 (4.75 oz, 135 g)	360	8	77	3	5	4½ S
Bagel, everything	1 (4 oz, 113 g)	300	10	59	3	4	4 S
Bagel, plain	1 (3.75 oz, 106 g)	290	10	59	2	4	3½ S
Bagel, whole-grain	1 (4.5 oz, 128 g)	370	13	70	4	4½	4 S, 1 LM
Baguette, French	1 (2 oz, 57 g)	150	5	30	1	2	2 S
Baguette, whole-grain	1 (2 oz, 57 g)	150	6	30	2	2	2 S
Blondie, macadamia nut	1 (99 g)	460	4	62	21	4	4 S, 3 F
Brownie, chocolate fudge	1 (99 g)	410	5	64	14	4	4 S, 2 F
Cake, Cinnamon Coffee	1 (120 g)	470	6	54	25	3½	3½ S, 4 F
Chowder, New England Clam	8 oz (227 g)	300	5	19	23	1	1 S, 5 F
Ciabatta bread	1 (6.25 oz, 177 g)	460	16	84	6	5½	5 S, 1 LM
Cookie, Chocolate Chipper	1 (92 g)	440	5	59	23	4	4 S, 3 F
Cookie, oatmeal raisin	1 (92 g)	370	5	57	14	4	4 S, 1 F
Cookie, shortbread	1 (71 g)	350	3	36	21	2½	2 S, 2 F
Focaccia bread	1 (2 oz, 57 g)	180	5	28	5	2	2 S
Irish soda bread	1 (2 oz, 57 g)	180	5	23	7	1½	1½ S, 1 F
Muffin, carrot walnut	1 (142 g)	440	7	62	19	4	4 S, 3 F
Muffin, wild bueberry	1 (128 g)	390	5	58	15	4	4 S, 2 F
Panini, Chicken, Bacon Dijon on Country bread	1 (347 g)	850	57	78	35	5	5 S, 3 HFM, 1 F
Panini, Frontega Chicken	1 (369 g)	860	46	80	39	5	5 S, 3 HFM, 1 F
Panini, Smokehouse Turkey on Three Cheese bread	1 (312 g)	720	51	66	29	4½	4 S, 5 MFM
Panini, Tomato and Mozzarella on Ciabatta bread	1 (340 g)	770	30	96	29	6½	6 S, 3 HFM
Panini, Turkey Artichoke on Focaccia bread	1 (397 g)	750	40	88	27	6	6 S, 4 LM, 1 F
Parfait, strawberry granola	1 (234 g)	280	9	41	12	3	2 WM
Salad, Asian Sesame Chicken	1 (11.25 oz, 319 g)	410	30	30	20	2	1 S, 3 V, 2 HFM, 1 F
Salad, BBQ Chopped Chicken	1 (411 g)	500	31	47	22	3	2 S, 3 V, 2 HFM, 1 F

INGREDIENT	SERVING	CALORIES	PRO G	CARB G	FAT G	CARB CHOICE	DIABETIC EXCHANGE
Salad, Caesar	1 (276 g)	390	12	25	27	1½	1 S, 2 V, 1 HFM, 4 F
Salad, Fuji Apple	1 (291 g)	400	7	32	29	2	1 FR, 3 V, 6 F
Salad, Greek	1 (383 g)	380	8	14	34	1	3 V, 1 HFM, 5 F
Salad dressing, Asian Sesame, reduced-sugar	1 (43 g)	90	0	6	8	½	½ S, 1 F
Salad dressing, BBQ Ranch	1 (43 g)	140	1	8	12	½	½ S, 2 F
Salad dressing, Caesar	1 (43 g)	150	1	2	16	0	3 F
Salad dressing, White Balsamic Apple	1 (43 g)	150	0	11	12	1	½ S, 2 F
Salad dressing, Greek and Herb	1 (43 g)	220	0	1	24	0	5 F
Sandwich, Asiago Cheese Bagel with Egg and Cheese	1 (184 g)	480	23	55	18	3½	3½ S, 2 HFM
Sandwich, Asiago Roast Beef on Asiago Cheese bread	1 (368 g)	690	48	64	27	4	4 S, 5 MFM
Sandwich, Bacon Turkey Bravo on Tomato Basil bread	1 (404 g)	840	51	87	32	6	6 S, 5 MFM
Sandwich, Chicken Caesar on Three-Cheese bread	1 (376 g)	710	43	66	32	4½	4 S, 5 MFM
Sandwich, Italian Combo on Ciabatta bread	1 (503 g)	1040	61	94	45	6	6 S, 6 MFM, 2 F
Sandwich, Napa Almond Chicken Salad on Sesame Semolina bread	1 (347 g)	680	29	87	26	6	6 S, 2 HFM
Sandwich, Sierra Turkey on Focaccia with Asiago Cheese	1 (383 g)	970	39	80	54	5	5 S, 5 HFM, 1 F
Sandwich, Smoked Ham and Swiss on Stone-Milled Rye bread	1 (390 g)	700	46	65	28	4	4 S, 5 MFM
Sandwich, Tuna Salad on Honey Wheat bread	1 (333 g)	750	20	64	47	4	4 S, 3 HFM, 3 F
Scone, orange	1 (149 g)	470	4	97	11	6½	6 S
Smoothie, mango, low-fat	16 oz (454 g)	230	6	51	2	3½	4 F
Soup, Broccoli Cheddar	8 oz (227 g)	190	8	16	10	1	1 S, 1 HFM
Soup, Chicken Noodle, low-fat	8 oz (227 g)	80	6	7	3	½	½ S, 1 VLM
Soup, French Onion with cheese and croutons	9.25 oz (262 g)	200	8	19	10	1	1 S, 1 V, 1 HFM
Olive Garden							
Capellini Pomodoro dinner	1 (602 g)	840	31	141	17	9½	9 S, 1 HFM
Linguine alla Marinara dinner	1 (482 g)	430	18	76	6	5	5 S, 1 VLM
Shrimp Primavera dinner	1 (747 g)	730	46	110	12	7	7 S, 2 MFM
Subway							
Salad, Veggie Delite, no dressing and croutons	1 (300 g)	50	3	10	1	½	2 V
Sandwich, Black Forest Ham, on wheat bread	6 in (226 g)	290	18	47	5	3	3 S, 2 VLM

INGREDIENT	SERVING	CALORIES	PRO G	CARB G	FAT G	CARB CHOICE	DIABETIC EXCHANGE
Sandwich, Breakfast, Western Egg with cheese	6 in (229 g)	450	27	48	19	3	3 S, 3 MFM
Sandwich, Chipotle Southwest Cheese Steak, on Italian bread	6 in (271 g)	450	24	48	20	3	3 S, 3 MFM
Sandwich, Club, on wheat bread	6 in (257 g)	320	26	47	5	3	3 S, 2 VLM
Sandwich, Cold Cut Combo, on wheat bread	6 in (252 g)	410	21	48	16	3	3 S, 3 LM
Sandwich, Double Meat Classic Tuna	6 in (315 g)	780	31	43	55	3	3 S, 5 HFM, 1 F
Sandwich, Double Meat Roast Beef	6 in (281 g)	360	29	46	7	3	3 S, 4 VLM
Sandwich, Italian BMT, on wheat bread	6 in (245 g)	450	22	48	20	3	3 S, 3 MFM
Sandwich, Meatball Marinara, on wheat bread	6 in (379 g)	580	24	70	23	4½	4 S, 1 V, 3 MFM
Sandwich, Oven Roasted Chicken Breast, on wheat bread	6 in (240 g)	320	23	49	5	3	3 S, 3 VLM
Sandwich, Roast Beef, on wheat bread	6 in (240 g)	310	26	46	5	3	3 S, 2 VLM
Sandwich, Savory Turkey Breast and Ham, on white bread	6 in (227 g)	280	19	45	5	3	3 S, 1 F
Sandwich, Seafood Sensation, on white bread	6 in (243 g)	440	15	49	22	3	3 S, 2 HFM
Sandwich, Tuna, on wheat bread	6 in (252 g)	530	21	46	30	3	3 S, 3 HFM
Sandwich, Veggie Delite, on wheat bread	6 in (169 g)	230	8	45	3	3	3 S
Soup, Roasted Chicken Noodle	10 oz (310 g)	80	6	12	2	1	1 S
Soup, Vegetable Beef	10 oz (310 g)	100	5	17	2	1	1 S
Taco Bell							
Burrito, Bean	1 (198 g)	370	13	56	10	4	3 S, 2 LM
Burrito, Cheesy Bean and Rice	1 (227 g)	480	13	60	21	4	4 S, 2 MFM
Burrito, Chicken	1 (177 g)	440	16	48	20	3	3 S, 2 HFM
Burrito, Chili Cheese	1 (156 g)	370	16	40	16	2½	2 S, 2 HFM
Burrito, Pacific Shrimp	1 (197 g)	450	16	48	22	3	3 S, 2 HFM
Burrito, 7 Layer	1 (283 g)	510	18	68	18	4½	4 S, 2 HFM
Burrito, Supreme Beef	1 (248 g)	420	17	52	15	3½	3 S, 2 HFM
Burrito, Supreme Chicken	1 (248 g)	390	21	51	12	3½	3 S, 2 MFM
Burrito, Supreme Steak, Fresco	1 (241 g)	330	16	49	8	3	3 S, 2 LM
Chalupa Baja Chicken	1 (153 g)	390	17	29	23	2	2 S, 2 HFM, 1 F
Chalupa Baja Steak	1 (153 g)	380	14	29	23	2	2 S, 2 HFM
Chalupa Supreme Beef	1 (153 g)	370	14	31	21	2	2 S, 2 HFM
Cinnamon Twists	1 (35 g)	170	1	26	7	2	2 S

CALORIE VALUES

INGREDIENT	SERVING	CALORIES	PRO G	CARB G	FAT G	CARB CHOICE	DIABETIC EXCHANGE
Crunchwrap Supreme	1 (254 g)	540	16	71	21	5	4 S, 2 HFM
Enchirito Chicken	1 (213 g)	350	22	34	14	2	2 S, 3 MFM
Frutista Freeze, Strawberry	1 (479 g)	230	0	57	0	4	3 S
Gordita, Baja Steak	1 (153 g)	310	14	28	15	2	2 S, 2 MFM
Gordita Supreme, Chicken	1 (153 g)	270	17	29	10	2	2 S, 2 LM
Mexican Pizza	1 (213 g)	540	21	47	30	3	3 S, 3 HFM
Mexican Rice	1 order (85 g)	130	2	21	4	1½	1½ S
Nachos	1 order (99 g)	330	4	31	20	2	2 S, 4 F
Nachos, BellGrande	1 order (305 g)	770	20	78	42	5	5 S, 3 HFM, 2 F
Nachos, Volcano	1 order (354 g)	1000	22	89	62	6	6 S, 3 HFM, 5 F
Potatoes, Cheesy Fiesta	1 (135 g)	270	4	28	16	2	2 S, 2 F
Quesadilla, Cheese	1 (142 g)	470	19	40	26	2½	2 S, 3 HFM
Salad, Fiesta Taco, with Shell	1 (463 g)	770	27	75	41	5	5 S, 4 MFM, 2 F
Taco, Chicken, Soft tortilla	1 (99 g)	200	12	19	8	1	1 S, 1 HFM
Taco, Fresco, Beef, Soft tortilla	1 (113 g)	180	8	22	7	1½	1 S, 1 HFM
Taco, Original, with Beef	1 (78 g)	179	7	15	10	1	1 S, 1 HFM
Taquitos, Chicken	1 (128 g)	320	18	37	11	2½	2 S, 2 MFM
Tostada	1 (170 g)	250	11	29	10	2	2 S, 1 HFM
Wendy's							
Bacon Deluxe, double	1 (354 g)	860	56	46	50	3	3 S, 8 MFM
Bacon Deluxe, single	1 (275 g)	640	37	46	35	3	3 S, 4 HFM
Baconator, single	1 (200 g)	610	33	43	34	3	3 S, 5 MFM
Baconator, double	1 (312 g)	970	62	44	60	3	3 S, 9 MFM, 1 F
Baconator, triple	1 (424 g)	1330	90	47	86	3	3 S, 11 HFM
Baked potato, with bacon and Cheese	1 (366 g)	460	19	67	13	4½	4 S, 2 MFM
Baked potato, with broccoli and cheese	1 (396 g)	330	10	69	2	4½	4 S
Boneless wings, Sweet & Spicy Asian	1 order (259 g)	550	31	67	18	4½	4 S, 4 LM
Cheeseburger, Junior	1 (109 g)	270	15	27	11	2	2 S, 1 VLM
Cheeseburger, Junior, Deluxe	1 (152 g)	300	15	29	14	2	2 S, 2 VLM
Chicken nuggets	10 (150 g)	470	23	21	32	1½	1 S, 3 HFM, 2 F
Chili, small	8 oz (227 g)	220	18	22	7	1½	1 S, 2 MFM
French fries, medium	5 oz (142 g)	410	4	56	19	4	3 S, 4 F
Frosty Float	1 (467 g)	380	7	75	7	5	5 S
Go Wrap, Homestyle Chicken	1 (126 g)	310	15	30	15	2	2 S, 2 MFM
Hamburger, Bacon and Blue	1 (252 g)	680	37	44	40	3	3 S, 5 MFM, 1 F
Hamburger, double, with cheese	1 (8 oz, 337 g)	750	50	44	42	3	3 S, 7 MFM
Hamburger, single	1 (4 oz, 241 g)	470	27	43	21	3	3 S, 4 M
Hamburger, Triple Stack	1 (188 g)	490	34	27	27	2	2 S, MFM, 1 F

INGREDIENT	SERVING	CALORIES	PRO G	CARB G	FAT G	CARB CHOICE	DIABETIC EXCHANGE
Hamburger, triple, with cheese	1 (12 oz, 434 g)	**1030**	73	45	62	3	3 S, 10 MFM, 1 F
Mandarin Chicken Salad, with Grilled Chicken Fillet	1 (402 g)	**540**	31	51	25	3½	1 S, 1 FR, 4 V, 4 MFM
Sandwich, Chicken Club	1 (265 g)	**620**	37	55	29	3½	3 S, 5 MFM
Sandwich, Premium Fish Filet	1 (188 g)	**500**	18	52	24	3½	3 S, 2 HFM, 1 F

CALORIE VALUES

Each recipe in *The Calories In, Calories Out Cookbook* includes both metric and US measures. For quick reference, the charts below list conversions for liquid (volume) and solid (weight) measurements, oven temperatures, and length. Liquid and solid conversions are almost always rounded off. To simplify the numbers, the conversions from ounces to grams were based on 1 ounce = 30 grams. The precise equivalent is 1 ounce = 28.35 grams, but rounding up by less than 2 grams should not affect the outcome of the recipes. Remember that all scales are different, so you might get slightly different values when you measure foods.

Measuring cups and spoons may vary from one country to another, but differences are generally small and rarely affect the outcome of a recipe. One notable exception is Australian tablespoons, which hold 20 ml or 4 teaspoons, not the usual 15 ml tablespoon holding 3 teaspoons used in North America, New Zealand, and the United Kingdom.

In this book, all cup and spoon measurements are level unless otherwise specified (e.g., "heaping teaspoon" or "scant cup"). When measuring dry ingredients, such as flour or sugar, I usually scoop the cup through the flour or sugar and then level it with the blunt side of a table knife or spatula. Some people spoon the flour or sugar into the measuring cup and then level it, which is fine, too. Herbs and fresh greens are loosely packed unless otherwise specified.

LIQUID MEASURES

US	OUNCES	METRIC
1 tablespoon	½ fl oz	15 ml
2 tablespoons	1 fl oz	30 ml
3 tablespoons	1½ fl oz	45 ml
¼ cup	2 fl oz	60 ml
⅓ cup	3 fl oz	80 ml
½ cup	4 fl oz	125 ml
⅔ cup	5 fl oz	160 ml
¾ cup	6 fl oz	180 ml
1 cup	8 fl oz	250 ml
2 cups (1 pint)	16 fl oz	500 ml
4 cups (1 quart)	32 fl oz	1 liter

SOLID MEASURES

US/OUNCES	METRIC
½ oz	15 g
1 oz	30 g
2 oz	60 g
4 oz	120 g
5 oz	150 g
6 oz	180 g
7 oz	210 g
8 oz	240 g
12 oz	360 g
16 oz	480 g

OVEN TEMPERATURES

FAHRENHEIT	CELSIUS	GAS MARK
250°	120°	½
275°	135°	1
300°	150°	2
325°	160°	3
350°	180°	4
375°	190°	5
400°	200°	6
425°	220°	7
450°	230°	8
475°	245°	9
500°	260°	

LENGTH

US/INCHES	METRIC/CM	US/INCHES	METRIC/CM
¼	0.6	13	33
½	1.25	14	35
¾	2	15	38
1	2.5	16	41
2	5	17	43
3	8	18	46
4	10	19	48
5	13	20	51
6	15	21	53
7	18	22	56
8	20	23	58
9	23	24 (2 feet)	60
10	25	25	62
11	28	26	65
12 (1 foot)	30	27	67

GLUTEN-FREE RECIPES

Recipes included on this list are gluten-free provided that you choose ingredients that are confirmed gluten-free by their manufacturer. Certain naturally gluten-free ingredients, such as some grains, condiments, and spice blends, may be cross-contaminated with gluten during production; if you follow a gluten-free diet, check all package labels carefully.

Recipes on this list that contain soy, hoisin, and/or oyster sauce can be made gluten-free provided you use gluten-free variants of these sauces. These recipes are identified as follows:

s = soy sauce   h = hoisin sauce   o = oyster sauce

0 TO 199 CALORIES PER SERVING

Customized Fruit Salad (page 44)

Rhubarb-Raspberry Sauce (page 46)

Blueberry-Plum Sauce (page 47)

Spiced-Up Hash Browns (page 50)

Spinach and Cheese Omelet (page 54)

Homemade Roasted Vegetable Stock (page 56)

Homemade Chicken Stock (page 57)

Thai-Style Hot-and-Sour Shrimp Soup (page 59)

Gently Cooked Gazpacho (page 60)

Quick Zucchini-Basil Soup (page 62)

Gingery Squash Soup (page 63)

Hearty Beet Soup (page 66)

Roasted Carrot and Fennel Soup (page 68)

Cauliflower, Watercress, and Parmesan Soup (page 69)

Thai-Style Chicken Soup with Coconut Milk (page 73)

Indian-Style Cucumber Yogurt Salad (page 75)

Tomato, Cucumber, and Radish Salad (page 76)

Hot-and-Sweet Cucumber, Carrot, and Red Bell Pepper Salad (page 77)

Lemony Dill Cabbage Slaw (page 78)

Creamy All-American Potato Salad (page 80)

Austrian-Style Potato Salad (page 82)

Caesar Salad with a Light Touch (page 83)

Tomato, Artichoke Heart, Feta, and White Bean Salad (page 84)

Broiled Portobello Mushrooms with Herbs (page 86)

Roasted Asparagus with Dill and Lemon Zest (page 88)

Napa Cabbage with Ginger and Oyster Sauce (page 89) s, o

Broiled Zucchini with Parmesan (page 90)

Greek-Style Broccoli (page 91)

Sautéed Baby Bok Choy and Red Bell Peppers (page 92) s

Roasted Cauliflower and Mushrooms with Pine Nuts (page 93)

Maple-Glazed Carrots (page 95)

Sautéed Kale with Beans and Balsamic Vinegar (page 97)

Roasted New Potatoes (page 98)

Brussels Sprouts with Parmesan and Pine Nuts (page 99)

Sweet-and-Sour Red Cabbage (page 101)

Smashed Potatoes with Fresh Herbs (page 102)

Polenta with Herbs and Cheese (page 103)

Sweet Potato Oven Fries (page 104)

Great Green Couscous (page 105)

Aromatic Brown Basmati Rice (page 107)

Grilled Vegetables (page 108)

The Best Roasted Ratatouille (page 112)

Paneer with Spinach, Tomatoes, and Spices (page 113)

Vegetarian Chili (page 115)

Tofu and Bok Choy with Chili Sauce (page 116) s, h

RESOURCES:
FOOD AND NUTRITION INFORMATION

Most all of the ingredients in *The Calories In, Calories Out Cookbook* can be found in well-stocked supermarkets, natural foods stores, Whole Foods stores, Trader Joe's stores, and/or specialty Asian and Indian stores, but the following purveyors, as well as amazon.com, are excellent resources.

Food Resources

SPICES AND SPECIALTY FOODS

Asianfoodgrocer.com
131 West Harris Avenue
South San Francisco, CA 94080
Tel: 888-482-2742

Igourmet.com
508 Delaware Avenue
West Pittston, PA 18643
Tel: 877-446-8763

Importfoods.com
PO Box 2054
Issaquah, WA 98027
Tel: 888-618-8424

Kalustyan's
123 Lexington Avenue
New York, NY 10016
Tel: 800-352-3451; 212-685-3451
www.kalustyans.com

Penzeys Spices
12001 West Capitol Drive
Wauwatosa, WI 53222
Tel: 800-741-7787
www.penzeys.com

The Spice House
Tel: 847-328-3711
www.thespicehouse.com

WHOLE GRAINS AND FLOURS

Anson Mills
1922-C Gervais Street
Columbia, SC 29201
Tel: 803-467-4122
www.ansonmills.com

Arrowhead Mills
The Hain Celestial Group
4600 Sleepytime Drive
Boulder, CO 80301
Tel: 800-434-4246
www.arrowheadmills.com

Bob's Red Mill
13521 SE Pheasant Court
Milwaukie, OR 97222
Tel: 800-349-2173; 503-654-3215
www.bobsredmill.com

Bob's Red Mill Whole Grain Store
5000 SE International Way
Milwaukie, OR 07222
Tel: 800-553-2258; 503-607-6455
www.bobsredmill.com

Eden Foods, Inc.
701 Tecumseh Road
Clinton, MI 49236
Tel: 888-424-3336; 517-456-7457
www.edenfoods.com

Hodgson Mill, Inc.
1100 Stevens Avenue
Effingham, IL 62401

Tel: 800-347-0105
www.hodgsonmill.com

King Arthur Flour
135 US Route 5 South
Norwich, VT 05055
Tel: 800-827-6836
www.kingarthurflour.com

Lundberg Family Farms
5311 Midway
PO Box 369
Richvale, CA 95974
Tel: 707-545-3280
www.lundberg.com

Sun Ridge Farms
423 Salinas Road
Royal Oaks, CA 95076
Tel: 831-786-7000
www.sunridgefarms.com

EQUIPMENT

OXO
1331 South Seventh Street
Second floor
Chambersburg, PA 17201
Tel: 800-545-4411
www.oxo.com

Sur la Table
Tel: 800-243-0852
www.surlatable.com

Williams-Sonoma
Tel: 877-812-6235
www.williams-sonoma.com

Nutrition Resources

There are numerous websites where you can find nutrition and physical activity information, to the point where the information can be overwhelming and difficult to sort through. The list below should make the search easy for you. It is a select list of reputable sites that is designed to assist you in learning more about healthy eating and physical activity.

NUTRITION

Academy of Nutrition and Dietetics (formerly the American Dietetic Association)
www.eatright.org

Centers for Disease Control and Prevention
www.cdc.gov/nutrition

National Institute of Diabetes and Digestive and Kidney Diseases: Nutrition
www2.niddk.nih.gov/HealthEducation/Health Nutrition.html

USDA ChooseMyPlate
www.choosemyplate.gov

PHYSICAL ACTIVITY

American College of Sports Medicine
www.acsm.org

Centers for Disease Control and Prevention
www.cdc.gov/physicalactivity/index.html

Physical Activity Guidelines for Americans, Department of Health and Human Services
www.health.gov/paguidelines

USDA ChooseMyPlate
www.choosemyplate.gov/physical-activity.html

FOOD AND PHYSICAL ACTIVITY TRACKERS (FOR JOURNALING)

USDA Super Tracker
www.supertracker.usda.gov/default.aspx

SOURCES AND FURTHER READING

SOURCES

Epigraph

Bharati, Veda. *Five Pillars of Sadhana*. Edited by Claudia Crawford. Rishikesh: Sadhana Mandir Trust, 1997.

A Cookbook for Everyone

Gilbert, Lynn and Gaylen Moore. Particular Passions: Julia Child (Women of Wisdom). Kindle Edition. Amazon Digital Services, Inc., 2012.

Understanding the World of Calories

U.S. Department of Agriculture and U.S. Department of Health and Human Services. Dietary Guidelines for Americans, 2010. 7th edition. Washington, DC: U.S. Government Printing Office, 2010. http://www.health.gov/dietaryguidelines/dga2010/dietaryguidelines2010.pdf.

Determining Your Calorie and Exercise Needs

Hollins, JF, CM Gullion, VJ Stevens, et al. "Weight loss during the intensive intervention phase of weight-loss maintenance trial." American Journal of Preventative Medicine. 35 (2008): 118–26. doi:10.1016/j.amepre.2008.04.013.

Frequently Asked Questions

Fitch, Cindy, and Kathryn Keim. "Use of Nutritive and Nonnutritive Sweeteners." Journal of the Academy of Nutrition and Dietetics. 112 (2012): 739–758. http://www.sciencedirect.com/science/article/pii/S2212267212003255.

Pasiakos, Stefan M., Jay J. Cao, Lee M. Margolis, et al. "Effects of high-protein diets on fat-free mass and muscle protein synthesis following weight loss: a randomized controlled trial." The Journal of the Federation of American Societies for Experimental Biology. (2013). doi:10.1096/fj.13-230227.

U.S. Department of Agriculture and U.S. Department of Health and Human Services. Dietary Guidelines for Americans, 2010. 7th edition. Washington, DC: U.S. Government Printing Office, 2010. http://www.health.gov/dietaryguidelines/dga2010/dietaryguidelines2010.pdf.

Institute of Medicine of the National Academies. Dietary Reference Intakes: Water, Potassium, Sodium, Chloride, and Sulfate. Washington, DC: The National Academies Press, 2004.

FURTHER READING

Aggarwal, Bharat B. and Deborah Yost. Healing Spices: How to Use 50 Everyday and Exotic Spices to Boost Health and Beat Disease. New York: Sterling, 2011.

Bladholm, Linda. The Asian Grocery Store Demystified: A Food Lover's Guide to All the Best Ingredients. Los Angeles: Renaissance Books, 1999.

Bowden, Jonny. The 150 Healthiest Foods on Earth: The Surprising, Unbiased Truth About What You Should Eat and Why. Massachusetts: Fair Winds Press, 2007.

Campbell, T. Colin, Thomes M. Campbell II, Howard Lyman, and John Robbins. The China Study: The Most Comprehensive Study of Nutrition Ever Conducted and the Startling Implications for Diet, Weight Loss, and Long-Term Health. Dallas: BenBella Books, 2004.

Campbell, T. Colin, and Howard Jacobson. Whole: Rethinking the Science of Nutrition. Dallas: BenBella Books, 2013.

Hemphill, Ian: The Spice and Herb Bible: A Cook's Guide. Ontario: Robert Rose Inc., 2002.

Nestle, Marion. Food Politics: How the Food Industry Influences Nutrition and Health. Berkeley: University of California Press, 2002.

———, and Malden Nesheim. Why Calories Count: From Science to Politics. Berkeley: University of California Press, 2011.

Ottolenghi, Yotam, and Jonathan Lovekin. Plenty: Vibrant Vegetable Recipes from London's Ottolenghi. San Francisco: Chronicle Books, 2011.

Panjabi, Camellia. 50 Great Curries of India. London: Kyle Books, 2005.

Pollan, Michael. Food Rules: An Eater's Manual. New York: Penguin, 2009.

———. In Defense of Food: An Eater's Manifesto. New York: Penguin, 2008.

———. The Omnivore's Dilemma: A Natural History of Four Meals. New York: Penguin, 2006.

Speck, Maria. Ancient Grains for Modern Meals. Berkeley: Ten Speed Press, 2011.

Swanson, Heidi. Super Natural Every Day: Well-Loved Recipes from My Natural Foods Kitchen. Berkeley: Ten Speed Press, 2011.

Thompson, David. Thai Food. Berkeley: Ten Speed Press, 2002.

ACKNOWLEDGMENTS

FROM CATHERINE JONES

I am truly blessed to work with Matthew Lore, my publisher. Every book starts with an idea, and for fifteen years, Matthew has always encouraged my ideas. Thank you for giving me the chance, once again, to share my recipes, knowledge, and passion for healthy living.

I am humbled by the dedication, talent, and positive energy of the entire crew at The Experiment. Their immense talents are paralleled by their resolute pursuit of perfection: Peter Burri, COO/CFO; Dan O'Connor, associate publisher; Batya Rosenblum, managing editorial assistant; Molly Cavanaugh, associate editor; and Anne Rumberger and Sarah Schneider, in the publicity, marketing, and sales department.

When I saw the proposed layout of the book I honestly had to catch my breath. The team at Neuwirth spun their magic to transform massive amounts of information into beautiful pages. A huge, heartfelt thanks to Pauline Neuwirth, interior designer, Beth Metrick, production director, and Sabrina Plomitallo-González, Beth's right hand gal. The cover by Susi Oberhelman is genius: a combination of art, message, and fun. Karen Giangreco brought the ebook edition to life. Thank you all!

My great friend and writing partner, Elaine Trujillo, is among the best nutritionists on this planet. Her advice and practical approach to healthy eating have fueled my creative energy over the decades. Thank you, Elaine, for compiling all of the nutritional data with your meticulous attention to detail. My thanks also to Malden Nesheim, PhD, for his stellar introduction, and to Walter Lefeber, my husband's former history professor at Cornell University, who connected me with Malden. I am profoundly grateful to Elisabeth Langworthy for her legal support over the past years, and to her assistant, Christina Galus.

I've said it before and I'll say it again, Judith Sutton is the top cookbook copy-editor in the business, bar none. When my manuscripts are with her, I can sleep at night. Our friendship dates back to 1987, when we met at La Varenne Cooking School in Paris. Suzanne Fass, proofreader extraordinaire, did a phenomenal job. A bow of thanks to you both.

Living in Malaysia while writing the bulk of this book allowed me to work with two special talents: Soo Phye, a truly gifted food photographer who captured the natural beauty of my food; and Rohani Jelani, an awesome food stylist as well as author, chef, and cooking teacher. Also, applause to Matt Greenland for shooting the veggie burger on the cover.

Behind this book there was a very special kitchen crew. Luan Wong, who helped me test recipes, is an extraordinary cook, equally artful at eastern and western fare. Many of the Chinese recipes included here are adapted from her repertoire. I so much appreciate all of my recipe testers. I loved your comments, every single one of them, especially the ones that made me laugh out loud: Yukiko Jacques, Dorothy Cabuhat, Carmen Wong, Brock Fox, Jennifer Lim, Ellen Moulier, Alice Moulier, Hilde Pearson and the Pearson Family, Martha Grove, Liz Renda,

Sharon Tan, Jessica Schnepple, Melissa Alshab, Allie Jones, Peggy Terry, Rana Burley, Lauren Hannon, Liz Abernethy, and Elaine Trujillo.

A deep well of gratitude goes to my younger brother, Mark Grove, who has no shortage of creative ideas. This book is for Mark, and his partner, Troy, too. To my beloved husband of almost twenty years, I say thank you for giving me the freedom and encouragement I need to pursue my passions. My beautiful children, Allie and Hale, make my life meaningful and exciting. Allie, your quest to be healthy keeps me on track. Don't ever change. Hale, your humor keeps me sane! I also want to thank my father, Brandon Grove, for travelling to Malaysia to live with us for a few months and gamely sampling just about every dish in this cookbook. My mother, Mary Abernethy, taught me the joys of the kitchen. A big thanks to my other brothers, Paul and Jack Grove and their families, and to my sister, Liz Abernethy.

Finally, I thank YOU! For buying this book and using it. It's not easy to put meals on the table every day, I know, but it's one of the greatest gifts you can give your family, friends, and yourself. Keep cooking!

FROM ELAINE TRUJILLO, MS, RDN

Catherine is an inspiration, whether cooking in the kitchen, writing at the keypad, or chatting over a cup of coffee. It was a pleasure and a gift to work with her again.

This book comes at a perfect time. Calorie awareness is in the spotlight and increasing attention is geared toward solving the obesity epidemic and the chronic diseases that often accompany it. We all need to be aware of our energy needs, and this book provides an excellent tool to do just that.

I am grateful to my colleagues, Colleen Spees, Maureen Leser, and Anu Kaur for their nutritional advice and support. My former student, Sasha Sutherland Nunez, was instrumental in cross-checking all the nutritional information, and I thank her. I was thrilled that Malden Nesheim, an esteemed colleague, did a brilliant job with the introduction. I also want to thank Nacho Montesinos for designing our website, and for all of his tech help. Donny Bliss, a friend and medical illustrator, created amazing illustrations to help readers understand the often confusing world of calories.

I wish to thank my extended family. They are a constant source of inspiration, humor, and love. My brother-in-law, Ernie Renda, shared his amazing collection of cocktails and beverages (those were the most fun to test!). My sister, Liz Renda, enthusiastically helped with recipe testing and reviewing content. My parents, Anthony and Clare Barbella, are my biggest supporters and fans. They are always behind my dreams. A deep gratitude to my three brothers, Frank, Don, and Brian Barbella and their families for their encouragement. Mil gracias a mi familia Mexicana—Mama Lupita, Papa Roberto Trujillo, and my brother-in-laws, Marco Antonio, Jose and Gustavo Trujillo.

I want to thank my son, Danny, and my daughter, Jacky, for always keeping things real and reminding me of what is important in life. Finally, I want to thank my life partner, my husband, Roberto, for making me dream big.

INDEX

Page numbers in *italics* refer to photos.

PLEASE SHARE YOUR CALORIES

There's a higher purpose behind *The Calories In, Calories Out Cookbook*. The main goal of this book is to make healthy eating a delicious and rewarding experience for you, your families, and friends, but beyond that, as your calorie awareness increases, we invite you to be part of the movement to end world hunger one calorie at a time.

While writing this book, we founded the nonprofit Share Your Calories (EIN: 27-0350125) to allow people to track their calories and share the extras through an incredible mobile app called the Share Your Calories App. It's the first-ever nonprofit weight-loss app with a social-giving component. Extra calories you cut from your daily intake can be converted into meals for hungry children at the rate of one penny per calorie.

We are proud to partner with Stop Hunger Now, an amazing nonprofit with a proven track record of providing hundreds of millions of freeze-dried meals to global school feeding programs and disaster relief. We encourage you to visit www.shareyourcalories.com to learn more and to download this free mobile app when it launches in 2015.

We firmly believe that world hunger can be conquered. Awareness is key, and from awareness comes action. Proper nourishment for children from school feeding programs leads to less disease, higher school attendance, and a chance at breaking the cycle of poverty. Let's work together to make this world a healthier place for everyone.

Catherine Jones   *Elaine Trujillo*

Take Action!

Please join the movement to increase calorie awareness and to end world hunger. Learn more at www.shareyourcalories.com and www.stophungernow.org. Check us out on Twitter @ShareYourCals and join the conversation with #shareyourcalories. Like our Share Your Calories Facebook page and follow our Share Your Calories boards on Pinterest. We look forward to hearing from you!

ABOUT THE AUTHORS

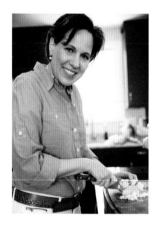

Catherine Jones, a graduate of Connecticut College and La Varenne Culinary School in Paris, France, is an award-winning cookbook author. Her books include *Eating for Pregnancy: The Essential Nutrition Guide and Cookbook for Today's Mothers-to-Be*, *Eating for Lower Cholesterol: A Balanced Approach to Heart Health with Recipes Everyone Will Love*, and *A Year of Russian Feasts*. She and Elaine Trujillo cofounded the nonprofit organization Share Your Calories and are in the process of creating an app of the same name for users to track their calories and share the extras through social giving. Please visit www.shareyourcalories.com. When not living overseas on assignment with her husband, US Ambassador Paul W. Jones, Catherine calls Bethesda, Maryland, home. She is the mother of two children.

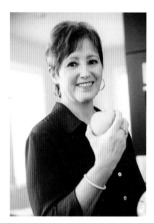

Elaine Trujillo, MS, RDN, is a leader in nutrition at the National Cancer Institute, National Institute of Health in Maryland; she previously worked at the Brigham and Women's Hospital, Harvard Medical School. She received a BS from the University of Delaware and an MS from Texas Woman's University. She is Chair of the Oncology Nutrition Dietetic Practice Group of the Academy of Nutrition and Dietetics, which in 2013 published *Oncology Nutrition for Clinical Practice*. She is a former Chair of Education and Research for the Maryland Academy of Nutrition and Dietetics. She uses a variety of approaches to share her views and findings about nutrition, including coauthoring, with Catherine Jones, *Eating for Lower Cholesterol: A Balanced Approach to Heart Health with Recipes Everyone Will Love* and authoring a textbook, *Nutritional Support in the Care of the Critically Ill*. She has also written numerous scientific journal articles and book chapters. She and her husband live in Maryland and have two children.

For more information, visit www.caloriesinandcaloriesout.com

Be in Touch!

Please check out our social media menu. We love connecting with our readers. We like to hear about your cooking adventures and we welcome any motivational tips you can share with us and fellow readers for a healthier life. Please join our conversation on Twitter, like us on Facebook, and follow us on Pinterest and Instagram. If you've got a cooking group going, we'd love to join you virtually on Skype to answer any cooking or nutrition questions, or just to be part of the fun. Please contact Catherine to set that up: catherinejonescooks@gmail.com

Twitter: @CalorieCookbook
Facebook: The Calories In Calories Out Cookbook
Pinterest: Calories In Calories Out Cookbook
Instagram: caloriesin_caloriesout